T0226424

Hematopoietic Neoplasms: Controversies in Diagnosis and Classification

Editors

TRACY I. GEORGE
DANIEL A. ARBER

SURGICAL PATHOLOGY CLINICS

surgpath.theclinics.com

Consulting Editor
JOHN R. GOLDBLUM

December 2013 • Volume 6 • Number 4

ELSEVIER

1600 John F. Kennedy Boulevard ● Suite 1800 ● Philadelphia, Pennsylvania, 19103-2899

http://www.theclinics.com

SURGICAL PATHOLOGY CLINICS Volume 6, Number 4
December 2013 ISSN 1875-9181, ISBN-13: 978-0-323-27786-0

Editor: Joanne Husovski
Developmental Editor: Donald Mumford

© **2013 Elsevier Inc. All rights reserved.**

This periodical and the individual contributions contained in it are protected under copyright by Elsevier, and the following terms and conditions apply to their use:

Photocopying
Single photocopies of single articles may be made for personal use as allowed by national copyright laws. Permission of the Publisher and payment of a fee is required for all other photocopying, including multiple or systematic copying, copying for advertising or promotional purposes, resale, and all forms of document delivery. Special rates are available for educational institutions that wish to make photocopies for non-profit educational classroom use. For information on how to seek permission visit www.elsevier.com/permissions or call: (+44) 1865 843830 (UK)/(+1) 215 239 3804 (USA).

Derivative Works
Subscribers may reproduce tables of contents or prepare lists of articles including abstracts for internal circulation within their institutions. Permission of the Publisher is required for resale or distribution outside the institution. Permission of the Publisher is required for all other derivative works, including compilations and translations (please consult www.elsevier.com/permissions).

Electronic Storage or Usage
Permission of the Publisher is required to store or use electronically any material contained in this periodical, including any article or part of an article (please consult www.elsevier.com/permissions). Except as outlined above, no part of this publication may be reproduced, stored in a retrieval system or transmitted in any form or by any means, electronic, mechanical, photocopying, recording or otherwise, without prior written permission of the Publisher.

Notice
No responsibility is assumed by the Publisher for any injury and/or damage to persons or property as a matter of products liability, negligence or otherwise, or from any use or operation of any methods, products, instructions or ideas contained in the material herein. Because of rapid advances in the medical sciences, in particular, independent verification of diagnoses and drug dosages should be made.

Although all advertising material is expected to conform to ethical (medical) standards, inclusion in this publication does not constitute a guarantee or endorsement of the quality or value of such product or of the claims made of it by its manufacturer.

Surgical Pathology Clinics (ISSN 1875-9181) is published quarterly by Elsevier Inc., 360 Park Avenue South, New York, NY 10010. Months of issue are March, June, September, and December. Business and Editorial Office: Elsevier Inc., 1600 John F. Kennedy Blvd., Ste. 1800, Philadelphia, PA 19103-2899. Accounting and Circulation Offices: Elsevier Inc., 3251 Riverport Lane, Maryland Heights, MO 63043. Periodicals postage paid at New York, NY and at additional mailing offices. Subscription prices are $200.00 per year (US individuals), $233.00 per year (US institutions), $100.00 per year (US students/residents), $250.00 per year (Canadian individuals), $266.00 per year (Canadian Institutions), $250.00 per year (foreign individuals), $266.00 per year (foreign institutions), and $120.00 per year (international & Canadian students/residents). Foreign air speed delivery is included in all *Clinics*' subscription prices. All prices are subject to change without notice. **POSTMASTER:** Send address changes to *Surgical Pathology Clinics*, Elsevier, 3251 Riverport Lane, Maryland Heights, MO 63043. Customer Service: 1-800-654-2452 (US). From outside the United States, call 1-314-447-8871. Fax: 1-314-447-8029. E-mail: JournalsCustomerServiceusa@elsevier.com (for print support) and JournalsOnlineSupport-usa@elsevier.com (for online support).

Reprints. For copies of 100 or more, of articles in this publication, please contact the Commercial Reprints Department, Elsevier Inc., 360 Park Avenue South, New York, NY 10010-1710. Tel. 212-633-3874; Fax: 212-633-3820; E-mail: reprints@elsevier.com.

Contributors

CONSULTING EDITOR

JOHN R. GOLDBLUM, MD
Chairman, Professor of Pathology, Department of Anatomic Pathology, Cleveland Clinics Lerner College of Medicine, Cleveland Clinic, Cleveland, Ohio

EDITORS

DANIEL A. ARBER, MD
Professor and Vice Chair of Pathology, Director of Anatomic Pathology and Clinical Laboratories, Department of Pathology, Stanford University Medical Center, Stanford University, Stanford, California

TRACY I. GEORGE, MD
Associate Professor of Pathology, Chief, Hematopathology Division, Department of Pathology, University of New Mexico School of Medicine, Albuquerque, New Mexico

AUTHORS

DANIEL A. ARBER, MD
Professor and Vice Chair of Pathology, Director of Anatomic Pathology and Clinical Laboratories, Department of Pathology, Stanford University Medical Center, Stanford University, Stanford, California

DAVID R. CZUCHLEWSKI, MD
Department of Pathology, University of New Mexico, Albuquerque, New Mexico

ANDREW L. FELDMAN, MD
Department of Laboratory Medicine and Pathology, Mayo Clinic, Rochester, Minnesota

KATHRYN FOUCAR, MD
Department of Pathology, University of New Mexico, Albuquerque, New Mexico

TRACY I. GEORGE, MD
Associate Professor of Pathology; Chief, Hematopathology Division, Department of Pathology, University of New Mexico School of Medicine, Albuquerque, New Mexico

DITA GRATZINGER, MD, PhD
Assistant Professor, Department of Pathology, Stanford University Medical Center, Stanford, California

PETER L. GREENBERG, MD
Professor Emeritus, Hematology Division; Director, MDS Center, Stanford University Medical Center, Stanford, California

ROBERT P. HASSERJIAN, MD
Associate Professor, Department of Pathology, Massachusetts General Hospital, Boston, Massachusetts

MATTHEW T. HOWARD, MD
Department of Laboratory Medicine and Pathology, Mayo Clinic, Rochester, Minnesota

ERIC D. HSI, MD
Robert J. Tomsich Pathology and Laboratory Medicine Institute, Cleveland Clinic, Cleveland, Ohio

RYAN C. JOHNSON, MD
Chief Resident, Department of Pathology, Stanford University School of Medicine, Stanford, California

WILLIAM G. MORICE, MD, PhD
Department of Laboratory Medicine and
Pathology, Mayo Clinic, Rochester,
Minnesota

JADEE L. NEFF, MD, PhD
Department of Laboratory Medicine and
Pathology, Mayo Clinic, Rochester,
Minnesota

ROBERT S. OHGAMI, MD, PhD
Department of Pathology, Stanford University
Medical Center, Stanford, California

KAAREN K. REICHARD, MD
Associate Professor of Pathology, Division
of Hematopathology, Mayo Clinic, Rochester,
Minnesota

HEESUN J. ROGERS, MD, PhD
Robert J. Tomsich Pathology and
Laboratory Medicine Institute, Cleveland
Clinic, Cleveland, Ohio

LAWRENCE M. WEISS, MD
Medical Director, Clarient Diagnostic Services,
Inc, Aliso Viejo, California

Contents

Preface: Why Is Hematopathology so Complicated?   ix

Daniel A. Arber and Tracy I. George

Clonal Relationships Between Malignant Lymphomas and Histiocytic/Dendritic Cell Tumors   619

Andrew L. Feldman

Tumors of histiocytic or dendritic cell origin appear to occur with increased frequency in patients with lymphoma. Recent molecular data have demonstrated clonal relationships between the lymphoma and the histiocytic/dendritic cell tumor in some of these cases. Clinical, pathologic, and experimental data suggest that this phenomenon probably represents transdifferentiation of the lymphoma clone to a histiocytic/dendritic cell lineage in most cases. Awareness of this entity is necessary to prompt comparative molecular studies in appropriate cases.

Distinguishing T-cell Large Granular Lymphocytic Leukemia from Reactive Conditions: Laboratory Tools and Challenges in Their Use   631

Jadee L. Neff, Matthew T. Howard, and William G. Morice

This article focuses on the challenges of diagnosing T-cell large granular leukemia and distinguishing it from benign reactive conditions, as well as more aggressive neoplasms of cytotoxic lymphocytes. No single laboratory method is sufficient to make the diagnosis, but instead a combination of flow cytometry, genetic studies, and bone marrow immunohistochemistry must be used.

Erythroleukemia and Its Differential Diagnosis   641

Robert P. Hasserjian

Acute erythroid leukemias encompass 2 main subtypes: acute erythroid leukemia (erythroid/myeloid subtype) and pure erythroid leukemia. This article reviews the main clinicopathologic features of the acute erythroid leukemias and the criteria used to diagnose them. In this article, the differential diagnosis between acute erythroid leukemias and their mimics is discussed and helpful morphologic clues and diagnostic tests that help arrive at the correct diagnosis are provided. The appropriate application of diagnostic criteria, including ancillary testing, such as immunophenotyping, cytogenetics, and molecular genetic testing, is essential to categorize bone marrow erythroid proliferations.

Early T-cell Precursor Acute Lymphoblastic Leukemia/Lymphoma   661

David R. Czuchlewski and Kathryn Foucar

Discrete diagnostic subtypes of T lymphoblastic leukemia/lymphoma (T-cell acute lymphoblastic leukemia/lymphoma) have historically not been widely recognized. A novel subset with distinctive immunophenotypic, molecular, and clinical features has been proposed. Termed *early T-cell precursor ALL (ETP-ALL)*, these cases seem to correspond to a very early stage of T-cell development. ETP-ALL is associated with a poor prognosis using standard protocols, and patients with ETP-ALL may benefit from intensified, alternative, or targeted therapies. Recognizing

ETP-ALL and distinguishing it from other forms of acute leukemia are important elements of an up-to-date diagnostic approach to precursor T-cell neoplasms.

Myeloid Neoplasms with inv(3)(q21q26.2) or t(3;3)(q21;q26.2)   677

Heesun J. Rogers and Eric D. Hsi

Acute myeloid leukemia (AML) with inv(3)(q21q26.2)/t(3;3)(q21;q26.2) [inv3/t(3;3)] is a distinct entity under the subgroup of AMLs with recurrent genetic abnormalities in the 2008 World Health Organization classification. Myelodysplastic syndrome (MDS) with inv3/t(3;3) has a high risk of progression to AML. AML and MDS with inv3/t(3;3) have a similarly aggressive clinical course with short overall survival and are commonly refractory to therapy. In this article, clinical and pathologic features and prognosis in AML and MDS with inv3/t(3;3) are reviewed, and other myeloid neoplasms with similar dysplastic features to be differentiated from AML and MDS with inv3/t(3;3) are discussed.

Update on Myelodysplastic Syndromes Classification and Prognosis   693

Dita Gratzinger and Peter L. Greenberg

Myelodysplastic syndromes (MDSs) are a collection of cytogenetically heterogeneous clonal bone marrow failure disorders derived from aberrant hematopoietic stem cells in the setting of an aberrant hematopoietic stem cell niche. Patients suffer from variably progressive and symptomatic bone marrow failure with a risk of leukemic transformation. Diagnosis of MDS has long been based on morphologic assessment and blast percentage as in the original French-American-British classification. The recently developed Revised International Prognostic Scoring System provides improved prognostication using more refined cytogenetic, marrow blast, and cytopenia parameters. With the advent of deep sequencing technologies, dozens of molecular abnormalities have been identified in MDS.

Atypical Phenotypes in Classical Hodgkin Lymphoma   729

Lawrence M. Weiss

Classical Hodgkin lymphoma has a characteristic immunophenotype in most cases, with expression of CD30, CD15, and PAX-5, and absence of CD45 and T-lineage markers. However, in a significant subset of cases, atypical staining patterns may be seen for one or more antigens, particularly negative staining for CD15 or staining for one or more B-lineage markers, such as CD20, CD79a, OCT-2, or BOB.1. The greatest pitfall is in the misinterpretation of other cells, such as immunoblasts or histiocytes, as Hodgkin cells.

Blastic Plasmacytoid Dendritic Cell Neoplasm: How do You Distinguish It from Acute Myeloid Leukemia?   743

Kaaren K. Reichard

BPDCN is a recently elucidated clinicopathologic entity. This disease typically involves the skin, with 30% to 40% of patients showing an additional concurrent leukemic component. Although BPDCN often exhibits cytologic features akin to acute lymphoblastic leukemia, the main differential diagnostic challenge, in the skin and in the bone marrow, is distinction from AML, in particular AML with monocytic differentiation.

The Differential Diagnosis of Eosinophilia in Neoplastic Hematopathology   767

Ryan C. Johnson and Tracy I. George

Eosinophilia in the peripheral blood is classified as primary (clonal) hematologic neoplasms or secondary (nonclonal) disorders, associated with hematologic or nonhematologic disorders. This review focuses on the categories of hematolymphoid neoplasms recognized by the 2008 World Health Organization *Classification of Tumours and Haematopoietic and Lymphoid Tissues* that are characteristically associated with eosinophilia. We provide a systematic approach to the diagnosis of these neoplastic proliferations via morphologic, immunophenotypic, and molecular-based methodologies, and provide the clinical settings in which these hematolymphoid neoplasms occur. We discuss recommendations that eosinophilia working groups have published addressing some of the limitations of the current classification scheme.

Challenges in Consolidated Reporting of Hematopoietic Neoplasms   795

Robert S. Ohgami and Daniel A. Arber

This article focuses on the challenges of generating comprehensive diagnostic reports in hematopathology. In particular, two main challenges that diagnosticians face are (1) interpreting and understanding the rapid advances in molecular and genetic pathology, which have gained increasing importance in classifications of hematopoietic neoplasms, and (2) managing the logistics of reporting ancillary studies and incorporating them effectively into a final synthesized report. This article summarizes many important genetic findings in hematopoietic neoplasms, which are required for accurate diagnoses, and discusses practical issues to generating accurate and complete hematopathology reports.

Index   807

SURGICAL PATHOLOGY CLINICS

FORTHCOMING ISSUES

Cytopathology
Tarik El Sheikh, *Editor*

Cutaneous Lymphoma
Antonio Subtil, *Editor*

Thyroid Pathology
Peter Sadow, *Editor*

Pathology Informatics
Anil Parwani, *Editor*

RECENT ISSUES

Gastrointestinal Pathology: Classification, Diagnosis, Emerging Entities
Jason L. Hornick, MD, PhD, *Editor*

Liver Pathology
Sanjay Kakar, MD, and Dhanpat Jain, MD, *Editors*

Placental Pathology
Rebecca N. Baergen, MD, *Editor*

Current Concepts in Molecular Oncology
Jennifer Hunt, MD, *Editor*

RELATED INTEREST

Experimental Hematology, Volume 40, Issue 8, August 2012, Pages 634–45.e10
The HDAC Inhibitor Givinostat Modulates the Hematopoietic Transcription Factors NFE2 and C-MYB in JAK2V617F Myeloproliferative Neoplasm Cells
Ariel Amaru Calzada, Katia Todoerti, Luca Donadoni, Anna Pellicioli, Giacomo Tuana, Raffaella Gatta, Antonino Neri, Guido Finazzi, Roberto Mantovani, Alessandro Rambaldi, Martino Introna, Luigia Lombardi, Josée Golay, AGIMM Investigators, *Editors*

**DOWNLOAD
Free App!**

Review Articles
THE CLINICS

NOW AVAILABLE FOR YOUR iPhone and iPad

Preface
Why Is Hematopathology so Complicated?

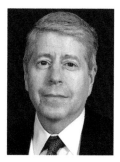 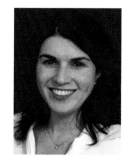

Daniel A. Arber, MD   Tracy I. George, MD

Editors

Hematopathology is well known for its complicated classification systems that seem to change every few years. Unfortunately, this trend will only continue and has spread to other areas of diagnostic pathology as we learn more about the complex diseases that we diagnose. Changes in classification systems, however, are usually driven by advances in the field. This volume of *Surgical Pathology Clinics* highlights selected topics in hematopathology that have seen critical advances in recent years and pose diagnostic challenges for the practicing pathologist. The first article focuses on the clonal link between malignant lymphoma and histiocytic tumors; a discovery that has further confirmed the plasticity of hematopoietic progenitor cells. In the second article, the clues to assist in the separation of reactive from leukemic large granular lymphocyte proliferations are discussed. This is followed by articles on erythroleukemia, myeloid neoplasms with inv(3)/t(3;3), and updates on myelodysplastic syndrome. These three articles highlight the difficulty of separating myelodysplastic syndromes from acute leukemia, the importance of specific genetic abnormalities in establishing these diagnoses and the role of genetic abnormalities in prognosis. Two "new" categories of acute leukemia, early precursor T-cell acute leukemia and blastic plasmacytoid dendritic cell tumors, are described and how to distinguish these acute leukemias from morphologic and immunophenotypic mimics, and the therapeutic implications of these diagnoses are reviewed. As new immunohistochemical markers and technology are used in pathology, this brings difficulties in the diagnosis of classic diseases such as Hodgkin lymphoma, discussed in article 7. In article 9, the differential diagnosis of eosinophilia in hematopathology is described, including diagnostic algorithms useful in identifying these rare neoplasms and the clinical implications of specific genetic abnormalities with respect to treatment. In the final article, the challenges of integrating ancillary testing into a comprehensive report is discussed and the importance of developing such a report is highlighted.

We hope this issue will serve as a practical guide for pathologists that can be used in daily practice. While we cannot make the classification of these tumors less complicated, we hope this series of articles will help the readers understand the selected disorders better. As with most tasks, it is the people that make such a series possible and we commend the authors on eloquently sharing their expertise with outstanding images, salient tables, and clear summaries.

Daniel A. Arber, MD
Department of Pathology
Stanford University
Stanford, CA 94305, USA

Tracy I. George, MD
Hematopathology Section
University of New Mexico School of Medicine
Albuquerque, NM 87131, USA

E-mail addresses:
darber@stanford.edu (D.A. Arber)
TracyGeorge@salud.unm.edu (T.I. George)

Surgical Pathology 6 (2013) ix
http://dx.doi.org/10.1016/j.path.2013.08.004
1875-9181/13/$ – see front matter © 2013 Elsevier Inc. All rights reserved.

surgpath.theclinics.com

Clonal Relationships Between Malignant Lymphomas and Histiocytic/Dendritic Cell Tumors

Andrew L. Feldman, MD

KEYWORDS

- Transdifferentiation • Histiocytic sarcoma • Dendritic cell tumor • Langerhans cell histiocytosis
- Transformation • Lineage plasticity • Clonality

KEY POINTS

- Some histiocytic/dendritic cell (H/DC) tumors in patients with lymphoma are clonally related to the underlying lymphoma; these H/DC tumor may arise synchronously or metachronously.
- The mechanism for this clonal relationship appears to be transdifferentiation of the lymphoma clone in most cases.
- The most commonly reported lymphomas are low-grade B-cell lymphomas, particularly follicular lymphomas and cases of chronic lymphocytic leukemia/small lymphocytic lymphoma.
- The most commonly reported H/DC tumor is histiocytic sarcoma.
- Diagnosis requires awareness of the entity, thorough immunophenotypic evaluation, and supporting evidence from comparative molecular studies.

ABSTRACT

Tumors of histiocytic or dendritic cell origin appear to occur with increased frequency in patients with lymphoma. Recent molecular data have demonstrated clonal relationships between the lymphoma and the histiocytic/dendritic cell tumor in some of these cases. Clinical, pathologic, and experimental data suggest that this phenomenon probably represents transdifferentiation of the lymphoma clone to a histiocytic/dendritic cell lineage in most cases. Awareness of this entity is necessary to prompt comparative molecular studies in appropriate cases.

INTRODUCTION

Tumors of histiocytic or dendritic cell (H/DC) origin appear to occur with increased frequency in patients with lymphoma.[1–3] Recent molecular data have demonstrated clonal relationships between the lymphoma and the H/DC tumor in some of these cases (Table 1). Most early data focused on clonal relationships between B or T lymphoblastic leukemias/lymphomas and H/DC tumors.[4–7] Because lymphoblastic neoplasms are tumors of precursor lymphoid cells, such tumors might retain some degree of lineage plasticity inherent to hematopoietic precursors in general. However, more recent data have established that clonal relationships also can be seen between lymphomas derived from mature lymphoid cells and H/DC tumors.[8] Experimental data also have demonstrated reprogramming of mature lymphocytes into H/DC cells.[9] These findings challenge the concept of lineage commitment in the traditional model of hematopoietic cell differentiation, and suggest mature lymphoid cells have more lineage plasticity than previously thought.

Clinical, pathologic, and experimental data suggest that this phenomenon probably represents transdifferentiation of the lymphoma clone to an

Disclosures: None.
Department of Laboratory Medicine and Pathology, Mayo Clinic, 200 First Street Southwest, Rochester, MN 55905, USA
E-mail address: feldman.andrew@mayo.edu

Surgical Pathology 6 (2013) 619–629
http://dx.doi.org/10.1016/j.path.2013.08.003
1875-9181/13/$ – see front matter © 2013 Elsevier Inc. All rights reserved.

Table 1
Reported examples of clonal relationships between lymphomas and H/DC tumors

| Lymphoma | H/DC Tumor (No. of Reported Cases) | | | | References |
	HS	IDCS	LCH	LCS	
Precursor lymphoid neoplasms:					
B-LBL	6	—	—	1	5,6,25,33–36
T-LBL	2	—	3	—	4,7,25,27
Mature lymphoid neoplasms:					
CLL/SLL	3	5	—	1	28,37,38
SMZL	1	—	—	—	39
HCL	—	—	—	2	40,41
FL	12	1	2	1	8,13,14,24,26,39,42,43
MCL	1	—	—	—	44
DLBCL	1	—	—	—	42

Abbreviations: B-LBL, B lymphoblastic leukemia/lymphoma; CLL/SLL, chronic lymphocytic leukemia/small lymphocytic lymphoma; DLBCL, diffuse large B-cell lymphoma; FL, follicular lymphoma; HCL, hairy cell leukemia; H/DC, histiocytic/dendritic cell; HS, histiocytic sarcoma; IDCS, interdigitating cell sarcoma; LCH, Langerhans cell histiocytosis; LCS, Langerhans cell sarcoma; MCL, mantle cell lymphoma; SMZL, splenic marginal zone lymphoma; T-LBL, T lymphoblastic leukemia/lymphoma.

H/DC lineage in most cases.[8,10] Transdifferentiation refers to the reprogramming of a cell of one lineage to another lineage, as assessed by a combination of morphologic, phenotypic, and in some cases functional characteristics (**Fig. 1**). Outside the laboratory setting, it is difficult to distinguish transdifferentiation from the alternate mechanism of dedifferentiation to a pluripotent precursor cell and redifferentiation to a different lineage.[11] Here, we use the term transdifferentiation for lack of clinical evidence of an intermediate, dedifferentiated component in the cases reported.[8,10]

MICROSCOPIC FEATURES

Microscopic features of reported cases of clonal relationships between lymphomas and H/DC tumors have not differed from those seen in each of the entities alone according to standard World Health Organization (WHO) criteria.[12] The classifications of the lymphoma and H/DC components in previous reports are shown in **Table 1**. The 2 components may occur metachronously or synchronously, and when synchronous may occur in the same or different anatomic sites.

Among precursor lymphoid neoplasms, both B and T precursor lymphoblastic leukemia/lymphoma have been seen (**Fig. 2**). These may have either a leukemic or lymphomatous presentation. Among mature lymphoid neoplasms, B-cell lymphomas have represented all the well-documented cases (see **Fig. 2**; **Figs. 3** and **4**). The most common reported subtypes have been follicular lymphoma

and chronic lymphocytic leukemia/small lymphocytic lymphoma (CLL/SLL). Cases with diffuse large B-cell lymphoma, hairy cell leukemia, splenic marginal zone lymphoma, and mantle cell lymphoma also have been reported. Most reported H/DC tumors have been histiocytic sarcomas, followed by Langerhans cell tumors (either Langerhans cell histiocytosis or Langerhans cell sarcoma) and interdigitating dendritic cell sarcomas.

DIFFERENTIAL DIAGNOSIS

Clonal relationships between lymphomas and H/DC tumors must be differentiated from sporadic occurrence of clonally unrelated neoplasms in the same patient. An apparent increase in the appearance of H/DC tumors among patients with lymphoma has been reported regardless of clonal relationship.[1–3] This may be due to increased tissue sampling in patients with cancer, treatment effects (including immunosuppression), genetic predisposition to both neoplasms, effects of lymphoma-derived cytokines, and reporting bias.[1,3]

H/DC tumors arising in patients with lymphoma also must be differentiated from conventional transformation of a low-grade (typically B-cell) lymphoma to a higher-grade process (usually diffuse large B-cell lymphoma). Morphologic similarities between some large-cell lymphomas and histiocytic proliferations are reflected in the older "histiocytic lymphoma" nomenclature. Although this differential diagnosis probably applies more to cases reported in the preimmunohistochemistry

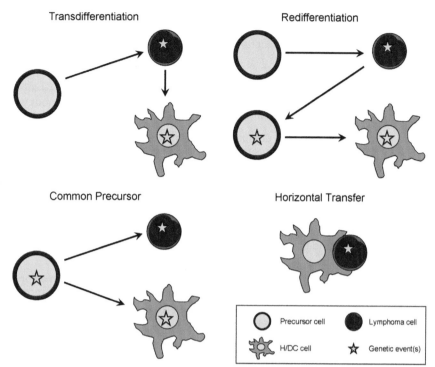

Fig. 1. Potential mechanisms for clonal relationships between lymphomas and H/DC tumors. Transdifferentiation represents a reprogramming of the lymphoma cell to a neoplastic cell of H/DC lineage. Genetic events acquired during lymphoid maturation (eg, immunoglobulin or T-cell receptor gene rearrangements) or lymphomagenesis (eg, chromosomal translocations) are passed on to the H/DC tumor. Redifferentiation implies an intermediate stage in which the lymphoma cell dedifferentiates to a pluripotent precursor and then redifferentiates to an H/DC tumor. A common pluripotent precursor that acquires genetic abnormalities may generate distinct tumors of lymphoid and H/DC origin. Horizontal transfer by cell fusion or engulfment of lymphoma DNA is a theoretic mechanism by which lymphoma-specific genetic abnormalities might be detected in H/DC cells from the same patient in the absence of a clonally related H/DC neoplasm.

literature, lymphomas occasionally may express markers seen in H/DC tumors, and may lose expression of traditional lymphoid markers due to an aberrant phenotype or treatment effect (eg, rituximab). In addition, rare patients with low-grade lymphomas may present with both a clonally related H/DC tumor and a conventional transformation event (diffuse large B-cell lymphoma).[13,14]

The differential diagnosis also includes lymphoma with a prominent reactive H/DC component. This occurs most frequently in classical Hodgkin lymphomas and peripheral T-cell lymphomas, including Lennert lymphoma and some cases of lymph node involvement by mycosis fungoides with pronounced dermatopathic change. In addition, Langerhans cell proliferations seen in lymphoma specimens can be quite extensive without necessarily representing a neoplastic (ie, clonal) process.[15,16] Conversely, cases of H/DC tumors with clonal *IGH* gene rearrangements and/or *IGH/BCL2* translocations should not be presumed to be transdifferentiated from an

underlying B-cell lymphoma unless the lymphoma is documented by other means, as these genetic findings have been seen in some sporadic H/DC tumors.[17–20]

When both lymphoma and an H/DC tumor occur synchronously at the same anatomic site, only one component may be recognized. If the H/DC tumor is cytologically bland (especially Langerhans cell histiocytosis), and particularly if the lymphoma is being diagnosed for the first time, the H/DC component may not be recognized as such. Conversely, minimal involvement by a low-grade lymphoma in the face of a new diagnosis of an H/DC tumor easily may be missed (see **Fig. 3**).

Finally, lymphoblastic transformation of chronic myelogenous leukemia should be considered separately from transdifferentiation as described here, although they have a common clonal origin (see **Fig. 1**). Rare examples of other clonal relationships between lymphoid neoplasms and myeloid leukemias, as well as the subject of bilineal leukemias, are not discussed here.[21,22]

Differential Diagnosis
CLONAL RELATIONSHIPS BETWEEN LYMPHOMAS AND H/DC TUMORS

Diagnosis	Important Points
Clonally related lymphoma and H/DC tumor	• H/DC tumor typically follows (or is synchronous with) lymphoma diagnosis
	• Comparative polymerase chain reaction and/or fluorescence in situ hybridization can support the clonal relationship
Clonally unrelated lymphoma and H/DC tumor	• H/DC tumors preceding the diagnosis of lymphoma are less likely to be clonally related
	• Discordant (or negative) comparative molecular studies do not exclude the possibility of a clonal relationship
Low-grade lymphoma with transformation to higher-grade lymphoma	• Lymphomas may express H/DC markers seen in tumors or lose expression of lymphoid markers due to an aberrant phenotype or treatment effect
	• Rare patients with low-grade lymphomas may present with both an H/DC tumor and conventional transformation
Lymphoma with prominent reactive H/DC cell proliferation	• Lymphomas may be accompanied by prominent collections of reactive H/DC cells
	• Further workup is merited if the H/DC cell proliferation is atypical
Sporadic H/DC tumor	• Sporadic H/DC tumors may have clonal immunoglobulin gene rearrangements and/or *IGH/BCL2* translocations; this should not be taken as evidence of an underlying lymphoma without further data

DIAGNOSIS

Diagnosis of clonally related lymphoma and H/DC tumor requires fulfillment of standard WHO criteria necessary to diagnose both processes separately as well as molecular data to support a clonal relationship between them.[12] Ideally, this involves integration of clinical, morphologic, immunophenotypic, and genetic data. Most cases of transdifferentiation begin as either a precursor lymphoblastic leukemia/lymphoma or a low-grade B-cell lymphoma, and suspicion should be raised in these settings. If the presence of an H/DC population cannot be explained by other clinicopathologic data, comparative molecular studies can be performed to determine its relationship to the lymphoma.

Most overtly malignant H/DC tumors will be recognized readily by morphology, although even histiocytic sarcoma occasionally may be difficult to identify due to numerous background inflammatory cells.[23] Other H/DC tumors may be more cytologically bland, such as Langerhans cell histiocytosis, and present a greater challenge. In some cases, these are clonally related to the underlying lymphoma.[7,24–27] In other cases, however, clonality studies suggest that even prominent Langerhans cell proliferations accompanying lymphomatous infiltrates may not be clonal themselves and perhaps should not be designated Langerhans cell histiocytosis.[15,16] Clonal relationships also have been reported between precursor lymphoblastic neoplasms and H/DC proliferations designated "atypical," but that did not fit into a well-defined WHO category of H/DC tumor.[25] Some of these atypical histiocytic lesions, as well as some cases of otherwise typical Langerhans cell histiocytosis, subsequently demonstrated aggressive clinical behavior.

H/DC tumors are rare and can mimic other malignancies morphologically. The initial evaluation may include a broad panel of nonhematopoietic immunohistochemical markers (eg, keratins). By the time the correct diagnosis is made, it may be relatively easy to miss a subtle atypical lymphoid infiltrate in the background, such as a few atypical follicles that represent low-grade follicular lymphoma (see **Fig. 3**) or a subtle infiltrate by CLL/SLL. Therefore, awareness of the phenomenon of transdifferentiation is critical, and all diagnoses of an H/DC tumor should be accompanied by careful morphologic evaluation for an atypical lymphoid infiltrate in the background and, if possible, a comprehensive clinical history. Any

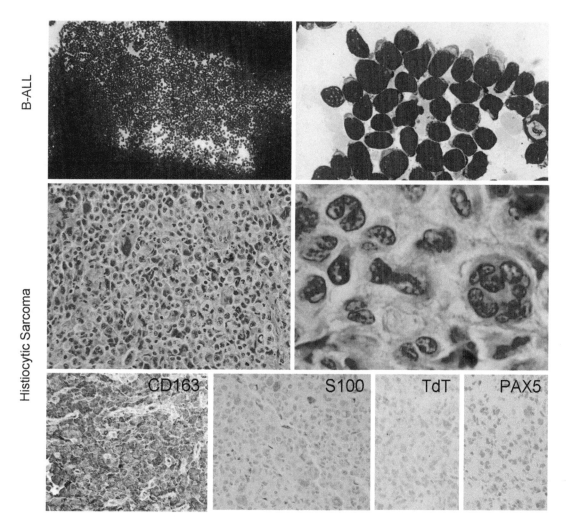

Fig. 2. Pathologic features of histiocytic sarcoma arising in the setting of precursor B lymphoblastic leukemia (B-ALL). The histiocytic sarcoma cells show marked nuclear pleomorphism and abundant eosinophilic cytoplasm. They express the histiocytic marker CD163, show focal expression of S100, and are negative for TdT and PAX5, which were expressed in the B-ALL. Subsequent studies demonstrated similar clonal rearrangements of immunoglobulin and T-cell receptor genes, as well as homozygous deletion of *CDKN2A* in both components.

suspicious lymphoid infiltrate should be evaluated immunophenotypically.

For cases with metachronous involvement, the order of presentation of the 2 components is important. In metachronous cases published to date, the lymphoma component has presented first, suggesting that H/DC tumors represent transdifferentiation of the lymphoma clone. Although the transdifferentiation model may not apply to all cases or an H/DC tumor might present in the setting of a clinically occult lymphoma, cases in which the H/DC is diagnosed following or simultaneously with the lymphoma should raise the greatest suspicion.

In general, both the lymphoma and the H/DC components show phenotypes similar to sporadic examples of each tumor type (see **Figs. 2–4**). Cases classified as histiocytic sarcoma often express S100 at least partially, suggesting a degree of dendritic cell differentiation (see **Fig. 3**).[8] Downregulation of PAX5 and expression of myeloid transcription factors, such as CEBPβ and PU.1, accompany transdifferentiation clinically and can induce it experimentally.[8,9,28] However, this transcription factor profile is common to H/DC cells in general, and is not a reliable means to distinguish transdifferentiated from sporadic H/DC tumors. Conversely, weak expression of PAX5, typically a B-cell–specific transcription factor, rarely may be seen in the H/DC component in cases of transdifferentiation (see **Fig. 4**); although PAX5 expression is not limited to B cells and

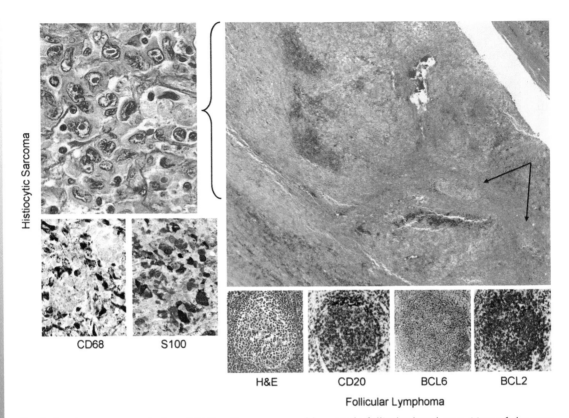

Fig. 3. Synchronous presentation of histiocytic sarcoma and low-grade follicular lymphoma. Most of the specimen is involved by a histiocytic sarcoma expressing CD68 and partially expressing S100, indicating a degree of dendritic cell differentiation. Only rare atypical follicles were present in the background (*arrows*), which on further staining were shown to express CD20, BCL6, and BCL2, typical of follicular lymphoma. Subsequent studies demonstrated *IGH/BCL2* in both components.

data in H/DC tumors are limited, this expression might raise suspicion for a clonal relationship.[24,29]

Definitive diagnosis of a clonal relationship between lymphomas and H/DC tumors relies on comparative molecular testing. The most widely available test to assess clonal relationship is comparative PCR testing for similar clonal immunoglobulin or T-cell receptor gene rearrangements (**Fig. 5**). This approach has limitations. Clonal rearrangements cannot always be detected in lymphoma samples for either technical or genetic reasons. In addition, detection of identical electrophoretic mobilities in PCR amplicons from the 2 samples does not always equate to identical sequences. Sequencing the amplicons can help verify the same clone, but is not available in many clinical laboratories. However, sequencing has provided support for transdifferentiation (rather than a common clonal precursor) as a mechanism by detecting evidence of somatic hypermutation in the immunoglobulin genes in H/DC tumors clonally related to B-cell lymphomas.[10] If the lymphoma and H/DC tumor are presenting synchronously at

the same anatomic site, it may not be possible to compare the 2 tumor cell populations by this method (see **Fig. 3**). Microdissection of the 2 components can be informative but generally is not available clinically.[24,26] Even if the lymphoma and H/DC tumor are presenting at different anatomic sites or are metachronous, care must be taken to exclude subtle lymphoma involvement in the H/DC tumor specimen, which could falsely give the impression that the same clone is present in the H/DC tumor. Finally, some sporadic H/DC tumors have been reported to have clonal immunoglobulin gene rearrangements.[17–20] The significance of this phenomenon is unknown; however, this should not be interpreted to indicate transdifferentiation unless a definitive diagnosis of B-cell lymphoma can be made using standard WHO criteria and there is molecular evidence to support a clonal relationship.

Fluorescence in situ hybridization (FISH) can be helpful in supporting a clonal relationship between lymphomas and H/DC tumors (**Fig. 6**). This technique also has limitations. A cytogenetic

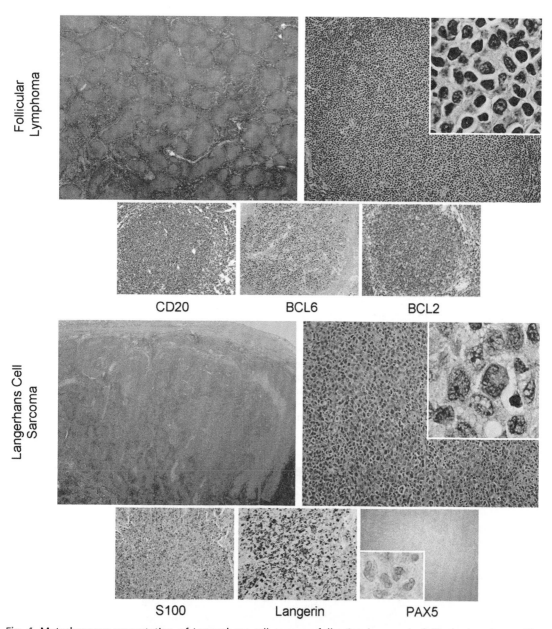

Fig. 4. Metachronous presentation of Langerhans cell sarcoma following low-grade follicular lymphoma. The original follicular lymphoma had a typical phenotype and no atypical H/DC cell population was present. The Langerhans cell sarcoma showed sinusoidal and diffuse growth patterns and was composed of markedly pleomorphic cells without eosinophils. The tumor cells expressed S100, langerin, CD1a (not shown), and, weakly, PAX5. Subsequent studies demonstrated similar clonal rearrangements of immunoglobulin genes as well as *IGH/BCL2* in both components.

abnormality detectable by clinically available FISH testing has to be present in at least one of the samples, typically the lymphoma sample. The most common example in the literature is identifying an *IGH/BCL2* translocation in both a follicular lymphoma and an H/DC tumor.[8,10] Unlike polymerase chain reaction (PCR)-based approaches, it usually is possible to distinguish H/DC tumor cells from background lymphoma cells based on a combination of location on the tissue section, nuclear morphology, and relative abundance of the 2 tumor cell populations (see **Fig. 6**). More precise identification can be used combining immunofluorescence with FISH, but this often is not available

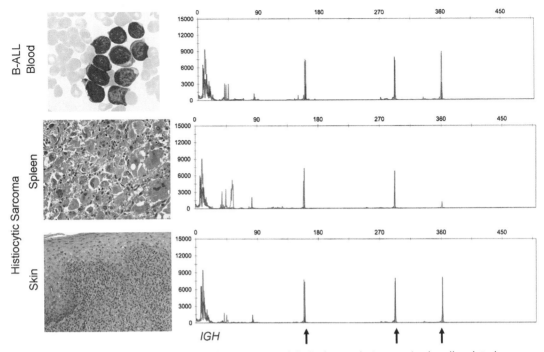

Fig. 5. Comparative PCR analysis of a case of the immunoglobulin heavy chain gene in clonally related precursor B-ALL followed by histiocytic sarcoma 4 months later. Three clonal peaks (*arrows*) are seen with the same sizes in the original B-ALL and in 2 subsequent histiocytic sarcoma specimens. The histiocytic sarcoma specimens showed no morphologic or phenotypic evidence of B-ALL, nor was there evidence of B-ALL in the blood or bone marrow at this time. (*Adapted from* McClure R, Khoury J, Feldman A, et al. Clonal relationship between precursor B-cell acute lymphoblastic leukemia and histiocytic sarcoma: a case report and discussion in the context of similar cases. Leuk Res 2010;34(2):e71–3; with permission.)

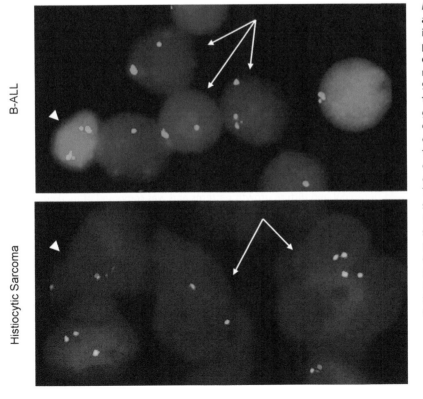

Fig. 6. Comparative FISH analysis of the case shown in Fig. 2. Green signals represent the centromere of chromosome 9 and red signals represent *CDKN2A* on 9q21. Arrowheads point to cells with a normal red/green signal pattern, indicating presence of 2 copies of *CDKN2A*. Arrows point to cells with green signals only, indicating homozygous deletion of *CDKN2A*. The same deletion is present in both the precursor B-ALL and the histiocytic sarcoma. The nuclear morphology of the H/DC tumor cells helps to exclude the possibility that the abnormal FISH signals correspond to residual B-ALL cells in the background.

clinically.[24] Rare sporadic H/DC tumors carry *IGH/BCL2* translocations, and presence of this translocation is not sufficient to assume the presence of underlying follicular lymphoma.[17,20]

As transdifferentiated macrophages and H/DC tumors (particularly histiocytic sarcoma) may retain phagocytic activity, engulfment of lymphoma cells or their apoptotic debris could theoretically lead to detection of lymphoma-specific DNA in an H/DC tumor (horizontal transfer; see **Fig. 1**).[6,9,23] This mechanism probably is not responsible for previously reported cases because there is no evidence that engulfed lymphoma DNA is passed on to the progeny of H/DC tumor cells, and because in many cases demonstration of a lymphoma-associated translocation in the H/DC tumor by FISH has not identified additional copies of the involved loci.

PROGNOSIS

Because relatively few cases of clonal relationships between lymphomas and H/DC tumors have been published, data on prognosis and management of this entity are limited. Aggressive clinical behavior has been reported in many cases, particularly histiocytic sarcomas. A recent review indicated a median survival of 6.5 months among cases originating from B-cell lymphomas.[10] Sporadic histiocytic sarcoma also has a poor prognosis.[23,30] The prognosis of B or T lymphoblastic leukemia/lymphoma clonally related to H/DC tumors other than histiocytic sarcoma has been suggested to be more favorable.[25] It has been suggested that transdifferentiation of a low-grade B-cell neoplasm, such as follicular lymphoma or CLL/SLL, might be considered a rare form of transformation analogous to the more common transformation to diffuse large B-cell lymphoma, which typically is associated with poor prognosis.[31,32] Because there are few prognostic data on transdifferentiation, particularly cases involving H/DC tumors typically associated with a less aggressive course (eg, Langerhans cell histiocytosis), transdifferentiation to an H/DC tumor is best considered a separate entity at this time.

REFERENCES

1. Egeler RM, Neglia JP, Arico M, et al. The relation of Langerhans cell histiocytosis to acute leukemia, lymphomas, and other solid tumors. The LCH-Malignancy Study Group of the Histiocyte Society. Hematol Oncol Clin North Am 1998;12(2):369–78.

2. Vasef MA, Zaatari GS, Chan WC, et al. Dendritic cell tumors associated with low-grade B-cell malignancies. Report of three cases. Am J Clin Pathol 1995;104(6):696–701.

3. Trebo MM, Attarbaschi A, Mann G, et al. Histiocytosis following T-acute lymphoblastic leukemia: a BFM study. Leuk Lymphoma 2005;46(12):1735–41.

4. van der Kwast TH, van Dongen JJ, Michiels JJ, et al. T-lymphoblastic lymphoma terminating as malignant histiocytosis with rearrangement of immunoglobulin heavy chain gene. Leukemia 1991;5(1):78–82.

5. Bouabdallah R, Abena P, Chetaille B, et al. True histiocytic lymphoma following B-acute lymphoblastic leukaemia: case report with evidence for a common clonal origin in both neoplasms. Br J Haematol 2001; 113(4):1047–50.

6. Feldman AL, Minniti C, Santi M, et al. Histiocytic sarcoma after acute lymphoblastic leukaemia: a common clonal origin. Lancet Oncol 2004;5(4): 248–50.

7. Feldman AL, Berthold F, Arceci R, et al. Clonal relationship between precursor T-lymphoblastic leukaemia/lymphoma and Langerhans-cell histiocytosis. Lancet Oncol 2005;6(6):435–7.

8. Feldman AL, Arber DA, Pittaluga S, et al. Clonally related follicular lymphomas and histiocytic/dendritic cell sarcomas: evidence for transdifferentiation of the follicular lymphoma clone. Blood 2008;111(12): 5433–9. PMCID: 2424145.

9. Xie H, Ye M, Feng R, et al. Stepwise reprogramming of B cells into macrophages. Cell 2004;117(5): 663–76.

10. Stoecker MM, Wang E. Histiocytic/dendritic cell transformation of B-cell neoplasms: pathologic evidence of lineage conversion in differentiated hematolymphoid malignancies. Arch Pathol Lab Med 2013;137(6): 865–70.

11. Cobaleda C, Jochum W, Busslinger M. Conversion of mature B cells into T cells by dedifferentiation to uncommitted progenitors. Nature 2007;449(7161): 473–7.

12. Swerdlow S, Campo E, Harris N, et al. WHO classification of tumours of haematopoietic and lymphoid tissues. In: Bosman F, Jaffe E, Lakhani S, et al, editors. World Health Organization classification of tumours. 4th edition. Lyon (France): International Agency for Research on Cancer; 2008.

13. Zhang D, McGuirk J, Ganguly S, et al. Histiocytic/dendritic cell sarcoma arising from follicular lymphoma involving the bone: a case report and review of literature. Int J Hematol 2009;89(4):529–32.

14. Wang E, Papalas J, Hutchinson CB, et al. Sequential development of histiocytic sarcoma and diffuse large b-cell lymphoma in a patient with a remote history of follicular lymphoma with genotypic evidence of a clonal relationship: a divergent (bilineal) neoplastic transformation of an indolent B-cell lymphoma in a single individual. Am J Surg Pathol 2011;35(3):457–63.

15. Christie LJ, Evans AT, Bray SE, et al. Lesions resembling Langerhans cell histiocytosis in association

with other lymphoproliferative disorders: a reactive or neoplastic phenomenon? Hum Pathol 2006; 37(1):32–9.

16. Benharroch D, Guterman G, Levy I, et al. High content of Langerhans cells in malignant lymphoma—incidence and significance. Virchows Arch 2010; 457(1):63–7.

17. Chen W, Lau SK, Fong D, et al. High frequency of clonal immunoglobulin receptor gene rearrangements in sporadic histiocytic/dendritic cell sarcomas. Am J Surg Pathol 2009;33(6):863–73.

18. Chen W, Wang J, Wang E, et al. Detection of clonal lymphoid receptor gene rearrangements in Langerhans cell histiocytosis. Am J Surg Pathol 2010; 34(7):1049–57.

19. Vos JA, Abbondanzo SL, Barekman CL, et al. Histiocytic sarcoma: a study of five cases including the histiocyte marker CD163. Mod Pathol 2005;18(5): 693–704.

20. Hayase E, Kurosawa M, Yonezumi M, et al. Aggressive sporadic histiocytic sarcoma with immunoglobulin heavy chain gene rearrangement and t(14;18). Int J Hematol 2010;92(4):659–63.

21. Szczepanski T, de Vaan GA, Beishuizen A, et al. Acute lymphoblastic leukemia followed by a clonally-unrelated EBV-positive non-Hodgkin lymphoma and a clonally-related myelomonocytic leukemia cutis. Pediatr Blood Cancer 2004;42(4):343–9.

22. Monma F, Nishii K, Ezuki S, et al. Molecular and phenotypic analysis of Philadelphia chromosome-positive bilineage leukemia: possibility of a lineage switch from T-lymphoid leukemic progenitor to myeloid cells. Cancer Genet Cytogenet 2006;164(2):118–21.

23. Grogan TM, Pileri SA, Chan JK, et al. Histiocytic sarcoma. In: Swerdlow S, Campo E, Harris N, et al, editors. WHO classification of tumours of haematopoietic and lymphoid tissues. Lyon (France): International Agency for Research on Cancer; 2008. p. 356–7.

24. West DS, Dogan A, Quint PS, et al. Clonally related follicular lymphomas and Langerhans cell neoplasms: expanding the spectrum of transdifferentiation. Am J Surg Pathol 2013;37(7):978–86.

25. Castro EC, Blazquez C, Boyd J, et al. Clinicopathologic features of histiocytic lesions following ALL, with a review of the literature. Pediatr Dev Pathol 2010;13(3):225–37.

26. Magni M, Di Nicola M, Carlo-Stella C, et al. Identical rearrangement of immunoglobulin heavy chain gene in neoplastic Langerhans cells and B-lymphocytes: evidence for a common precursor. Leuk Res 2002; 26(12):1131–3.

27. Rodig SJ, Payne EG, Degar BA, et al. Aggressive Langerhans cell histiocytosis following T-ALL: clonally related neoplasms with persistent expression of constitutively active NOTCH1. Am J Hematol 2008;83(2):116–21.

28. Shao H, Xi L, Raffeld M, et al. Clonally related histiocytic/dendritic cell sarcoma and chronic lymphocytic leukemia/small lymphocytic lymphoma: a study of seven cases. Mod Pathol 2011;24(11):1421–32.

29. Feldman AL, Dogan A. Diagnostic uses of Pax5 immunohistochemistry. Adv Anat Pathol 2007;14(5): 323–34.

30. Pileri SA, Grogan TM, Harris NL, et al. Tumours of histiocytes and accessory dendritic cells: an immunohistochemical approach to classification from the International Lymphoma Study Group based on 61 cases. Histopathology 2002;41(1):1–29.

31. Wong E, Dickinson M. Transformation in follicular lymphoma: biology, prognosis, and therapeutic options. Curr Oncol Rep 2012;14(5):424–32.

32. Jain P, O'Brien S. Richter's transformation in chronic lymphocytic leukemia. Oncology 2012;26(12):1146–52.

33. Dictor M, Warenholt J, Gyorgy C, et al. Clonal evolution to histiocytic sarcoma with the BCR/ABL rearrangement 14 years after acute lymphoblastic leukemia. Leuk Lymphoma 2009;50(11):1892–5.

34. Kumar R, Khan SP, Joshi DD, et al. Pediatric histiocytic sarcoma clonally related to precursor B-cell acute lymphoblastic leukemia with homozygous deletion of CDKN2A encoding p16INK4A. Pediatr Blood Cancer 2011;56(2):307–10.

35. McClure R, Khoury J, Feldman A, et al. Clonal relationship between precursor B-cell acute lymphoblastic leukemia and histiocytic sarcoma: a case report and discussion in the context of similar cases. Leuk Res 2010;34(2):e71–3.

36. Ratei R, Hummel M, Anagnostopoulos I, et al. Common clonal origin of an acute B-lymphoblastic leukemia and a Langerhans' cell sarcoma: evidence for hematopoietic plasticity. Haematologica 2010;95(9): 1461–6.

37. Fraser CR, Wang W, Gomez M, et al. Transformation of chronic lymphocytic leukemia/small lymphocytic lymphoma to interdigitating dendritic cell sarcoma: evidence for transdifferentiation of the lymphoma clone. Am J Clin Pathol 2009;132(6):928–39.

38. Wetzler M, Kurzrock R, Goodacre AM, et al. Transformation of chronic lymphocytic leukemia to lymphoma of true histiocytic type. Cancer 1995;76(4): 609–17.

39. Wang E, Hutchinson CB, Huang Q, et al. Histiocytic sarcoma arising in indolent small B-cell lymphoma: report of two cases with molecular/genetic evidence suggestive of a 'transdifferentiation' during the clonal evolution. Leuk Lymphoma 2010;51(5):802–12.

40. Muslimani A, Chisti MM, Blenc AM, et al. Langerhans/dendritic cell sarcoma arising from hairy cell leukemia: a rare phenomenon. Ann Hematol 2012; 91(9):1485–7.

41. Furmanczyk PS, Lisle AE, Caldwell RB, et al. Langerhans cell sarcoma in a patient with hairy cell leukemia: common clonal origin indicated by identical

immunoglobulin gene rearrangements. J Cutan Pathol 2012;39(6):644–50.

42. Bassarova A, Troen G, Fossa A, et al. Transformation of B cell lymphoma to histiocytic sarcoma: somatic mutations of PAX-5 gene with loss of expression cannot explain transdifferentiation. J Hematop 2009; 2(3):135–41.

43. Zeng W, Meck J, Cheson BD, et al. Histiocytic sarcoma transdifferentiated from follicular lymphoma presenting as a cutaneous tumor. J Cutan Pathol 2011;38(12):999–1003.

44. Hure MC, Elco CP, Ward D, et al. Histiocytic sarcoma arising from clonally related mantle cell lymphoma. J Clin Oncol 2012;30(5):e49–53.

.

Distinguishing T-cell Large Granular Lymphocytic Leukemia from Reactive Conditions

Laboratory Tools and Challenges in Their Use

Jadee L. Neff, MD, PhD, Matthew T. Howard, MD,
William G. Morice, MD, PhD*

KEYWORDS

- T-LGL • Neoplasms of cytotoxic lymphocytes • Differential diagnosis • KIR flow cytometry
- Intrasinusoidal bone marrow infiltrates • Large granular lymphocytes

KEY POINTS

- The differential diagnosis of T-cell large granular leukemia (T-LGL) includes benign reactive expansions, hepatosplenic T-cell lymphoma, and aggressive natural killer (NK) cell leukemia.
- A diagnosis of T-LGL may be made if 2 of the following conditions are demonstrated: phenotypically abnormal T-cells with NK cell antigen expression, clonal T-cell gene rearrangements, or intrasinusoidal bone marrow cytotoxic lymphocyte infiltrates.

ABSTRACT

This article focuses on the challenges of diagnosing T-cell large granular leukemia and distinguishing it from benign reactive conditions, as well as more aggressive neoplasms of cytotoxic lymphocytes. No single laboratory method is sufficient to make the diagnosis, but instead a combination of flow cytometry, genetic studies, and bone marrow immunohistochemistry must be used.

INTRODUCTION

In the 1970s, cases with an increase in circulating lymphocytes having granulated cytoplasm and unexplained cytopenias were first reported; these lymphocytes were subsequently recognized as T-cell lineage and eventually the moniker T-cell large granular leukemia (T-LGL) was coined.[1,2] Early disease definitions emphasized peripheral blood granular lymphocyte counts and demonstration of T-cell clonality. Subsequent studies characterizing T-LGL reflect the evolution of immunophenotyping and molecular genetic tools available for the evaluation of this enigmatic condition. T-LGL is now recognized as a clonal cytotoxic T-cell disorder with abnormalities of pan T-cell antigen expression and high levels of NK-cell associated antigen expression.[3] The bone marrow pathology of T-LGL is typified by intrasinusoidal LGL infiltration, as demonstrated by immunohistochemistry.[4,5] At the molecular level, an activating STAT3 gene mutation has been found in approximately 50% of T-LGLs.[6,7] Although these attributes describe T-LGL in a broad sense, it remains problematic to determine how these individual features combine to make the diagnosis for individual patients. The challenge in rendering a T-LGL diagnosis is heightened by the recognition that many of the T-LGL

Disclosures: None.
Department of Laboratory Medicine and Pathology, Mayo Clinic, 200 First Street SW, Rochester, MN 55905, USA
* Corresponding author.
E-mail address: morice.william@mayo.edu

"disease features" are also found in the physiologic response of cytotoxic T cells.[8,9] Added to this is the proclivity of T-LGL to arise in association with autoimmune phenomena or other potential stimulants of cellular immunity, such as clonal B-cell disorders.[10,11] All of these elements on the one hand make it imperative to distinguish T-LGL from reactive T-cell expansion, and on the other make it more problematic to do so.

GROSS AND MICROSCOPIC FEATURES

Apart from splenomegaly, which is variably present and usually mild, T-LGL has minimal gross pathologic abnormalities. Microscopically, T-LGL is characterized by lymphoid cells with small, bland nuclei and cytoplasm that, despite the name, is variably abundant and variably granulated. In most cases, these cells will comprise greater than 50% of the circulating lymphocytes; however, they are indistinguishable from normal/reactive granular lymphocytes, and if there is significant cytologic atypia, other potential diagnoses should be considered (**Fig. 1**). Given the difficulties in the morphologic distinction of normal and abnormal cells, in the past an absolute granular lymphocyte count of greater than 2×10^9/L was a diagnostic criterion.[12] However, it has been established that not all T-LGLs meet this threshold, and patients may also be receiving drugs that lower the lymphocyte count (such as corticosteroids) due to the frequent association with autoimmune conditions. For these reasons, absolute LGL counts are no longer part of the diagnostic criteria and this is not routinely used by most laboratories.

As in the peripheral blood, morphologic recognition of marrow involvement by T-LGL is challenging. In bone marrow aspirates, the cytoplasmic features of the granular lymphocytes are difficult to appreciate, and, when combined with the bland nuclear features, make these cells essentially impossible to recognize. In the bone

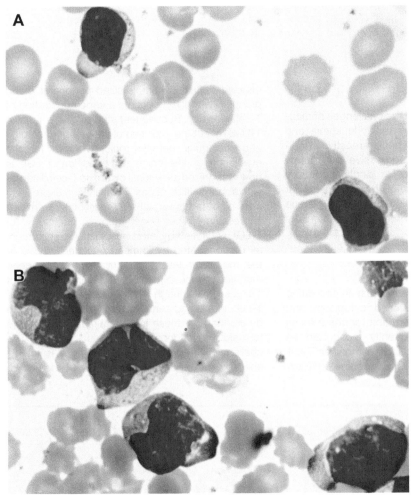

Fig. 1. Peripheral smears of T-LGL (*A*) and hepatosplenic T-cell lymphoma (HSTCL) (*B*). Note the relatively bland cytology in T-LGL (*A*) compared with the marked atypia in this case of HSTCL (*B*). (Wright Giemsa stain, ×400).

marrow, the most readily identified histologic feature is the presence of benign interstitial lymphoid aggregates, which are frequently associated but are an entirely nonspecific finding and are not populated by the abnormal cells.[4,5] Rather than populating the lymphoid aggregates, the abnormal lymphocytes are found in the bone marrow sinusoids. However, unlike other aggressive cytotoxic T-cell disorders that involve marrow sinusoids, such as hepatosplenic T-cell lymphoma (HSTCL), T-LGL does not distend or distort the marrow microvascular structures, rendering these bland cells nearly undetectable on histologic examination (**Fig. 2**).

DIFFERENTIAL DIAGNOSIS

The differential diagnosis of T-LGL includes both benign, reactive expansions of cytotoxic lymphocytes, and aggressive neoplasms of cytotoxic lymphocytes that can involve the blood and bone marrow, such as HSTCL and aggressive NK-cell leukemia.

T-LGL and physiologic cytotoxic T-cell responses appear closely related, and T-LGL may, in some instances, represent a distorted cytotoxic T-cell response to chronic stimulation with varying degrees of clonal "purity."[13] As such, distinguishing between these 2 can be extremely challenging

Fig. 2. Bone marrow biopsies stained with granzyme B showing intrasinusoidal infiltrates of T-LGL (*A*) and HSTCL (*B*). Unlike HSTCL, which distends the marrow sinusoids (*B*), T-LGL sinusoidal infiltrates are distributed single-file and can be subtle (*A*). (TIA-1 stain, ×400).

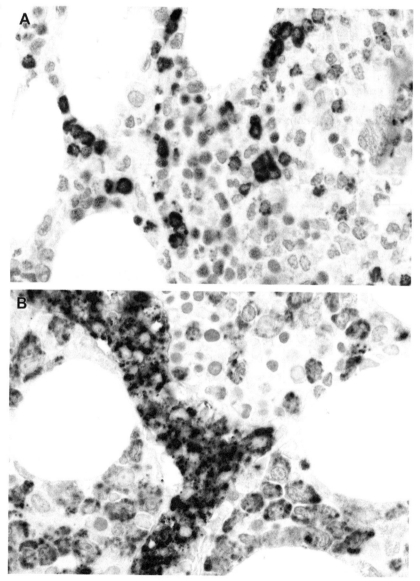

and requires a comprehensive approach with appropriate use of the full armamentarium of available laboratory tools. Morphology is particularly unreliable for making this distinction, as are T-cell receptor gene rearrangements when used in isolation (**Fig. 3**, see **T-LGL Key Features**). Flow cytometry is particularly helpful, as it can reveal if an increase in granular lymphocytes is composed of a variety of T-cell and NK-cell subsets, as expected of reactive conditions, or a more homogeneous population, as is seen in T-LGL. Extensive evaluation of NK-cell associated antigens (such as KIR) is valuable in this regard, as the varied composition of reactive cytotoxic lymphocytes may be difficult to appreciate with routine T-cell phenotyping (**Fig. 4**).[14,15] Flow cytometry can also reveal phenotypic abnormalities useful in establishing a T-LGL diagnosis; it is important to remember, however, that many of these can also be found in normal gamma/delta T cells and, therefore, caution should be exercised when attempting to determine if an increase in this cell type is reactive or indicative of T-LGL.[16] *STAT3* mutational analysis may also help confirm a T-LGL diagnosis, although it is not present in all cases.[6,7] If peripheral blood findings are inconclusive, bone marrow examination should be strongly considered, both to evaluate for other potential causes of any cytopenias and to allow for the immunohistochemical studies, which can be helpful in establishing the diagnosis.[17]

The distinction of T-LGL from aggressive malignancies of cytotoxic lymphocytes is usually less problematic, as the latter usually presents with B-symptoms and pronounced organomegaly. Therefore, correlation with the clinical features is a critical first step, although there are pathologic features that can also aid in the distinction. Aggressive NK-cell leukemia and related conditions typically occur in Asian populations, have destructive tissue infiltration with cytologic atypia, and are Epstein-Barr virus (EBV)-positive, all features that distinguish them from T-LGL.[18] Distinguishing T-LGL from HSTCL on pathologic grounds can be more difficult, as both can be cytologically bland, have a modest peripheral blood involvement, infiltrate marrow sinusoids, and are EBV-negative.[19] The proclivity of HSTCL to occur in young males and be gamma/delta T-cell lineage is helpful but nonspecific. Although both entities express NK-associated antigens, there are differences that can aid in their

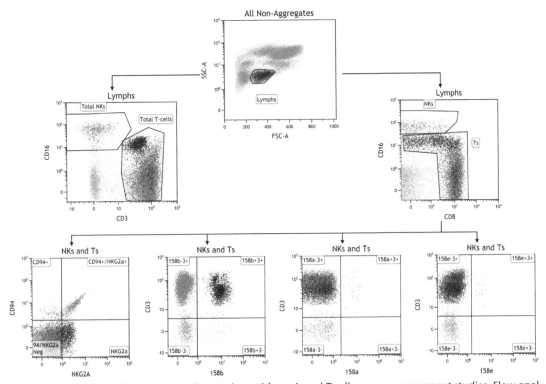

Fig. 3. Peripheral blood flow cytometry in a patient with equivocal T-cell gene rearrangement studies. Flow analysis revealed a small subset of T cells with CD16 coexpression and aberrant KIR CD158b restriction (*blue*), supporting a diagnosis of T-LGL. The majority population of normal T cells (*red*) likely masked the clonality of the abnormal population in the T-cell gene rearrangement studies.

T-LGL Key Features

Clinical Features

- Usually affects middle age or older adults.

- No proclivity to occur in specific geographic regions or affect specific ethnic groups or gender.

- 20% to 30% of cases associated with rheumatoid arthritis or other autoimmune conditions.

- 10% to 20% of cases associated with other clonal hematolymphoid disorders, including monoclonal B-cell lymphocytosis.

Peripheral Blood Features

- Typically, more than 50% of lymphocytes have granules, although there is frequently only a minimal increase in the absolute LGL cell count.

- Unexplained neutropenia is present in approximately two-thirds of cases.

- Anemia also common but may be slightly less often seen than neutropenia. Thrombocytopenia is uncommon and rarely occurs as the sole cytopenia.

Bone Marrow Features

- Although often hypercellular, the marrow may be normocellular or hypocellular.

- Left-shifted granulopoiesis and left-shifted and megaloblastoid erythropoiesis are relatively common; abnormalities in megakaryopoiesis are infrequent.

- The abnormal T-LGL cells are essentially impossible to recognize by routine morphology.

- Immunohistochemistry for CD8 and the cytotoxic granule proteins TIA-1 and granzyme B reveals disease-associated intrasinusoidal infiltration in up to 80% of cases.

Flow Cytometry

- Studies can be performed on the peripheral blood or bone marrow aspirate.

- Routine T-cell immunophenotyping will reveal a relative increase in CD8-positive T cells with an inverted peripheral blood CD4:CD8 ratio in most cases.

- NK cells often decreased (both relative proportion and absolute number).

- Abnormally diminished or absent expression of CD5 and/or CD7 present in 80% to 90%; abnormalities of CD2 and CD3 much less frequent.

- NK-cell–associated antigens CD16 and CD57 expressed in 80% or more of cases, although isolated CD57 expression has low diagnostic specificity.

- Assessment of other NK cell antigens including KIR helpful in one-third of cases.

T-Cell Clonality

- Clonality can be demonstrated by either T-cell receptor (TCR) gene rearrangement studies or flow cytometric assessment of TCR beta chain variable region family expression.

- A number of studies suggest that T-LGL is an "oligoclonal" disorder, and changes in or evolution of clone composition in T-LGL may be seen if followed longitudinally.

- Physiologic T-cell repertoires may be oligoclonal and therefore yield TCR gene rearrangement patterns indistinguishable from those seen in T-LGL.

- Abnormal patterns of KIR expression or detectable STAT3 mutation may serve as surrogate markers of clonality.

- Given challenges in establishing T-cell clonality and oligoclonal nature of disease, a diagnosis of T-LGL can be rendered in the absence of documented T-cell clonality if the clinical context is appropriate, other pathologic criteria are satisfied, and the process inexplicably persists.

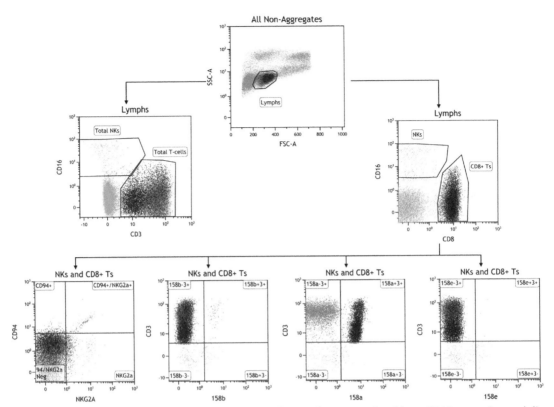

Fig. 4. Peripheral blood flow cytometry showing a population of CD8+ T cells with no CD16 expression and dim CD3 expression (*blue*). Further analysis for expression of the NK-associated antigens CD94 and the KIR receptors revealed abnormal expression of the KIR CD158a, supporting a diagnosis of T-LGL. Background CD8-positive T cells (*red*) show no KIR expression.

distinction; in particular, uniform expression of CD56 and coexpression of multiple KIR antigens is common in HSTCL and rare in T-LGL.[20] Bone marrow histology and cytogenetic studies can also be helpful as, unlike T-LGL, HSTCL tends to distend and distort marrow sinusoids (see **Fig. 2**) and have recurrent cytogenetic abnormalities, including trisomy 8 and isochromosome 7q.

DIAGNOSIS

Given the number of conditions that can cause either cytopenias or lymphocytosis, evaluation for T-LGL should be limited to cases with either unexplained cytopenias or persistent lymphocytosis. As a first step in the laboratory evaluation, the peripheral smear should be reviewed to screen for features of myelodysplasia or other lymphoproliferative disorders as potential underlying causes and to assess for granular lymphocyte cytology.

If T-LGL remains a diagnostic consideration, flow cytometric immunophenotyping should be performed. At a minimum, these studies should include assessment of pan T-cell and NK-cell

antigens to screen for features such as loss of CD5 or CD7, or aberrant coexpression of CD16, which is present in most cases.[14,20,21] Although most T-LGL cases are CD57-positive, CD57 is also expressed by normal memory T-cells and therefore has limited diagnostic specificity unless used in a multiparametric approach.[22] Other NK-cell associated antigens such as KIR can be helpful in making the diagnosis, as in some cases routine phenotyping may not reveal abnormalities beyond an abnormal CD4:CD8 ratio. If the clinical features are appropriate, and abnormal T cells are detected by flow cytometry, then T-cell clonality assessment (by polymerase chain reaction or TCR-Vbeta flow cytometry) should be performed, as a positive (clonal) result will allow for an unequivocal T-LGL diagnosis. However, peripheral blood T-cell clonality can be detected in a variety of conditions, including healthy subjects, and therefore these studies should not be used to screen for T-LGL in the absence of correlative flow cytometry.[23,24] STAT3 mutation may also be considered for diagnostic evaluation of T-LGL, although a negative study does not exclude the diagnosis, and the specificity of this finding in the absence of more traditional T-LGL assessments is unknown.

If the peripheral blood studies are inconclusive for the presence of T-LGL, then bone marrow examination should be considered to both exclude potential secondary causes, such as marrow involvement by other hematopoietic malignancy, and to help confirm a T-LGL diagnosis. Peripheral blood flow cytometry and molecular genetic studies do not necessarily need to be repeated on the bone marrow specimen. However, bone marrow immunohistochemistry with antibodies to CD8 and the cytotoxic granule proteins TIA-1 and granzyme B is required. In most T-LGLs, interstitial clusters or intrasinusoidal staining of CD8 and TIA-1 positive cells will be present; granzyme B reveals similar patterns but is slightly less sensitive.[4] These immunohistochemical findings are strongly disease associated; it should be remembered that lineage (T cell vs NK cell) cannot be established by this method and that these marrow immunohistochemistry findings may not be easily seen in all cases (**Fig. 5**).

Fig. 5. Bone marrow biopsy stained with CD8 (*A*) and granzyme B (*B*) showing a nonspecific pattern of marrow involvement. Cytotoxic T cells are slightly increased, but there is no distinct intrasinusoidal distribution pattern. This patient's T-LGL was diagnosed by classic receptor abnormalities demonstrated by flow cytometry and positive T-cell clonality demonstrated in T-cell gene rearrangement studies. (×200).

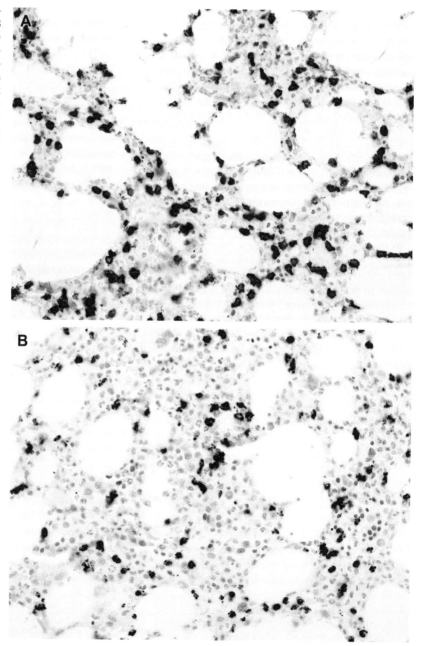

From a practical perspective, the presence of any 2 of these 3 abnormalities (phenotypically aberrant T cells, T-cell clonality/*STAT3* mutation, and intrasinusoidal marrow infiltrates) should be considered sufficient to render a T-LGL diagnosis. If, however, the diagnosis remains in doubt, then repeat evaluation is prudent after a period of 6 months to 1 year to establish persistence and exclude an unusual self-limited reactive process.

PROGNOSIS

In most instances, T-LGL is a clinically indolent condition with excellent long-term survival. Treatment is predicated on the presence of either symptomatic anemia or neutropenia. In the past, patients with isolated neutropenia frequently received treatment only after neutropenic infection, although prophylactic therapy is now advocated in this setting, and it appears that most patients with T-LGL will require treatment over time.[17,25] Most T-LGLs respond with single-agent treatment using methotrexate or cyclophosphamide, often combined with a short course of corticosteroids. Purine analogues or anti-CD52 monoclonal antibodies may be used in refractory cases; splenectomy or corticosteroid single-agent therapy does not have established efficacy.

In the vast majority of T-LGLs, morbidity and mortality is attributable to the disease-associated cytopenias rather than uncontrollable tumor burden or tissue infiltration. There are isolated descriptions of "aggressive" T-LGL or "transformed T-LGL," with more overt malignant clinical behavior.[26] Given the paucity of such cases, their relationship to clinically indolent T-LGL is unclear. Interestingly, many of these clinically aggressive cases are described as CD56-positive, a relatively infrequent occurrence in indolent T-LGL, raising the possibility that some are actually peripheral blood involvement by other malignancies, such as HSTCL.

REFERENCES

1. McKenna RW, Arthur DC, Gajl-Peczalska KJ, et al. Granulated T cell lymphocytosis with neutropenia: malignant or benign chronic lymphoproliferative disorder? Blood 1985;66(2):259–66.

2. Loughran TP Jr, Starkebaum G. Large granular lymphocyte leukemia. Report of 38 cases and review of the literature. Medicine (Baltimore) 1987;66(5):397–405.

3. Swerdlow SH, Campo E, Harris NL, et al. WHO classification of tumours of haematopoietic and lymphoid tissues. In: Bosman FT, Jaffe ES, Lakhani SR, et al,

editors. World Health Organization Classification of Tumours. 4th edition. Lyon (France): IARC Press; 2008. p. 272–3.

4. Morice WG, Kurtin PJ, Tefferi A, et al. Distinct bone marrow findings in T-cell granular lymphocytic leukemia revealed by paraffin section immunoperoxidase stains for CD8, TIA-1, and granzyme B. Blood 2002; 99(1):268–74.

5. Osuji N, Beiske K, Randen U, et al. Characteristic appearances of the bone marrow in T-cell large granular lymphocyte leukaemia. Histopathology 2007;50(5): 547–54.

6. Jerez A, Clemente MJ, Makishima H, et al. STAT3 mutations unify the pathogenesis of chronic lymphoproliferative disorders of NK cells and T-cell large granular lymphocyte leukemia. Blood 2012;120(15): 3048–57.

7. Koskela HL, Eldfors S, Ellonen P, et al. Somatic STAT3 mutations in large granular lymphocytic leukemia. N Engl J Med 2012;366(20):1905–13.

8. Vivier E, Anfossi N. Inhibitory NK-cell receptors on T cells: witness of the past, actors of the future. Nat Rev Immunol 2004;4(3):190–8.

9. Narni-Mancinelli E, Vivier E, Kerdiles YM. The 'T-cell-ness' of NK cells: unexpected similarities between NK cells and T cells. Int Immunol 2011;23(7): 427–31.

10. Bareau B, Rey J, Hamidou M, et al. Analysis of a French cohort of patients with large granular lymphocyte leukemia: a report on 229 cases. Haematologica 2010;95(9):1534–41.

11. Howard MT, Bejanyan N, Maciejewski JP, et al. T/NK large granular lymphocyte leukemia and coexisting monoclonal B-cell lymphocytosis-like proliferations. An unrecognized and frequent association. Am J Clin Pathol 2010;133(6): 936–41.

12. Loughran TP Jr, Starkebaum G. Clinical features in large granular lymphocytic leukemia. Blood 1987; 69(6):1786.

13. Clemente MJ, Wlodarski MW, Makishima H, et al. Clonal drift demonstrates unexpected dynamics of the T-cell repertoire in T-large granular lymphocyte leukemia. Blood 2011;118(16):4384–93.

14. Lundell R, Hartung L, Hill S, et al. T-cell large granular lymphocyte leukemias have multiple phenotypic abnormalities involving pan-T-cell antigens and receptors for MHC molecules. Am J Clin Pathol 2005;124(6):937–46.

15. Morice WG, Kurtin PJ, Leibson PJ, et al. Demonstration of aberrant T-cell and natural killer-cell antigen expression in all cases of granular lymphocytic leukaemia. Br J Haematol 2003;120(6): 1026–36.

16. Roden AC, Morice WG, Hanson CA. Immunophenotypic attributes of benign peripheral blood gamma-delta T cells and conditions associated with their

increase. Arch Pathol Lab Med 2008;132(11): 1774–80.

17. Lamy T, Loughran TP Jr. How I treat LGL leukemia. Blood 2011;117(10):2764–74.

18. Cheung MM, Chan JK, Wong KF. Natural killer cell neoplasms: a distinctive group of highly aggressive lymphomas/leukemias. Semin Hematol 2003;40(3): 221–32.

19. Cooke CB, Krenacs L, Stetler-Stevenson M, et al. Hepatosplenic T-cell lymphoma: a distinct clinicopathologic entity of cytotoxic gamma delta T-cell origin. Blood 1996;88(11):4265–74.

20. Morice WG, Macon WR, Dogan A, et al. NK-cell-associated receptor expression in hepatosplenic T-cell lymphoma, insights into pathogenesis. Leukemia 2006;20(5):883–6.

21. Loughran TP Jr. Clonal diseases of large granular lymphocytes. Blood 1993;82(1):1–14.

22. Ohgami RS, Ohgami JK, Pereira IT, et al. Refining the diagnosis of T-cell large granular lymphocytic leukemia by combining distinct patterns of antigen expression with T-cell clonality studies. Leukemia 2011;25(9):1439–43.

23. Lantelme E, Granziero L, Angman L, et al. Clonal predominance, but preservation of a polyclonal reservoir, in the normal alpha beta T-cell repertoire. Hum Immunol 1997;53(1):49–56.

24. Pannetier C, Even J, Kourilsky P. T-cell repertoire diversity and clonal expansions in normal and clinical samples. Immunol Today 1995;16(4):176–81.

25. Lamy T, Loughran TP Jr. Clinical features of large granular lymphocyte leukemia. Semin Hematol 2003;40(3):185–95.

26. Alekshun TJ, Tao J, Sokol L. Aggressive T-cell large granular lymphocyte leukemia: a case report and review of the literature. Am J Hematol 2007;82(6):481–5.

Erythroleukemia and Its Differential Diagnosis

Robert P. Hasserjian, MD

KEYWORDS

- Erythroleukemia • Erythroid • Myelodysplastic syndrome • Acute myeloid leukemia

ABSTRACT

Acute erythroid leukemias encompass 2 main subtypes: acute erythroleukemia (erythroid/myeloid subtype) and pure erythroid leukemia. This article reviews the main clinicopathologic features of the acute erythroid leukemias and the criteria used to diagnose them. In this article, the differential diagnosis between acute erythroid leukemias and their mimics is discussed and helpful morphologic clues and diagnostic tests that help arrive at the correct diagnosis are provided. The appropriate application of diagnostic criteria, including ancillary testing, such as immunophenotyping, cytogenetics, and molecular genetic testing, is essential to categorize bone marrow erythroid proliferations.

Acronyms and Abbreviations: Erythroleukemia	
AEL	Acute erythroleukemia
AML	Acute myeloid leukemia
AML, NOS	Acute myeloid leukemia, not otherwise specified
AML-RGA	AML with recurrent genetic abnormalities
FAB	French-American-British (classification)
JMML	Juvenile myelomonocytic leukemia
MDS	Myelodysplastic syndrome
MPN	Myeloproliferative neoplasm
MDS/MPN	Myelodysplastic/myeloproliferative neoplasm
MPO	Myeloperoxidase
PCV	Polycythemia vera
PEL	Pure erythroid leukemia
RARS	Refractory anemia with ring sideroblasts
RARS-T	Refractory anemia with ring sideroblasts and marked thrombocytosis
RAEB	Refractory anemia with excess blasts
RCMD	Refractory cytopenia with multilineage dysplasia
RCUD	Refractory cytopenia with unilineage dysplasia

ACUTE ERYTHROID LEUKEMIA, ERYTHROID/MYELOID SUBTYPE (ACUTE ERYTHROLEUKEMIA)

DEFINITION

The erythroid/myeloid subtype of acute erythroid leukemia (acute erythroleukemia [AEL]) is a malignant myeloid proliferation characterized by impaired maturation of the myeloid series, with excess myeloblasts occurring in a background of expanded maturing erythropoiesis. In the prior French-American-British (FAB) classification, acute erythroid leukemias were designated as the "M6" type of acute myeloid leukemia (AML), with AEL specifically termed by some investigators as the "M6A" variant.[1,2] According to the 2008 World Health Organization (WHO) classification, AEL is considered to represent a subtype of AML, not otherwise specified (AML, NOS).[3] Its definition is as follows:

1. Erythroid precursors comprise most (50% or greater) nucleated bone marrow cells.
2. Myeloblasts comprise 20% or more of the nonerythroid nucleated bone marrow cells.
3. Criteria for another WHO AML subtype are not fulfilled.
   a. Absence of one of the specific cytogenetic abnormalities of AML with recurrent genetic

The author declares no conflicts of interest relevant to the topic.
Department of Pathology, Massachusetts General Hospital, 55 Fruit Street, Boston, MA 02114, USA
E-mail address: rhasserjian@partners.org

Surgical Pathology 6 (2013) 641–659
http://dx.doi.org/10.1016/j.path.2013.08.006
1875-9181/13/$ – see front matter © 2013 Elsevier Inc. All rights reserved.

Key Features
ACUTE ERYTHROID LEUKEMIA

1. Acute myeloid leukemia subtype characterized by an expansion of bone marrow myeloblasts in a background of increased erythropoiesis.

2. Many similarities to myelodysplastic syndromes, including frequent cytopenic presentation with no or few circulating blasts, trilineage dysplasia, and frequent evolution from a prior myelodysplastic syndrome.

3. Prognosis largely driven by the cytogenetic findings: most karyotypes are abnormal, with frequent losses of chromosomes 5 and 7, whereas a minority of cases have normal karyotype and display more indolent clinical behavior.

4. Differential diagnosis with other types of acute myeloid leukemia as well as erythroid-predominant myelodysplastic syndromes and reactive erythroid hyperplasias.

abnormalities (AML-RGA): no t(15;17), inv(16)/t(16;16), t(8;21), inv(3)/t(3;3), t(6;9), t(9;11), or t(1;22).

b. No history of cytotoxic chemotherapy or radiotherapy.

c. If myeloblasts comprise 20% or more of all nucleated cells, diagnostic features of AML with myelodysplasia-related changes are absent (see Differential Diagnosis section later in this article).

Since the blast percentage is derived only from the nonerythroid cells, which may be relatively sparse given the expanded erythroid population, a careful cell count of at least 500 cells from well-prepared bone marrow aspirate smears must be performed.[3] The WHO classification general guidelines state that lymphocytes and plasma cells should also be excluded in deriving the nonerythroid blast count,[4] although this exclusion is not specifically stated in the WHO definition of AEL and is not followed in practice by many hematopathologists. One possible approach would be to exclude such cells only if neoplastic (ie, in cases with a concurrent lymphoma or plasma cell neoplasm), but there is no consensus on this practice.[5]

CLINICAL FEATURES

AEL usually affects older adults, with a median age ranging from 51 to 67 years and a male:female ratio of approximately 3:2.[6–10] It is an uncommon subtype of AML, comprising 1.6% to 4.5% of adult AML cases in most published studies and registries.[11,12] It appears to be even less common in infants and children, comprising only 1% to 2% of all pediatric AMLs and representing the least common AML FAB subtype in children.[13–15] AEL rarely can occur as a congenital leukemia[16] and rare familial cases have also been reported.[17]

Compared with other patients with AML, patients with AEL more often present with cytopenias; leukocytosis is seen in fewer than 10% of patients. Anemia, thrombocytopenia, and neutropenia are each present in three-quarters of the patients, and about one-half of patients are pancytopenic.[7,10] Organomegaly and extramedullary myeloid sarcomas, which can characterize some other AML subtypes, are relatively uncommon in AEL.[8,9,18] Similar to adults, children with AEL also present with cytopenias, whereas hepatosplenomegaly appears to be more common in pediatric patients.[13]

About two-thirds of patients with AEL present de novo, whereas one-third evolve from a prior myelodysplastic syndrome (MDS). Rare cases of AEL have been reported to occur as progression of a myeloproliferative neoplasm or as blast transformation of chronic myelogenous leukemia.[19,20] Evolution from a prior myelodysplastic/myeloproliferative neoplasm, such as chronic myelomonocytic leukemia, appears to be exceedingly rare. Some investigators have noted a high proportion of cases following exposure to occupational toxins, such as solvents (benzene, toluene) and petroleum products.[9,21]

DIAGNOSIS: BLOOD AND BONE MARROW MORPHOLOGY

On examination of the peripheral smear, about one-half of patients have circulating myeloblasts, but these are often few in number compared with other types of AML. Circulating nucleated red blood cells are present in 50% to 75% of patients, with a median level of 5 per 100 white blood cells.[6,7] Although nonspecific, red cell morphologic abnormalities are more commonly seen in patients with AEL than in other AML types. Abnormalities include schistocytes, dacrocytes, and basophilic stippling; frequent "pincered" erythrocytes with globular cytoplasmic budding were described in one series.[6] Neutrophil hypogranulation and/or pseudo-Pelger-Huët forms are seen in about one-third of cases.

The bone marrow in AEL is typically hypercellular for age (median 80%), with de novo cases having higher cellularity than cases following MDS (Fig. 1A).[7] By definition, at least 50% of the

Fig. 1. AEL. (*A*) The bone marrow biopsy is typically markedly hypercellular, with a predominance of erythroid elements at various stages of maturation in a haphazard arrangement in the marrow; myeloblasts are difficult to enumerate, as they can resemble the numerous large early erythroid forms in biopsy sections (H&E, ×200). (*B*) In the aspirate smear, erythroid elements predominate (at least 50% of the cells) and show dysplastic features, such as binucleation and nuclear irregularities. A myeloblast (*arrow*) with a slightly irregular nucleus and more dispersed chromatin is also present (Wright-Giemsa, ×1000). (*C*) Case of myelodysplastic syndrome contrasting myeloblasts and a pronormoblast. The myeloblasts are smaller with more dispersed chromatin and paler cytoplasm; the pronormoblast cytoplasm is deeply basophilic (Wright-Giemsa, ×1000).

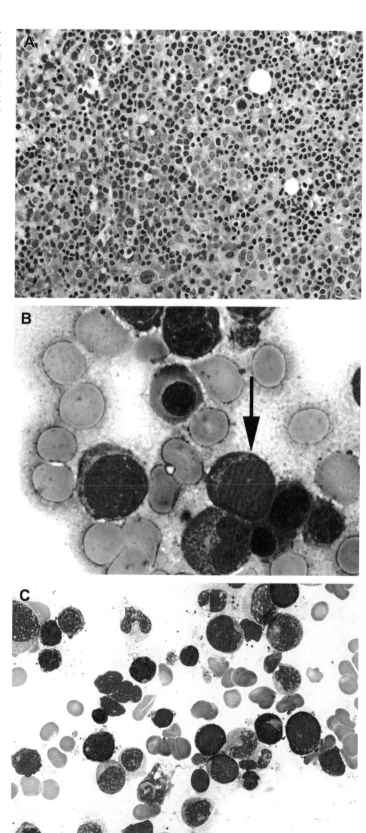

D

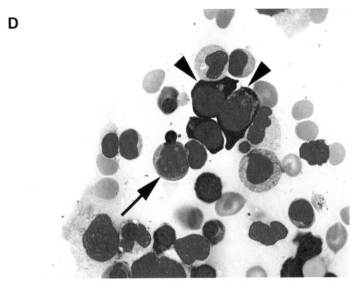

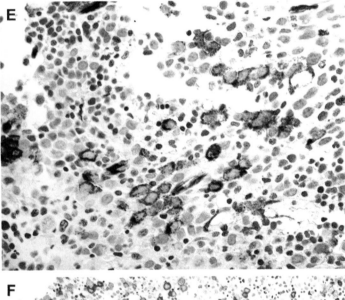

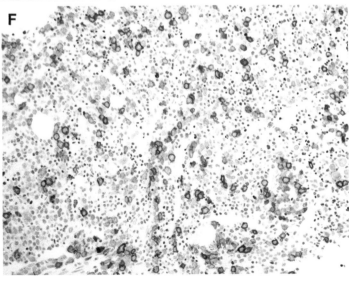

Fig. 1. (continued). AEL. (*D*) Case of autoimmune hemolytic anemia illustrating a myeloblast (*arrow*) and pronormoblasts (*arrowheads*). The myeloblast has basophilic cytoplasm, but it also has finer chromatin and paler, more scant cytoplasm compared with the larger erythroblasts (Wright-Giemsa, ×1000). (*E*) CD34 immunostain of AEL, showing small clusters of CD34-positive myeloblasts in a background of CD34-negative maturing erythroids (×400). (*F*) CD117 immunostain of AEL, which is positive in both early erythroblasts (larger cells with paler staining) and myeloblasts (smaller cells with darker staining) (×200).

nucleated cells on the bone marrow aspirate smears (median 63%) are erythroid elements, but unlike cases of pure erythroid leukemia (see later in this article), these show a full spectrum of maturation (see Fig. 1B). Some cases may have a striking erythroid predominance (up to 90% of bone marrow cells), and criteria for AEL may be fulfilled with only a small number of myeloblasts, given the paucity of nonerythroid cells. As mentioned previously, accurate diagnosis in such cases requires careful examination of a well-prepared aspirate smear that allows distinction between pronormoblasts and myeloblasts and precise counting of the latter. Pronormoblasts are large cells (20–25 μm in diameter) with a round to slightly oval nucleus, fine chromatin, and scant to moderate amounts of deeply basophilic cytoplasm. Compared with pronormoblasts, myeloblasts are smaller, with finer chromatin and more scant, pale cytoplasm, and often display nuclear irregularity or indentation (see Fig. 1B–D). Auer rods are infrequent, but may be occasionally seen in the myeloblasts of AEL, particularly in pediatric cases.[22] Some investigators have described "hybrid" cells in some cases showing morphologic features intermediate between an erythroblast and a myeloblast: round nuclei and basophilic cytoplasm with azurophilic peroxidase-containing granules.[23]

Morphologic dysplasia is usually prominent in AEL and can be seen in all hematopoietic lineages.[21,24] Dysplasia in the erythroid lineage is nearly ubiquitous in AEL and is manifested most often by megaloblastoid nuclear:cytoplasmic asynchrony; nuclear irregularities, binucleation, and cytoplasmic coarse basophilic stippling are also frequent (see Fig. 1B). In a small subset of cases, the dysplasia may be subtle or manifested only by nuclear:cytoplasmic asynchrony.[6] About one-third of AEL cases have ring sideroblasts on iron staining of the bone marrow aspirate, but this finding has neither diagnostic nor prognostic significance. Megakaryocytic dysplasia, characterized by small, hypolobated forms, is seen in about three-quarters of cases and myeloid lineage dysplasia in about one-half of cases.[7,8] The frequent morphologic dysplasia, cytopenic presentation, common evolution from antecedent MDS, and shared cytogenetic aberrations (see later in this article) suggest that AEL is biologically closely related to MDS.

DIAGNOSIS: CYTOCHEMISTRY AND IMMUNOPHENOTYPE

Cytochemical stains are usually not required to diagnose AEL. When cytochemical stains are performed on bone marrow aspirate smears, the myeloblasts are usually positive for myeloperoxidase (MPO), but only occasionally for nonspecific esterase.[8] A periodic acid-Schiff (PAS) stain performed on aspirate smears shows abnormal diffuse staining in most erythroid cells in greater than 90% of AEL cases; coarse granular staining characteristic of pure erythroid leukemia (PEL) is less common in AEL and is generally limited to cases with increased pronormoblasts.[6,23] By flow cytometry, the myeloblasts express typical myeloid-associated antigens, such as CD13, CD33, CD117, and MPO,[12] but may be CD34-negative in a significant subset of cases.[25] When positive, CD34 immunostaining can be used to highlight the expanded myeloblast population in the bone marrow biopsy (see Fig. 1E). However, care must be taken with CD117, which stains early erythroid elements that can be difficult to distinguish from the myeloblasts and may result in an overestimation of myeloblasts in the biopsy (see Fig. 1F). The erythroid cells are positive for CD71, CD36, glycophorin, and hemoglobin, and they are CD34-negative.[12] The platelet/megakaryocytic marker CD41 may be expressed on myeloblasts in AEL[26] and aberrant CD7 expression in myeloblasts is seen in about one-quarter of cases.[27]

In cases with bone marrow fibrosis or suboptimal aspirate smears, the erythroid percentage may appear to be less than 50% in the aspirate due to hemodilution. In such cases, if clear erythroid predominance is observed in the biopsy section (particularly if supported by immunostains such as hemoglobin, glycophorin, and/or CD71) and CD34+ myeloblasts are found to comprise greater than 20% of the nonerythroid cells by immunohistochemistry, it is reasonable to diagnose AEL.[8] However, flow cytometry percentages should not be used to establish a diagnosis of AEL; variable loss of nucleated erythroid elements and even myeloblasts during sample processing and variable expression of CD34 on the myeloblasts can lead to erroneous overdiagnosis or underdiagnosis.

DIAGNOSIS: GENETICS

An abnormal karyotype is present in 50% to 76% of adult AEL cases, with 31% to 37% having a complex karyotype.[25,28,29] Deletions or losses of chromosomes 5 and/or 7 are the most common findings, seen in 45% to 65% of cases, whereas trisomy 8 is seen in a significant subset of cases.[27] Although AEL shares these genetic features with therapy-related AML, deletions/losses of chromosome 5 are more common and deletions/losses of chromosome 7 are less common in AEL than in therapy-related AML.[8] An abnormal karyotype is reported in 50% of pediatric cases, but losses/deletions of chromosomes 5 and 7 appear to be less common than in adult AEL.[22] The translocation t(1;16)(p31;q24) causing NFIA-CBFA2T5 fusion is the only balanced cytogenetic abnormality specific to AEL, but it is present in only a small minority of cases and is associated with young age and aggressive disease.[30] The expanded erythroid proliferation in AEL is presumed to be neoplastic, deriving from the same abnormal stem cell as the myeloblasts. Evidence for this includes the often marked dysplasia seen in the erythroid lineage, as well as cytochemical and immunophenotypic abnormalities observed in the proliferating erythroblasts that are not seen in reactive erythroid hyperplasia.[23,26]

An NPM1 mutation is reported to occur in between 1.6% to 26.0% of AEL cases.[25,31,32] The reasons for this wide variability in reported incidence are uncertain, but this may reflect variation in the proportion of normal karyotype cases in the tested cohorts or possibly the inclusion of higher blast count cases that would be classified as AML-MRC according to WHO, and may have higher rates of NPM1 mutation. It is unclear if NPM1 mutated AML cases fulfilling AEL morphologic criteria should be classified within the provisional WHO category of AML with mutated NPM1 or be classified as AEL; NPM1 has not been associated with favorable outcome in AEL, but this may relate to the small number of cases studied. FLT3-ITD and TKD mutations are relatively uncommon in AEL, occurring in 3% to 6% of studied cases, whereas RAS mutations have been reported to occur in 4% of cases.[7,12,25,33] In one study, AEL was found to have a significantly lower incidence of NPM1 and RAS mutations compared with AML lacking erythroid predominance, suggesting underlying genetic differences between AML cases with and without a prominent erythroid proliferation. CEBPA mutations occur in approximately 7% of AEL cases, comparable to or somewhat lower than in other types of AML, NOS.[31] JAK2 mutations appear to be exceedingly rare in AEL.[34]

As of yet, no specific cytogenetic or molecular genetic finding common to AEL has been found, and any possible genetic basis that drives the exuberant erythroid proliferation is unknown. Although GATA1 mutations are associated with acute megakaryoblastic leukemia in patients with Down syndrome and the GATA1 protein appears to contribute to leukemogenesis in murine erythroleukemia models, GATA1 gene mutations have not been found in AEL.[35]

DIFFERENTIAL DIAGNOSIS

MYELODYSPLASTIC SYNDROME WITH ERYTHROID PREDOMINANCE

About 15% of MDS cases have 50% or greater erythroid elements.[36] Most of these cases are lower-grade MDS (refractory cytopenia with unilineage dysplasia [RCUD], refractory cytopenia with multilineage dysplasia [RCMD], and refractory anemia with ring sideroblasts [RARS]).[25,36] It is very important to distinguish low-grade MDS cases from AEL, as the latter have an inferior prognosis and may warrant more aggressive therapy. Cases that challenge this differential are those with extreme erythroid proliferation (80%–90%), in which only 2% to 5% of myeloblasts could fulfill criteria for AEL (Fig. 2A, B). In practice, extreme erythroid hyperplasia is uncommon in MDS with erythroid predominance, which has a median erythroid percentage of 60%.[36] Conversely, myeloblasts in most AEL cases (even those with very high erythroid percentages), usually comprise at least 5% of all cells. In cases with marked erythroid predominance, examination of CD34 and erythroid marker immunostains on the bone marrow biopsy may be helpful to document the increase in myeloblasts as a proportion of the nonerythroid cells: RCUD and RARS typically have only rare CD34+ cells that do not form clusters. Erythroid dysplasia is usually more marked in AEL compared with MDS with erythroid predominance. In difficult cases with borderline blast counts, it may be reasonable to wait and repeat the marrow to confirm the diagnosis, particularly in patients who have received growth factors that can influence the proportion of myeloid and erythroid elements, such as granulocyte colony-stimulating factor and erythropoietin.

Approximately one-third of erythroid-predominant MDS cases are classified as refractory anemia with excess blasts (RAEB) where myeloblasts comprise 5% or more of all marrow cells, but fewer than 20% of the nonerythroid cells. Distinguishing these cases from AEL may be problematic when the blast and/or erythroid percentages are borderline (for example, 5% blasts and 70% erythroids, or 12% blasts and 45% erythroids). In these cases, small changes in the blast and/or erythroid count, which lie within the range of statistical or interobserver variability, may lead to different diagnoses. Recent studies suggest that this distinction may not be relevant, as the outcome of erythroid-predominant RAEB resembles that of AEL in both adults and children, irrespective of the type of therapy administered.[7,22,25] Erythropoietin therapy administered to patients with RAEB may transiently increase the bone marrow erythroid percentage,

Fig. 2. Differential diagnosis of AEL. (*A*) RAEB with erythroid predominance, showing similar features to AEL (compare with Fig. 1A) on the bone marrow biopsy. Small, dysplastic megakaryocytes are present (H&E, ×400). (*B*) The bone marrow aspirate smear shows predominantly maturing erythroid elements, along with dysplastic myeloid cells. Careful enumeration of myeloblasts is required to confirm that they comprise fewer than 20% of the nonerythroid cells (Wright-Giemsa, ×400). (*C*) Prominent reactive erythroid hyperplasia and profound myeloid hypoplasia in the bone marrow biopsy from a patient presenting with anemia and agranulocytosis due to viral infection (H&E, ×400).

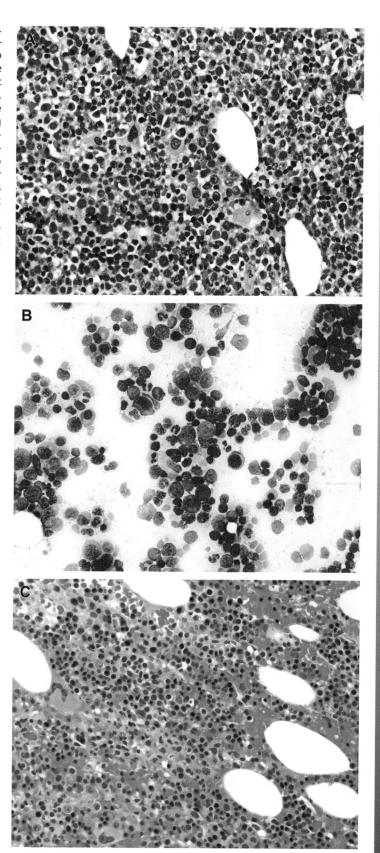

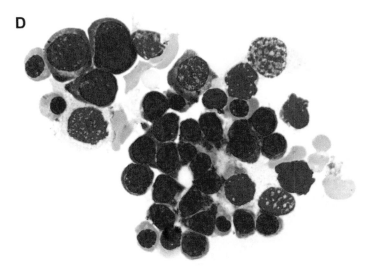

Fig. 2. (*continued*). Differential diagnosis of AEL. (*D*) The aspirate smear (same case as in *Panel C*) shows marked erythroid hyperplasia, including many pronormoblasts and some with irregular nuclei; myeloblasts were very rare and comprised fewer than 20% of the nonerythroid cells. On clinical follow-up, the patient's cytopenias resolved spontaneously (Wright-Giemsa, ×1000). (*E*) Bone marrow biopsy from a patient with polycythemia vera. Although erythroid elements are increased, there is a population of enlarged megakaryocytes with bulbous nuclei that would be unusual for AEL (H&E, ×400). (*F*) Bone marrow from a patient with RARS-T. Erythroid hyperplasia is similar to AEL (which may also contain ring sideroblasts), but the megakaryocytes are enlarged and clustered with bulbous nuclei; this patient also had a *JAK2* mutation (H&E, ×400).

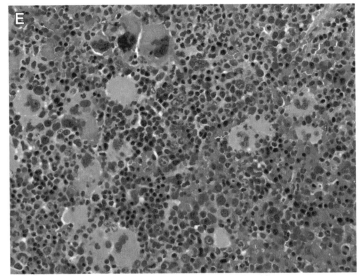

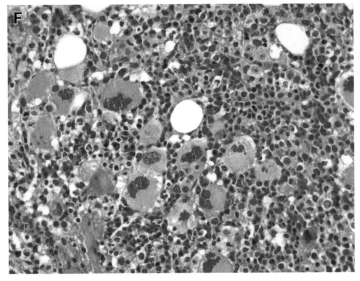

fulfilling criteria for AEL; these patients appear to share pathologic and cytogenetic features with AEL, and exhibit a similar or inferior prognosis.[27] In these borderline cases of RAEB versus AEL, the decision to treat as AML or as MDS should probably be based on the clinical characteristics (such as stability of counts) and karyotype-risk grouping, rather than the diagnostic category assigned according to the calculated blast percentage.

It is important to note that if criteria for AEL are not met and an erythroid-predominant myeloid neoplasm is classified as MDS, the 2008 WHO classification recommends that blasts be enumerated as a percentage of all nucleated marrow cells, rather than the nonerythroid cells.[4] Thus, the method of deriving the blast percentage differs between myeloid neoplasms with 50% or greater erythroid elements, depending on whether they are classified as AEL or MDS.

Reactive Conditions

The myeloblast count in reactive conditions, even with extreme erythroid hyperplasia, generally should not exceed 20% of the nonerythroid elements. However, caution should be exercised in cases of reactive erythroid hyperplasia with marked myeloid hypoplasia, where misclassification of even a small percentage of large cells (such as early erythroid forms) as myeloblasts could lead to an erroneous diagnosis of AEL (see **Fig. 2**C, D). It is also important to elicit any history of growth factor therapy, which could transiently increase the bone marrow myeloblast percentage. Although erythropoietin therapy may transiently increase erythroid elements, the bone marrow erythroblast percentage usually does not exceed 50%.[37]

Myeloproliferative Neoplasms and Myelodysplastic/Myeloproliferative Neoplasms

It is uncommon for myeloproliferative neoplasms (MPN) or myelodysplastic/myeloproliferative neoplasm (MDS/MPN) cases to show erythroid predominance, with the exception of polycythemia vera (PCV) and the provisional MDS/MPN entity

Differential Diagnosis of Acute Erythroleukemia	
AEL vs	**Helpful Distinguishing Feature(s) of AEL**
Low-grade myelodysplastic syndromes • RARS • RCUD • RCMD	Myeloblasts usually at least 5% of all cells, and must comprise at least 20% of the nonerythroid cells Marked erythroid dysplasia
High-grade myelodysplastic syndromes • RAEB	Based entirely on bone marrow myeloblast count (≥20% of the nonerythroid cells) and erythroid count (≥50% of all nucleated cells) in the aspirate smear
Reactive erythroid hyperplasias	Myeloblasts usually at least 5% of all nucleated cells, and must comprise at least 20% of the nonerythroid cells PAS positivity in erythroblasts
Myeloproliferative and myelodysplastic/myeloproliferative neoplasms	Marked erythroid dysplasia JAK2 mutation absent Presence of peripheral cytopenias and absence of thrombocytosis or erythrocytosis
AML with myelodysplasia-related changes and >50% bone marrow erythroid cells	If blasts are ≥20% of total cells, there is • No history of MDS or MDS/MPN • Absence of significant multilineage dysplasia • Absence of MDS-related cytogenetic abnormalities
Therapy-related AML	No prior history of cytotoxic chemotherapy or radiotherapy
AML with recurrent cytogenetic abnormalities	Absence of subtype-defining cytogenetic abnormality
Pure erythroid leukemia	Evidence of maturation in the erythroid lineage; pronormoblasts are usually <30% of all erythroid cells Myeloblasts are increased (≥20%) as a proportion of the nonerythroid cells

refractory anemia with ring sideroblasts and marked thrombocytosis (RARS-T). The enlarged, clustered megakaryocytes of PCV (see **Fig. 2**E) and RARS-T (see **Fig. 2**F) differ from the small, MDS-like megakaryocytes seen in AEL. By definition, thrombocytosis is present in RARS-T and is common in PCV, whereas thrombocytosis is not seen in AEL. Finally, the *JAK2* mutation is nearly ubiquitous in PCV and is present in many cases of RARS-T, whereas the *JAK2* mutation is rare in AEL. Juvenile myelomonocytic leukemia (JMML), a rare MDS/MPN, may present with an erythroid-predominant bone marrow picture.[22] However, JMML presents with leukocytosis and monocytosis and usually lacks erythroid and megakaryocytic dysplasia.

Other Types of Acute Myeloid Leukemia

As mentioned in the definition (see previously), AML-RGA cases are excluded from the AEL category according to the 2008 WHO classification. Erythroid predominance is uncommon in most types of AML-RGA, but it may be occasionally seen in AML with t(6;9) or AML with t(3;3)/inv(3). Between 14% and 30% of cases fulfilling the morphologic criteria for AEL occur following cytotoxic therapy and are classified as therapy-related MDS/AML.[10,25] Conversely, about 11% of therapy-related AML cases have morphologic features of AEL, which is a higher proportion than in de novo disease.[38] Thus, it is critical that the pathologist elicit any history of chemotherapy or radiotherapy, which would preclude classification as AEL. Finally, when myeloblasts comprise greater than 20% of all cells, AML cases are diagnosed as AML-MRC irrespective of erythroid predominance if they follow a documented diagnosis of MDS or MDS/MPN, have multilineage dysplasia (≥50% dysplastic cells in 2 or 3 hematopoietic lineages), or have one of the MDS-related cytogenetic abnormalities that define AML-MRC.[39]

PROGNOSIS AND PREDICTIVE FACTORS

The median survival of AEL is reported to be poor in some prior studies, ranging from 3 to 9 months.[10] However, when conforming to the WHO classification by excluding cases that are considered therapy-related AML or AML-MRC, median survival of patients with AEL is 11 to 19 months.[7,12,25,27] One recent study found that AEL has a prognosis identical to other types of AML, NOS.[31] Given the variable blast count of AEL, some have suggested that cases with low absolute blast count may have more favorable prognosis, akin to MDS.[40] However, several studies have shown that the cytogenetic profile is more important than blast count in such cases and that blast count is not associated with outcome in AEL.[7,8,21,25] In a multivariable analysis including AEL as well as erythroid-predominant AML-MRC, RAEB, and therapy-related AML, karyotype risk grouping was the main factor associated with prognosis. These results suggest that the prevalence of high-risk cytogenetics accounts for the adverse outcome of erythroid-predominant AML cases following MDS or cytotoxic therapy. Likewise, AEL cases with adverse cytogenetics have an aggressive course, even if their absolute blast count is low.[7] Conversely, the median survival of AEL with normal karyotype is reported to be 30 months or longer.[7,25] Older age, lower hemoglobin level, Eastern Cooperative Oncology Group performance status of 3 or 4, low albumin, high ferritin, and elevated LDH have also been associated with adverse outcome in AEL. The International Prognostic Scoring System (IPSS), which incorporates cytogenetic risk group, cytopenias, and blast percentage, successfully risk-stratifies patients with AEL, further supporting a relationship of AEL to MDS.[29] There are no data as of yet regarding application of the recently revised IPSS (IPSS-R) to AEL. Some investigators have suggested that increased pronormoblasts, although not included along with myeloblasts in deriving the nonerythroid blast percentage, are associated with a poorer prognosis in AEL.[41] Of note, when AEL recurs, 75% of cases relapse as "conventional" AML with fewer than 50% erythroid elements.[27] As with other types of AML, relapse in AEL requires that bone marrow blasts comprises 5% or greater of all nucleated cells.

Given the highly variable prognosis of AEL, it is not surprising that varied treatment approaches have been used. Patients with adverse cytogenetics appear to benefit from allogeneic bone marrow transplantation, and the 5-year survival of AEL patients treated with allogeneic stem cell transplantation was more than 50% in one series.[11] It is uncertain if patients with AEL who are not transplant candidates benefit from induction chemotherapy over less-intensive approaches similar to MDS.[7,29]

PURE ERYTHROID LEUKEMIA

DEFINITION

The PEL subtype of acute erythroid leukemia is a highly aggressive acute leukemia characterized by an expansion of growth-arrested primitive erythroblasts (pronormoblasts), but with no significant increase in myeloblasts. Its specific definition has evolved from the original "M6B" designation proposed by Kowal-Vern and colleagues,[42] which considered pronormoblasts to be blast equivalents and required that they comprise greater than 30% of the marrow cells. The 2008 WHO classification is more strict, in that the undifferentiated pronormoblasts must comprise greater than 80% of the bone marrow cells. PEL thus fundamentally differs from AEL in that the proliferating neoplastic cell is the pronormoblast rather than the myeloblast.

Rare leukemias with morphologic features of PEL have been reported to evolve from patients with a history of CML and carry a t(9;22) rearrangement; these cases should be classified as blast crisis of CML rather than as PEL.[28] Similarly, cases following exposure to cytotoxic therapy are classified as therapy-related AML.

Key Features
PURE ERYTHROID LEUKEMIA

1. Rare, highly aggressive subtype of acute myeloid leukemia characterized by a proliferation of primitive pronormoblasts, lack of erythroid maturation, and no significant increase in myeloblasts.

2. Often develops from a prior myelodysplastic syndrome, but can also develop de novo.

3. Almost always shows a highly complex karyotype with multiple abnormalities, often including losses of chromosomes 5 and/or 7, associated with a highly aggressive clinical course and poor patient outcome.

4. Differential diagnosis with megaloblastic anemia and other hematologic and nonhematologic neoplasms.

CLINICAL FEATURES

PEL is far rarer than AEL, and is in effect a rare subgroup of an already rare AML subtype. In the relatively few series that clearly distinguish PEL from AEL, PEL comprises only 3% to 14% of all acute erythroid leukemia cases and thus represents fewer than 1% of all AML cases.[6,10,43] Given its rarity, most reports of PEL are of single cases or small series. In one recent report of 18 cases (including 4 cases of therapy-related or post-CML disease that would be excluded by 2008 WHO classification criteria), the median age was 68 years and the male:female ratio was 2:1. PEL appears to be similarly rare in children.[44] About

half of the cases in adults occur as transformation of a prior MDS.[43]

DIAGNOSIS: PERIPHERAL BLOOD AND BONE MARROW MORPHOLOGY

Circulating neoplastic pronormoblasts with basophilic cytoplasm are present in the blood smear in most patients, but more mature circulating nucleated erythroid cells, which are commonly seen in AEL, are less prevalent in PEL.[44] Similar to AEL, leukocytosis is rare.[45] In a significant subset of cases, neoplastic pronormoblasts may infiltrate tissues such as the liver or spleen or form an extramedullary mass of malignant erythroblasts ("erythroblastic sarcoma").[44–46]

The bone marrow is typically hypercellular for age, with a median cellularity of approximately 80%.[43] The marrow cellularity is mostly or entirely replaced by sheets of pronormoblasts (**Fig. 3A**). According to the WHO classification, pronormoblasts (the most primitive stage of erythroid maturation) must comprise at least 80% of nucleated cells in the bone marrow aspirate smears. This number has been challenged in some recent publications, which advocate making the diagnosis with lower percentages if the primitive erythroblasts infiltrate as diffuse sheets in the bone marrow biopsy.[43] The neoplastic pronormoblasts in PEL are usually large, with abundant, vacuolated cytoplasm and occasional multinucleation; the cytoplasmic vacuoles are often large and located at the peripheral aspect of the cytoplasm (see **Fig. 3B–D**). Some cases have smaller pronormoblasts, with smooth, basophilic cytoplasm (see **Fig. 3C**). In contrast to AEL, the myeloid lineage, while reduced, shows intact maturation and there is no increase in myeloblasts (see **Fig. 3D**).[45] The degree of dysgranulopoiesis and dysmegakaryopoiesis in PEL appears similar to or somewhat less than AEL.[43] Ring sideroblasts are present in about half of the cases. When present in extramedullary tissues such as liver or spleen, the neoplastic pronormoblasts often occur within vascular sinusoids.

DIAGNOSIS: CYTOCHEMISTRY AND IMMUNOPHENOTYPE

The blasts in PEL show intense globular or granular "block" positivity with PAS stain of the aspirate smears (see **Fig. 3E**) and are negative for MPO and nonspecific esterase.[10,43] By both immunohistochemistry and flow cytometry, the immature pronormoblasts in PEL are negative for CD34, CD45, and MPO. Immunostaining for E-cadherin shows membrane staining in more than 90% of PEL cases

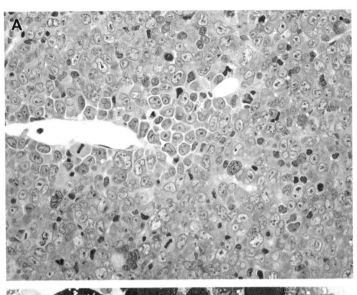

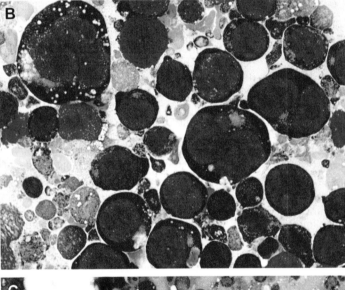

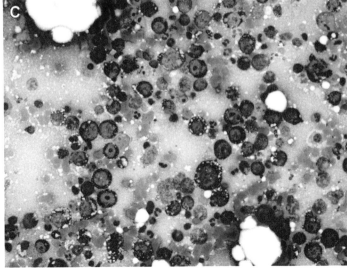

Fig. 3. PEL. (*A*) The bone marrow biopsy is markedly hypercellular, with sheets of large, primitive pronormoblasts with vesicular nuclei and prominent nucleoli (H&E, ×400). (*B*) In the bone marrow aspirate smear, the pronormoblasts include enlarged, bizarre multinucleated forms, often with cytoplasmic vacuoles and deeply basophilic cytoplasm; like normal pronormoblasts, these cells have perinuclear hofs (Wright-Giemsa, ×1000). (*C*) Pronormoblasts in some cases may be smaller and more monotonous, but retain cytoplasmic basophilia; mature erythroid forms are rare (Wright-Giemsa, ×400).

Fig. 3. (*continued*). PEL. (*D*) Myeloid elements, although reduced, show normal maturation and there is no increase in myeloblasts (Wright-Giemsa, ×1000). (*E*) PAS stain of the bone marrow aspirate shows granular cytoplasmic staining in the neoplastic pronormoblasts (×1000). (*F*) E-cadherin immunostain is strongly positive in the pronormoblasts (×400). ([*E*] *Courtesy of* Sa A. Wang, MD, Anderson Cancer Center, Houston, TX.)

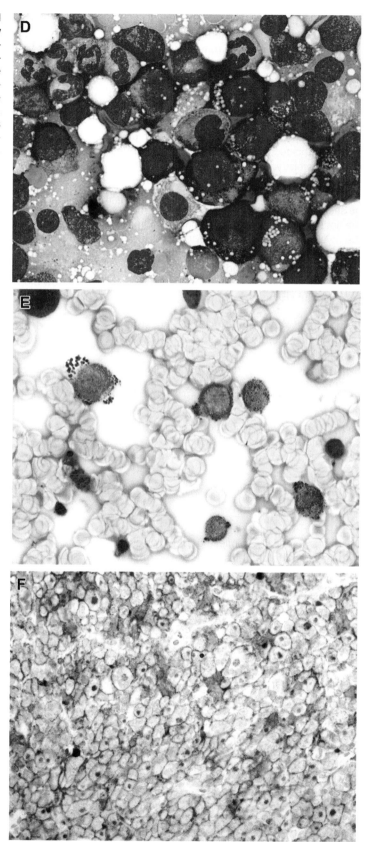

(see **Fig. 3**F), but glycophorin, hemoglobin, and Glut-1, markers that preferentially stain more mature erythroid elements, may be weak or stain only a subset of the pronormoblasts.[43] Ferritin H has recently been shown to mark primitive erythroblasts, including those in acute erythroid leukemias and may prove useful.[47] By flow cytometry, the pronormoblasts are positive for CD36 and CD71 and may show more reliable staining for glycophorin by this technique as compared with immunohistochemistry. Unlike the blasts of most AML subtypes, the neoplastic pronormoblasts in PEL are HLA-DR negative.[44,45] Variable staining can be seen with CD33 and CD117, but these markers are not specific for the erythroid lineage. Similar to the myeloblasts in MDS and AML-MRC, the pronormoblasts in PEL may aberrantly express T-cell markers, such as CD7 and CD2.[44,45]

DIAGNOSIS: GENETICS

An abnormal karyotype is seen in almost all reported PEL cases, and the abnormal karyotype is typically complex, with a median of 12 abnormalities. The most common abnormalities involve chromosomes 5, 7, 17, and 19.[43,45] Only 6 PEL cases to date have been studied for the prevalence of AML-associated gene mutations: 1 case had an *NPM1* mutation and no *FLT3* or *NRAS* mutations were detected in this small series.[25]

DIFFERENTIAL DIAGNOSIS

Myelodysplastic Syndromes

Cases of RARS may occasionally show marked left-shift, potentially mimicking PEL, which can also have ring sideroblasts. However, erythroid lineage dysplasia in PEL is usually much more prominent than in RARS, and erythroid maturation is arrested. Coarse granular PAS staining of erythroblasts in the aspirate smear is usually not seen in RARS. In borderline cases, cytogenetics may be helpful, as PEL almost always has a complex, abnormal karyotype, whereas the karyotype in most RARS cases is normal.[6]

Reactive Erythroid Hyperplasia

The most important reactive disorder that may mimic PEL is florid reactive erythroid hyperplasia with left-shifted and/or megaloblastoid erythroid maturation. In particular, megaloblastic anemia (Vitamin B12 of folate deficiency) may similarly present with profound cytopenias and a prominent bone marrow erythroid hyperplasia. It is important to note that although some reactive conditions associated with erythroid hyperplasia may be associated with circulating erythroid precursors, these are usually mature normoblasts; the presence of numerous circulating pronormoblasts should raise suspicion for PEL. Acquired or congenital hemolytic anemias may show prominent dyserythropoiesis and left-shifted erythroid maturation and cases with toxin effect (such as alcohol) may contain vacuolated pronormoblasts. However, the erythroid cells in these conditions will show sequential maturation through all stages (**Fig. 4**A–B). The pronormoblasts in megaloblastic anemia are often larger than the neoplastic pronormoblasts in PEL, with more condensed nuclear chromatin and less prominent nucleoli; giant band forms and hypersegmented neutrophils can be a clue to this diagnosis (see **Fig. 4**C, D). In the bone marrow biopsy, the neoplastic pronormoblasts of PEL form diffuse sheets in the bone marrow biopsy rather than being dispersed among maturing erythroid and myeloid elements.[5] On PAS staining of the aspirate smears, normal erythroid elements are negative, whereas the neoplastic erythroblasts of PEL show coarse granular PAS staining.[48] In difficult cases lacking clinical history, assessment of vitamin B12, folate, and methylmalonic acid levels may be required to exclude megaloblastic anemia.

Other Types of Acute Leukemia

Some cases of AEL may show increased pronormoblasts, raising the question of PEL. Indeed, some investigators have proposed the existence of a "hybrid" type of erythroleukemia with features of both AEL (increased myeloblasts) and PEL (>30% pronormoblasts), so-called "M6C."[2] However, M6C is not recognized as an entity by WHO, which would classify these cases as AEL if myeloblasts are ≥20% of the nonerythroid cells, irrespective of any degree of erythroid maturation arrest. Primitive cases of AML (with minimal differentiation, FAB M0) or ALL may be confused with PEL, as their blasts may also have basophilic cytoplasm. Compared with AML or ALL blasts, the blasts of PEL are usually larger with more deeply basophilic and often vacuolated cytoplasm, and can be shown to express E-cadherin or an erythroid-specific marker, such as hemoglobin or glycophorin. Differentiating PEL from acute megakaryoblastic leukemia is more problematic, as PEL can partially express CD41 or CD61. Both erythroblasts and megakaryoblasts express erythropoietin and thrombopoietin receptors and they exhibit some similarities in immunophenotype and in transcription factor expression profiles. Thus, it is not surprising that some AML cases may lie on the border between PEL and

Fig. 4. Differential diagnosis of PEL. (*A*) Autoimmune hemolytic anemia on bone marrow biopsy shows numerous left-shifted erythroid forms, including clusters of pronormoblasts (Giemsa stain, ×400). Although these form large clusters, they do not form sheets and occur amid numerous mature erythroid forms (Wright-Giemsa, ×1000). (*B*) In the aspirate smear, erythroid elements are prominently increased, but exhibit a full spectrum of maturation. (*C*) Megaloblastic anemia on bone marrow biopsy, with clusters of large primitive erythroid elements, including some with irregular nuclei (H&E, ×400).

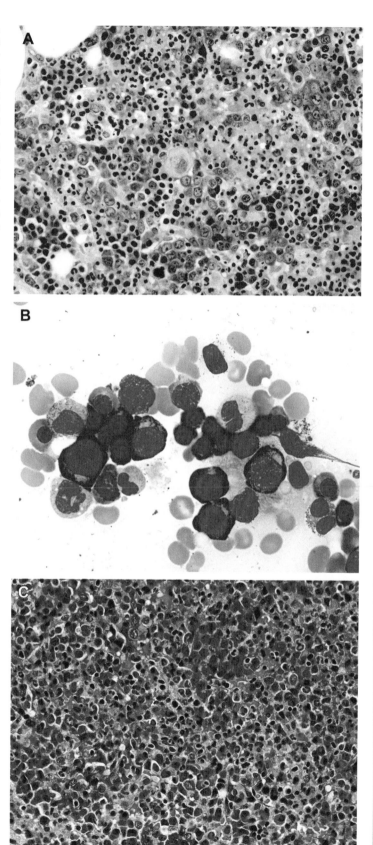

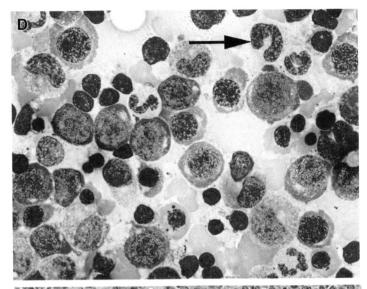

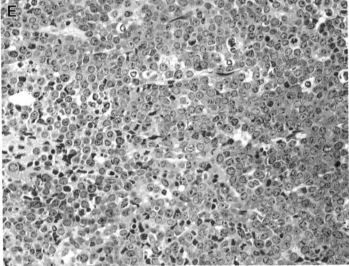

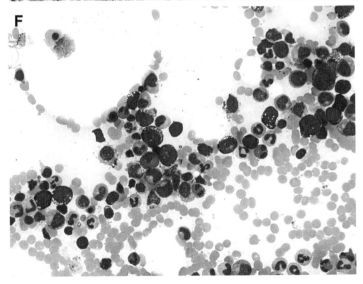

Fig. 4. (continued). Differential diagnosis of PEL. (*D*) In the aspirate smear, erythroid elements are left-shifted and megaloblastoid, contain occasional cytoplasmic vacuoles, and exhibit some dysplastic features; however, maturation is intact. One clue to the diagnosis is the presence of giant band forms (*arrow*) (Wright-Giemsa, ×1000). (*E*) Diffuse large B-cell lymphoma extensively involving the bone marrow. There are sheets of large cells with multiple nucleoli that resemble pronormoblasts, mimicking PEL (compare with **Fig. 3A**) (H&E, ×400). (*F*) Burkitt lymphoma in bone marrow aspirate smear from an HIV+ patient presenting with pancytopenia. There are scattered large cells with deeply basophilic cytoplasm and cytoplasmic vacuoles, reminiscent of PEL pronormoblasts. Flow cytometry, immunohistochemistry, and cytogenetics in this case confirmed the diagnosis of Burkitt lymphoma (Wright-Giemsa, ×400).

Differential Diagnosis of Pure Erythroid Leukemia	
PEL vs	Helpful Distinguishing Feature(s) of PEL
Myelodysplastic syndromes with erythroid predominance and left-shift	Lack of significant maturation of erythroid series Prominent dyserythropoiesis with highly dysplastic and vacuolated pronormoblasts Markedly complex karyotype
Megaloblastic anemia and reactive erythroid hyperplasias	Prominently dysplastic and vacuolated pronormoblasts Abnormal karyotype in almost all cases Normal B12 and folate levels and no clinical evidence of hemolysis
AML with minimal maturation	CD34-negative and E-cadherin–positive blasts
ALL	TdT-negative and CD34-negative blasts lacking expression of B-cell or T-cell markers
Acute megakaryoblastic leukemia	Markedly complex karyotype and lack of t(1;22) Not typically associated with Down syndrome
Burkitt lymphoma	Negativity for B-cell markers and surface immunoglobulin Lack of t(8;14) on karyotype

megakaryoblastic leukemia. It is uncertain how such cases should be classified.[12,13]

Other Neoplasms Involving the Bone Marrow

The sheetlike infiltration of the bone marrow by PEL and the negativity of blasts for CD34 and myeloid markers may lead to erroneous classification as a nonacute leukemia. High-grade B-cell lymphomas, such as Burkitt lymphoma, can present as leukemia with large cells with vacuolated, basophilic cytoplasm infiltrating the bone marrow and circulating in the blood (see **Fig.** 4E, F). Plasmablastic plasma cell myeloma shares some morphologic features (large cells with prominent nucleoli and basophilic cytoplasm) and immunophenotypic features (negativity for CD45) with PEL. Application of a full panel of flow cytometry immunophenotyping and/or immunohistochemistry, including erythroid markers, such as CD71, glycophorin, or hemoglobin, as well as E-cadherin, is critical in making the correct diagnosis in such cases. Solid tumors, including epithelioid vascular tumors and small blue-cell tumors of childhood, also may mimic PEL morphologically.

PROGNOSIS

PEL has a dismal prognosis, with a median survival of only 3 months in one recent series. This extremely short survival is significantly inferior to both AEL and erythroid-predominant AML-MRC, even after taking into account the adverse cytogenetics inherent to PEL.[43] The neoplastic erythroblasts in PEL have been found to express P-glycoprotein, the product of the multidrug-resistance gene (MDR-1), which may in part contribute to its resistance to therapy and poor prognosis.[49]

REFERENCES

1. Bennett JM, Catovsky D, Daniel MT, et al. Proposed revised criteria for the classification of acute myeloid leukemia. A report of the French-American-British Cooperative Group. Ann Intern Med 1985;103(4): 620–5.
2. Kowal-Vern A, Mazzella FM, Cotelingam JD, et al. Diagnosis and characterization of acute erythroleukemia subsets by determining the percentages of myeloblasts and proerythroblasts in 69 cases. Am J Hematol 2000;65(1):5–13.
3. Arber DA, Brunning RD, Orazi A, et al. Acute myeloid leukaemia, not otherwise specified. In: Swerdlow SH, Campo E, Harris NL, et al, editors. WHO classification of tumours of haematopoietic and lymphoid tissues. Lyon (France): International Agency for Research on Cancer; 2008. p. 130–9.
4. Vardiman JW, Bruno RD, Arber DA, et al. Introduction and overview of the classification of the myeloid neoplasm. In: Swerdlow S, Campo E, Harris N, et al, editors. WHO classification of tumours of haematopoietic and lymphoid tissues. 4th edition. Lyon (France): International Agency for Research on Cancer (IARC); 2008. p. 18–30.
5. Wang SA, Hasserjian RP. Erythroid proliferations in myeloid neoplasms. Hum Pathol 2012;43(2):153–64.
6. Domingo-Claros A, Larriba I, Rozman M, et al. Acute erythroid neoplastic proliferations. A biological study based on 62 patients. Haematologica 2002;87(2): 148–53.
7. Hasserjian RP, Zuo Z, Garcia C, et al. Acute erythroid leukemia: a reassessment using criteria

refined in the 2008 WHO classification. Blood 2010; 115(10):1985–92.

8. Olopade OI, Thangavelu M, Larson RA, et al. Clinical, morphologic, and cytogenetic characteristics of 26 patients with acute erythroblastic leukemia. Blood 1992;80(11):2873–82.

9. Park S, Picard F, Azgui Z, et al. Erythroleukemia: a comparison between the previous FAB approach and the WHO classification. Leuk Res 2002;26(5): 423–9.

10. Santos FP, Faderl S, Garcia-Manero G, et al. Adult acute erythroleukemia: an analysis of 91 patients treated at a single institution. Leukemia 2009; 23(12):2275–80.

11. Fouillard L, Labopin M, Gorin NC, et al. Hematopoietic stem cell transplantation for de novo erythroleukemia: a study of the European Group for Blood and Marrow Transplantation (EBMT). Blood 2002;100(9): 3135–40.

12. Zuo Z, Polski JM, Kasyan A, et al. Acute erythroid leukemia. Arch Pathol Lab Med 2010;134(9): 1261–70.

13. Barnard DR, Alonzo TA, Gerbing RB, et al. Comparison of childhood myelodysplastic syndrome, AML FAB M6 or M7, CCG 2891: report from the Children's Oncology Group. Pediatr Blood Cancer 2007;49(1): 17–22.

14. Pession A, Masetti R, Rizzari C, et al. Results of the AIEOP AML 2002/01 multicenter prospective trial for the treatment of children with acute myeloid leukemia. Blood 2013;122(2):170–8.

15. Webb DK, Harrison G, Stevens RF, et al. Relationships between age at diagnosis, clinical features, and outcome of therapy in children treated in the Medical Research Council AML 10 and 12 trials for acute myeloid leukemia. Blood 2001;98(6):1714–20.

16. van Dongen JC, Dalinghaus M, Kroon AA, et al. Successful treatment of congenital acute myeloid leukemia (AML-M6) in a premature infant. J Pediatr Hematol Oncol 2009;31(11):853–4.

17. Novik Y, Marino P, Makower DF, et al. Familial erythroleukemia: a distinct clinical and genetic type of familial leukemias. Leuk Lymphoma 1998;30(3–4): 395–401.

18. Keifer J, Zaino R, Ballard JO. Erythroleukemic infiltration of a lymph node: use of hemoglobin immunohistochemical techniques in diagnosis. Hum Pathol 1984;15(11):1090–3.

19. Bennett JM, Catovsky D, Daniel MT, et al. The chronic myeloid leukaemias: guidelines for distinguishing chronic granulocytic, atypical chronic myeloid, and chronic myelomonocytic leukaemia. Proposals by the French-American-British Cooperative Leukaemia Group. Br J Haematol 1994;87(4): 746–54.

20. Santos FP, Kantarjian HM, Jain N, et al. Phase 2 study of CEP-701, an orally available JAK2 inhibitor, in patients with primary or post-polycythemia vera/essential thrombocythemia myelofibrosis. Blood 2010;115(6):1131–6.

21. Park S, Picard F, Guesnu M, et al. Erythroleukaemia and RAEB-t: a same disease? Leukemia 2004;18(4): 888–90.

22. Honda Y, Manabe A, Tsuchida M, et al. Clinicopathological characteristics of erythroblast-rich RAEB and AML M6a in children. Int J Hematol 2008; 88(5):524–9.

23. Atkinson J, Hrisinko MA, Weil SC. Erythroleukemia: a review of 15 cases meeting 1985 FAB criteria and survey of the literature. Blood Rev 1992;6(4):204–14.

24. Mazzella FM, Alvares C, Kowal-Vern A, et al. The acute erythroleukemias. Clin Lab Med 2000;20(1): 119–37.

25. Bacher U, Haferlach C, Alpermann T, et al. Comparison of genetic and clinical aspects in patients with acute myeloid leukemia and myelodysplastic syndromes all with more than 50% of bone marrow erythropoietic cells. Haematologica 2011;96(9): 1284–92.

26. Cuneo A, Van Orshoven A, Michaux JL, et al. Morphologic, immunologic and cytogenetic studies in erythroleukaemia: evidence for multilineage involvement and identification of two distinct cytogenetic-clinicopathological types. Br J Haematol 1990;75(3):346–54.

27. Kasyan A, Medeiros LJ, Zuo Z, et al. Acute erythroid leukemia as defined in the World Health Organization classification is a rare and pathogenetically heterogeneous disease. Mod Pathol 2010;23(8): 1113–26.

28. Lessard M, Struski S, Leymarie V, et al. Cytogenetic study of 75 erythroleukemias. Cancer Genet Cytogenet 2005;163(2):113–22.

29. Liu CJ, Hong YC, Yang CF, et al. Clinicopathologic features and outcome of acute erythroid leukemia based on 2008 revised World Health Organization classification. Leuk Lymphoma 2012;53(2):289–94.

30. Micci F, Thorsen J, Panagopoulos I, et al. High-throughput sequencing identifies an NFIA/CBFA2T3 fusion gene in acute erythroid leukemia with t(1;16)(p31;q24). Leukemia 2013;27(4):980–2.

31. Walter RB, Othus M, Burnett AK, et al. Significance of FAB subclassification of "acute myeloid leukemia, NOS" in the 2008 WHO classification: analysis of 5848 newly diagnosed patients. Blood 2013; 121(13):2424–31.

32. Zuo Z, Medeiros LJ, Chen Z, et al. Acute myeloid leukemia (AML) with erythroid predominance exhibits clinical and molecular characteristics that differ from other types of AML. PLoS One 2012; 7(7):e41485.

33. Thiede C, Steudel C, Mohr B, et al. Analysis of FLT3-activating mutations in 979 patients with acute myelogenous leukemia: association with FAB subtypes

and identification of subgroups with poor prognosis. Blood 2002;99(12):4326–35.

34. Frohling S, Lipka DB, Kayser S, et al. Rare occurrence of the JAK2 V617F mutation in AML subtypes M5, M6, and M7. Blood 2006;107(3):1242–3.

35. Wechsler J, Greene M, McDevitt MA, et al. Acquired mutations in GATA1 in the megakaryoblastic leukemia of Down syndrome. Nat Genet 2002;32(1): 148–52.

36. Wang SA, Tang G, Fadare O, et al. Erythroid-predominant myelodysplastic syndromes: enumeration of blasts from nonerythroid rather than total marrow cells provides superior risk stratification. Mod Pathol 2008;21(11):1394–402.

37. Sikole A, Stojanovic A, Polenakovic M, et al. How erythropoietin affects bone marrow of uremic patients. Am J Nephrol 1997;17(2):128–36.

38. Kantarjian HM, Keating MJ, Walters RS, et al. Therapy-related leukemia and myelodysplastic syndrome: clinical, cytogenetic, and prognostic features. J Clin Oncol 1986;4(12):1748–57.

39. Arber DA, Brunning RD, Orazi A, et al. Acute myeloid leukaemia with myelodysplasia-related changes. In: Swerdlow SH, Campo E, Harris NL, et al, editors. WHO classification of tumours of haematopoietic and lymphoid tissues. 4th edition. Lyon (France): International Agency for Research on Cancer (IARC); 2008. p. 124–6.

40. Selby DM, Valdez R, Schnitzer B, et al. Diagnostic criteria for acute erythroleukemia. Blood 2003; 101(7):2895–6.

41. Mazzella FM, Kowal-Vern A, Shrit MA, et al. Acute erythroleukemia: evaluation of 48 cases with reference to classification, cell proliferation, cytogenetics, and prognosis. Am J Clin Pathol 1998;110(5):590–8.

42. Kowal-Vern A, Cotelingam J, Schumacher HR. The prognostic significance of proerythroblasts in acute erythroleukemia. Am J Clin Pathol 1992;98(1):34–40.

43. Liu W, Hasserjian RP, Hu Y, et al. Pure erythroid leukemia: a reassessment of the entity using the 2008 World Health Organization classification. Mod Pathol 2011;24(3):375–83.

44. Wang HY, Huang LJ, Liu Z, et al. Erythroblastic sarcoma presenting as bilateral ovarian masses in an infant with pure erythroid leukemia. Hum Pathol 2011;42(5):749–58.

45. Garand R, Duchayne E, Blanchard D, et al. Minimally differentiated erythroleukaemia (AML M6 'variant'): a rare subset of AML distinct from AML M6. Groupe Francais d'Hematologie Cellulaire. Br J Haematol 1995;90(4):868–75.

46. Hasserjian RP, Howard J, Wood A, et al. Acute erythremic myelosis (true erythroleukaemia): a variant of AML FAB-M6. J Clin Pathol 2001;54(3):205–9.

47. Wang W, Grier DD, Woo J, et al. Ferritin H is a novel marker of early erythroid precursors and macrophages. Histopathology 2013;62(6):931–40.

48. Park S, Picard F, Dreyfus F. Erythroleukemia: a need for a new definition. Leukemia 2002;16(8):1399–401.

49. Mazzella FM, Kowal-Vern A, Shrit MA, et al. Effects of multidrug resistance gene expression in acute erythroleukemia. Mod Pathol 2000;13(4):407–13.

Early T-cell Precursor Acute Lymphoblastic Leukemia/ Lymphoma

David R. Czuchlewski, MD*, Kathryn Foucar, MD

KEYWORDS

- Acute lymphoblastic leukemia • Acute lymphoblastic lymphoma • Early T-cell precursor • Prognosis

KEY POINTS

- Discrete diagnostic subtypes of T lymphoblastic leukemia/lymphoma (T-ALL) have historically not been widely recognized. Recently, a novel subset of T-ALL with distinctive immunophenotypic, molecular, and clinical features has been proposed.
- Termed ETP-ALL, these cases seem to correspond to a very early stage of T-cell development. ETP-ALL shows a characteristic immunophenotype that includes absence of several antigens typically associated with T-cell lineage.
- Cases of ETP-ALL also show nonspecific expression of myeloid and stem cell antigens.
- ETP-ALL is associated with a poor prognosis using standard T-ALL treatment protocols, and patients with ETP-ALL may benefit from intensified, alternative, or targeted therapies.
- Emerging data suggest that ETP-ALL is a specific subtype of T-ALL associated with unique diagnostic and therapeutic challenges.
- Recognizing ETP-ALL and distinguishing it from other forms of acute leukemia, such as acute leukemia of ambiguous lineage, are important elements of an up-to-date diagnostic approach to precursor T-cell neoplasms.

ABSTRACT

Discrete diagnostic subtypes of T lymphoblastic leukemia/lymphoma (T-cell acute lymphoblastic leukemia/lymphoma, T-ALL) have historically not been widely recognized. Recently, a novel subset with distinctive immunophenotypic, molecular, and clinical features has been proposed. Termed early T-cell precursor acute lymphoblastic leukemia (ETP-ALL), these cases seem to correspond to a very early stage of T-cell development. ETP-ALL is associated with a poor prognosis using standard protocols, and patients with ETP-ALL may benefit from intensified, alternative, or targeted therapies. Recognizing ETP-ALL and distinguishing it from other forms of acute leukemia are important elements of an up-to-date diagnostic approach to precursor T-cell neoplasms.

OVERVIEW

T-ALL is a neoplasm of immature blasts committed to T-lineage differentiation. The neoplastic cells express antigens (and patterns of antigens in combination) associated with immaturity and T-cell lineage. Immunophenotypic characterization, typically performed by flow cytometric analysis, is critical in the diagnosis of T-ALL. Broad immunophenotypic subsets of T-ALL have been described, largely corresponding to stages of normal T-cell maturation within the thymus (**Table 1**). Recurrent genetic/cytogenetic abnormalities associated with T-ALL have also been identified.[1] However, the World Health Organization 2008 Classification of Tumours of Haematopoietic and Lymphoid Tissues does not define specific diagnostic subtypes of T-ALL on immunophenotypic, molecular, or other grounds.[2] The

The authors have no relevant conflicts of interest to disclose.
Department of Pathology, University of New Mexico, Albuquerque, NM 87131, USA
* Corresponding author. 1001 Woodward Place Northeast, TriCore Reference Laboratories, Albuquerque, NM 87102.
E-mail address: DCzuchlewski@salud.unm.edu

surgpath.theclinics.com

Acronyms and Abbreviations	
AIEOP	Associazione Italiana Ematologia Oncologia Pediatrica
AML	Acute myeloid leukemia
BPDC	Blastic plasmacytoid dendritic cell
cCD3	Cytoplasmic CD3
CGH	Comparative genomic hybridization
DN	Double negative
ETP	Early thymic precursor or early T-lineage progenitor
ETP-ALL	Early T-cell precursor acute lymphoblastic leukemia
MPAL	Mixed-phenotype acute leukemia
MPO	Myeloperoxidase
NK	Natural killer
sCD3	Surface CD3
SNP	Singlenucleotide polymorphism
T-ALL	T-cell acute lymphoblastic leukemia/ lymphoma
TCR	T-cell receptor
TdT	Terminal deoxynucleotidyl transferase
WHO	World Health Organization

growing emphasis on ETP-ALL as a recognizable and clinically relevant subset of T-ALL[3–5] is, therefore, a novel development. Similar observations relating to other types of hematolymphoid malignancies have in the past led to the establishment of distinct diagnostic subcategories.

STAGES OF T-CELL DEVELOPMENT AND THE EARLY T-CELL PRECURSOR

ETP-ALL is closely associated with a very early stage of T-cell maturation.[6] T-cell development begins in the bone marrow as hematopoietic stem cells give rise to progenitor cells either committed to or primed for T-cell lineage.[7] These cells then journey via the peripheral blood to the thymus, where they complete their development.[8]

This process is reflected in changes in immunophenotype as the cells sequentially express different patterns of antigens, and in anatomic location as the cells migrate from the thymic cortex to the medulla. The prothymocyte represents the earliest well-characterized intrathymic precursor cell.[8] Prothymocytes express CD7, variable CD34, and terminal deoxynucleotidyl transferase (TdT) but not surface CD3 (sCD3), CD4, CD8, or CD1a.[2,4] Cytoplasmic CD3 (cCD3) also begins to be expressed at this stage.[2,9,10] Because these cells are negative for both CD4 and CD8, they are also known as double negative (DN). Based on esoteric patterns of antigen expression, typically studied in the mouse, the DN prothymocyte stage may be further subdivided into DN1, DN2, DN3, and DN4 phases.[11,12] The DN1 stage is also referred to as the early thymic precursor or early T-lineage progenitor (ETP).[8,11] ETPs express CD117 and retain the capacity (at least under experimental conditions) for differentiation along multiple lineages, including natural killer (NK), dendritic cell, myeloid, and erythroid, underscoring their primitive nature.[7,8,11,13–16] ETPs are rare, representing only 0.01% of total thymocytes.[8] Under the influence of Notch signaling, ETPs continue their maturation toward more differentiated stages of T-cell development, eventually giving rise to cortical thymocytes (CD1a+, sCD3−, CD4+, and CD8+) and, finally, medullary thymocytes (CD1a−, sCD3+, and either CD4+ or CD8 +).[2,8,10]

Cases of T-ALL generally show immunophenotypic profiles that recapitulate these broad stages of normal thymic maturation, including pro-T, cortical T, and medullary T (see Table 1).[1,2] T-ALL corresponding to early stages of maturation has been associated with inferior prognosis.[17] In 2009, Coustan-Smith and colleagues[6] at St. Jude Children's Research Hospital hypothesized that some cases of T-ALL might correspond specifically to the ETP stage of maturation and that, owing to the primitive and multipotent nature of the ETP, such cases might show inferior response

Table 1
Immunophenotype of T-ALL according to stages of thymic differentiation

Stage of Maturation	CD1a	CD34	CD2	cCD3	sCD3	CD4	CD5	CD7	CD8
Pro-T	−	±	−	+	−	−	−	+	−
Pre-T	−	±	+	+	−	−	±	+	−
Cortical T	+	−	+	+	−	+	±	+	+
Medullary T	−	−	+	+	+	±[a]	±	+	±[a]

[a] At the medullary stage, T cells express either CD4 or CD8 but not both.
Data from Refs.[1–4]

to standard lymphoid-directed T-ALL therapies. Gene expression profiling of blasts from a series of T-ALL patients identified a subset of T-ALL cases that clustered with the known expression profile of normal ETPs (**Fig. 1**). Strikingly, these patients shared a clinically aggressive disease with distinctly inferior outcome (**Fig. 2**). Both the existence of an ETP-ALL subgroup and its association with exceptionally poor prognosis were concurrently confirmed in a separate validation cohort from the Associazione Italiana Ematologia Oncologia Pediatrica (AIEOP).[6] A unique immunophenotype was also found to characterize this ETP-ALL subgroup (summarized in **Box 1**). This immunophenotypic description has been adopted by most subsequent workers as definitional for ETP-ALL.[18–21]

EPIDEMIOLOGY AND PRESENTING CLINICAL FEATURES

ETP-ALL accounts for approximately 12% to 15% of all cases of pediatric T lymphoblastic leukemia (range 5%–17%).[6,21–23] A similar proportion of T lymphoblastic lymphoma cases show the ETP immunophenotype.[24] Among children, the average age of onset seems to be approximately 12 years, with a majority of cases occurring in patients older than age 10.[6,22] A survey of a large cohort of adult T-ALL patients identified the ETP immunophenotype in a somewhat higher proportion of cases.[25] In all age groups, there is a male predominance, with a male-to-female ratio of 4:1.[6,22,25] Approximately one-fourth of cases have been associated with a mediastinal mass.[6,22,25] The presenting white blood cell count varies[6] and has been reported as significantly lower than generic cases of T-ALL in some studies[21,23] but not others.[25] Central nervous system involvement is seen in approximately 12% of cases.[6,22,25]

FLOW CYTOMETRY

Although ETP-ALL seems to be associated with distinct clinical and molecular findings, the characteristic flow cytometric immunophenotype is the true key to the diagnosis. As originally established by Coustan-Smith and colleagues[6] and presented in **Box 1**, the definition requires

1. Absence of CD1a and CD8 expression (less than 5% positive blasts) and
2. Weak to absent CD5 expression (less than 75% of blasts positive) and
3. Positive expression (in greater than 25% of blasts) of 1 or more of the following myeloid or stem cell–associated markers: CD117, CD34, HLA-DR, CD13, CD33, CD11b, and/or CD65[6]

All of these criteria must be fulfilled to consider a case ETP-ALL.[6] In addition, this immunophenotypic definition of ETP-ALL presumes the presence of cCD3 expression by flow cytometric

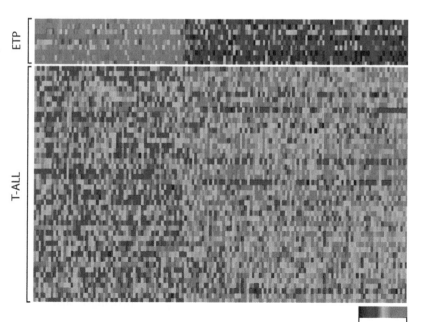

Fig. 1. Gene expression profiling of pediatric ETP-ALL and non–ETP-ALL shows distinct clustering of the ETP-ALL cases in this heat map of the top 150 differentially expressed genes. (*Adapted from* Coustan-Smith E, Mullighan CG, Onciu M, et al. Early T-cell precursor leukemia: a subtype of very high-risk acute lymphoblastic leukemia. Lancet Oncol 2009;10:149; with permission.)

ETP

T-ALL

-3   3

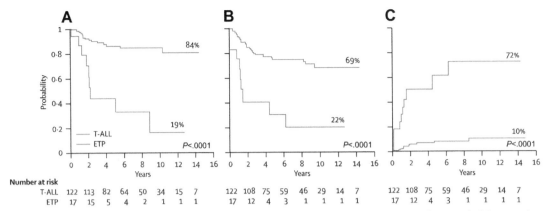

Fig. 2. Kaplan-Meier plots comparing ETP-ALL and non–ETP-ALL in terms of (A) overall survival, (B) event-free survival, and (C) the cumulative incidence of remission failure or hematological relapse show the distinctly inferior outcomes typical of ETP-ALL. (*Reproduced from* Coustan-Smith E, Mullighan CG, Onciu M, et al. Early T-cell precursor leukemia: a subtype of very high-risk acute lymphoblastic leukemia. Lancet Oncol 2009;10:152; with permission.)

analysis and absence of myeloperoxidase (MPO) expression (eg, less than 3% blasts positive by cytochemistry). In the authors' experience, rare cases of ETP-ALL can show limited expression of B-lineage antigens, although the World Health Organization (WHO) 2008 requirements for a bi-phenotypic acute leukemia of ambiguous lineage are not fulfilled; a similar case of B-lineage antigen expression in ETP-ALL has also been reported in the literature.[26] Representative flow cytometric histograms of ETP-ALL are shown in **Fig. 3**. Individual components of this overall immunopheno-type may be seen in a wide variety of entities (discussed later). Thus, a comprehensive immuno-phenotypic evaluation and an emphasis on pat-terns of overall expression, rather than specific individual markers, are most helpful in these cases. Although the Coustan-Smith immunophe-notypic definition has been widely accepted in subsequent studies,[18–21,25] at least 1 report used an alternative set of markers to identify cases.[22]

This seems, however, to have been done primarily to work around a lack of data on some of the markers described above. Given that ETP-ALL cases were originally identified by gene expression signatures similar to normal ETP cells, it is not surprising that the immunophenotype of ETP-ALL also follows that seen in these normal counterparts.

MOLECULAR AND GENETIC FINDINGS

Key molecular and genetic features of ETP-ALL are summarized in **Box 2**.

GENE EXPRESSION

ETP-ALL was identified largely through gene expression profiling experiments seeking to un-cover cases of expression profiles reminiscent of normal ETP cells. Thus, at the level of mRNA transcripts, ETP-ALL is intrinsically distinct from unselected T-ALL cases. The profile includes up-regulation of *KIT*, *GATA2*, and *CEBPA* expression in addition to underexpression of *CD3*, *CD4*, *CD8*, *RAG1*, and *ZAP70*.[6] *LYL1* and *ERG*, which encode transcription factors expressed in the early thymocyte stage of development, are also overexpressed.[6] The original gene expression work has been supplemented by additional comparisons of ETP-ALL to acute myeloid leuke-mia (AML), normal stem cells, normal granulocyte macrophage precursors, and B lymphoblastic leukemia. The ETP-ALL cases show significant overlap with early and/or stem cell–like features in all of these comparisons, consistent with the hypothesis that ETP-ALL corresponds to a very early and/or multipotent hematopoietic progenitor cell.[19]

Box 1
Immunophenotypic definition of ETP-ALL

To be considered ETP-ALL, a case of T-ALL must fulfill all of the following criteria[6,a]:

- Absence of CD1a and CD8 expression

- Weak to absent CD5 expression (<75% of blasts positive)

- Expression (positive in >25% of blasts) of one or more of the following myeloid or stem cell–associated markers: CD117, CD34, HLA-DR, CD13, CD33, CD11b, and/or CD65

[a] Assuming that blasts are cCD3 positive and MPO negative.

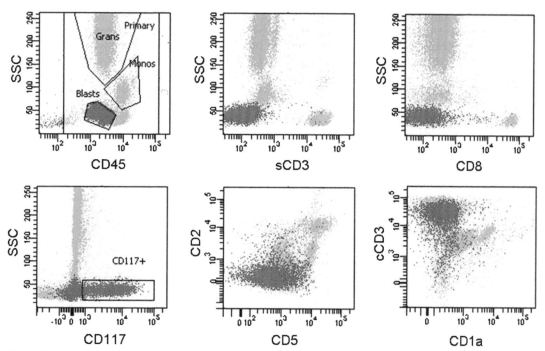

Fig. 3. Flow cytometric analysis reveals the characteristic immunophenotypic pattern of ETP-ALL. (*Top row*) Blasts are dim CD45 positive and negative for sCD3 and CD8. (*Bottom row*) Greater than 25% of blasts are positive for CD117, <75% of blasts are positive for CD5, and cCD3 is expressed in the absence of CD1a. Grans, background granulocytes; Monos, background monocytes; SSC, side scatter.

Box 2
Key molecular genetic features of ETP-ALL

- Gene expression signature distinct from non–ETP-ALL and similar to normal ETP precursor cells

- Increased structural genomic variability compared with non–ETP-ALL

- Slightly more common del(13q) on karyotype

- Moderate burden of somatic, nonsynonymous, coding mutations

- Spectrum of mutations partially reminiscent of myeloid neoplasms

- Mutations involve genes bearing on cytokine receptor and RAS signaling, hematopoietic differentiation, and epigenetic modification

- Clonal T-cell receptor (TCR) gene rearrangement(s) in most cases

- Absence of biallelic *TRG* VJ recombination in some, but not all, ETP-ALL

STRUCTURAL REARRANGEMENTS

ETP-ALL has been assessed for structural genetic alterations using a variety of traditional and novel techniques, including conventional cytogenetic analysis (karytotype), copy number detection via single nucleotide polymorphism (SNP) microarray analysis, and sequence-based rearrangement detection via whole genome sequencing. Approximately 80% of ETP-ALL cases show clonal cytogenetic abnormalities on karyotype; the detected abnormalities vary widely, with no pattern of specific recurrent anomalies, although del(13q) is found more common in ETP-ALL than in typical T-ALL.[6] SNP microarray analysis shows significantly more structural aberration and, on average, larger regions of gain or loss in ETP-ALL compared with non–ETP-ALL.[6] A next generation study uncovered an average of 15 structural variations in ETP-ALL, most of which interrupted coding genes and many of which generated fusion genes (*ETV6-INO80D*, *NUP214-SQSTM1*, etc).[19] *NF1* deletion has been documented in a case of ETP-ALL associated with in vitro sensitivity to the signaling inhibitor tipifarnib.[18] *TCF1*, which encodes a transcription factor relevant in early T-cell development, is deleted (with concurrent decreased expression) in some cases of ETP-ALL.[27] The pattern of structural rearrangements in up to 25% of ETP-ALL cases suggests the occurrence of *chromothripsis* (chromosome shattering), a recently recognized phenomenon in which a very large number of rearrangements occur within a localized choromosomal region.[19]

SOMATIC MUTATIONS

Next-generation sequencing has revealed a complicated mutational landscape in cases of ETP-ALL. The numeric burden of acquired, non-silent, coding mutations in ETP-ALL is similar to that seen in AML.[5] Mutations in pediatric ETP-ALL have been divided into 3 broad classes. More than two-thirds of ETP-ALL cases harbor acquired mutations affecting genes relating to cytokine receptor and/or RAS signaling (eg, *NRAS, KRAS, FLT3, BRAF,* and *IL7R*).[5,19] A majority of cases also carry mutations affecting genes relating to hematopoietic development (eg, *GATA3, ETV6, RUNX1,* and *IKZF1*).[5,19] Finally, approximately half of cases show mutations in genes tied to epigenetic modification (eg, *EZH2*).[5,19] The molecular alterations in adult ETP-ALL seem slightly different from pediatric cases, with frequent mutations *DNMT3A* and *NOTCH1* in addition to *FLT3*.[28,29] Several of these genes could possibly be amenable to targeted therapy.[28,29] The spectrum of mutations in ETP-ALL is similar in many respects to that seen in myeloid neoplasms, underscoring the subtle myeloid features of ETP-ALL. Somatic mutations inactivating several genes that encode DNA mismatch and repair proteins have been detected in some cases of ETP-ALL, a finding that may correlate with the high degree of chromosomal instability typical of ETP-ALL.[19]

MICRO RNA PROFILING

Global microRNA profiling highlights the distinct features of ETP-ALL. In comparison with non–ETP-ALL, miR-221 and miR-222 are up-regulated in ETP cases, whereas miR-363 and miR-576-3p are down-regulated.[30] The functional significance of these findings remains unclear. At least one target of miR-222 may have a role in granulocytic differentiation and apoptosis.[30]

T-CELL RECEPTOR GENE REARRANGEMENTS

ETP-ALL has been assessed for evidence of clonal T-cell receptor (TCR) gene rearrangements. In one analysis, approximately 90% of ETP-ALL cases showed evidence of clonal rearrangement, as detected in at least 1 TCR locus (*TRB, TRG,* and/or *TRD*).[6] The high proportion of ETP-ALL cases with TCR gene rearrangements (relative to the normal human prothymocyte, in which TCR rearrangements are rare) has led some investigators to question whether the ETP phenotype could perhaps arise in neoplasms corresponding to stages of T-cell development slightly later than the true ETP stage.[31,32] Absence of biallelic deletions at the *TRG* locus (as detected by array comparative genomic hybridization, corresponding to a lack of VJ recombination at this site) is a feature associated with, but not specific for, ETP-ALL.[32]

DIFFERENTIAL DIAGNOSIS

The differential diagnosis of ETP-ALL can be approached from several perspectives: disorders with overlapping immunophenotypic features, the differential diagnosis in patients presenting with a leukemic blood and bone marrow picture, and the differential diagnosis of blastic infiltrates in extramedullary sites, including mediastinum (Fig. 4, Tables 2–4).

Table 2 and Fig. 4 highlight the comparison of immunophenotypic features between ETP-ALL, other T-cell leukemias, mixed-phenotype acute leukemia (MPAL), and other blastic neoplasms. As expected, more mature T-ALL shows many immunophenotypic similarities with ETP-ALL in terms of phenotype. Other neoplasms (listed in Table 2) show some immunophenotypic overlap with ETP-ALL especially when expression of a single or a few antigens is considered. AML cases are typically readily distinguishable from ETP-ALL by expression of multiple myeloid antigens and cytochemical/flow cytometric MPO positivity. For NK-cell neoplasms, the detection of Epstein-Barr virus is essential, whereas CD123 and other dendritic cell antigens highlight blastic plasmacytoid dendritic cell (BPDC) tumors. Other useful immunophenotypic features for individual neoplasms are listed in Table 2.

In blood, bone marrow, and extramedullary tissues sites, ETP-ALL has generic morphologic features, including blastic chromatin, generally scant cytoplasm, and abundant mitotic activity. This morphologic profile can be seen in other blastic neoplasms, although some morphologic features may be helpful in the recognition of specific neoplasms. Cytoplasmic granules may be seen in both AML and NK-cell neoplasms; Auer rods and greater than 3% MPO cytochemical positivity in blasts are both convincing features of myeloid differentiation. The cytologic and morphologic features of other blastic neoplasms

Fig. 4. An algorithmic approach to the differential diagnosis of ETP-ALL is illustrated. This simplified approach assumes that blasts have been identified with flow cytometric expression of cCD3 but not sCD3.

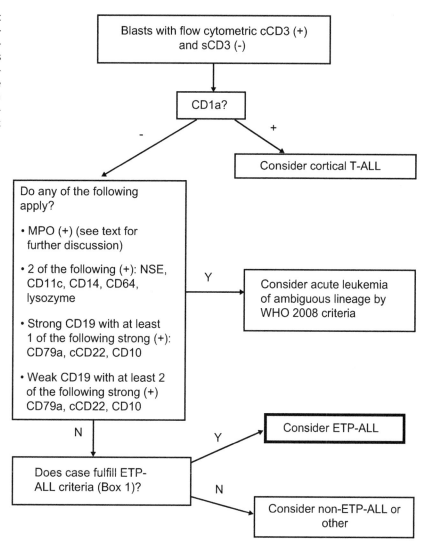

are not generally distinctive enough to permit diagnosis without immunophenotyping.

Particularly challenging are mediastinal biopsies, because lymphocyte-rich thymoma can mimic ALL (see Table 4). Cytokeratin immunohistochemical staining is essential to highlight often inconspicuous, elongated thymic epithelial cells in mediastinal biopsies.

Finally, expression of 2 antigens in particular—MPO and CD5—should be subjected to heightened scrutiny in potential cases of ETP-ALL. First, MPO expression is critical in distinguishing ETP-ALL from MPAL. As an example illustrating this point, a high rate of FLT3 mutation has been proposed as a feature of ETP-ALL[28]; however, other evidence suggests that FLT3 mutation is rare in well-defined T-ALL but is associated with acute leukemia of ambiguous lineage[33,34] [mixed

phenotype acute leukemia (MPAL), T/myeloid, NOS]: Hoehn and colleagues[33] applied an appropriate 3% cutoff for MPO positivity by cytochemistry, with cases fulfilling this criterion properly considered MPAL.[6,35] In difficult cases, cytochemistry for MPO should be performed in addition to flow cytometric analysis for best assessment of this critical antigen. Second, CD5 expression has been noted to be a potentially problematic area of interpretation in ETP-ALL. Gutierrez and colleagues[32] identified several cases of aggressive T-ALL with the gene expression profile and immunophenotype fulfilling all criteria for ETP-ALL except for diminished CD5 expression. Rare similar cases were also seen in the original ETP-ALL cohorts studied by Coustan-Smith and colleagues.[6] Because CD5 expression is generally present in ETP-ALL but

Table 2
Differential diagnosis ETP-all based on immunophenotypic features

Neoplasm	CD34	CD117	HLA-DR	Myeloid (13,33,11b)	CD65	Cytochem MPO	CYTO CD3	TdT	CD1a	Surface CD3	CD5	CD2	CD7	CD4	CD8	CD56	Comments
ETP-ALL	+ or	+ or	+ or	+ or	+	−	+	V	−	−	−/Weak	−	−	−	−	−	Notes 1 or more of columns 1-5 required
MPAL	Vª	V	V	MPO + Monocytic +	−	+−	+	V	−	Rare +	−	−	V	−	−	−	Complex criteria with multiple combinations for "mixed"
T-ALL Pro-T stage	+/−	−	−	−	−	−	+	+	−	−	−	−	+	−	−	−	Earliest T-ALL thymic stage
AUL	+	+	V	−	−	−	−	V	−	−	−	−	V	−	−	−	Lack specific myeloid, B, T lineage antigens
AML	+	+/−	+	+	+	+	Rare +	Rare +	−	−	−	−	−/+	Often +	−	OCC +	Wide range in IP
Blastic PDCT	−	−	+	Often +	−	−	−	Rare +	−	−	−	V	V	+	−	+	Also express CD43 and CD123
NK	−	−	+	Usually −	−	−	+	Rare +	−	−	V	+	+	−	+	+	TIA-1 and EBER also positive

Abbreviations: ALL, Acute Lymphoblastic Leukemia; AML, Acute Myeloid Leukemia; AUL, Acute Undifferentiated Leukemia; BPDCT, Blastic Plasmacytoid Dendritic Cell Tumor; MPAL, Mixed Phenotype Acute Leukemia; NK, Natural Killer; V, Variable.
ª Not required for specific diagnosis.

Table 3
Differential diagnosis of ETP-ALL in blood and bone marrow

Disease	Key Features/Comments
ETP-ALL	Indistinguishable from other types of ALL Blastic nuclear chromatin, variable usually high nuclear-to-cytoplasmic ratio
ALL	ALL of B-cell and T-cell types have overlapping morphologic features with ETP-ALL
AML	Usually distinguishable from ALL based on nuclear-to-cytoplasmic ratio, cytoplasmic granules, and Auer rods May be indistinguishable from ALL; cytochemical MPO stain essential
MPAL	No distinctive morphologic features; defined by immunophenotypic features
Other blastic neoplasms	BPDCs have many features mimicking lymphoblasts • Cytoplasm may exhibit shaggy projections and cytoplasmic vacuoles are common

expressed only on a subset of blasts (less than 75%) and/or at diminished intensity, precise assessment of CD5 pattern and intensity is essential in these cases. It is possible that interpretation of CD5 may be a source of difficulty in the flow cytometric work-up of ETP-ALL.[32]

PROGNOSIS AND TREATMENT

ETP-ALL is associated with poor response to treatment and decreased survival. When given standard therapy directed at T-lymphoblasts, these patients have a delayed rate of clearance of blasts and a high rate of minimal residual disease, including at the end of induction.[6] These patients are more likely to relapse than those with non–ETP-ALL (72% vs 10%), and ETP-ALL overall survival at 10 years is only 19% (vs 84% for non–ETP-ALL). Multivariate

analysis indicated that the ETP phenotype is decisively the strongest predictor of outcome in T-ALL compared with standard clinical parameters for risk stratification. These findings were initially reproduced in the AIEOP cohort,[6] and the high-risk nature of both pediatric and adult ETP-ALL has been confirmed in subsequent studies.[21–23,25,29] Cases of ETP lymphoblastic lymphoma show a similar poor prognosis (**Figs. 5–7**).[24]

The unfavorable outcome seen in ETP-ALL with standard intensive chemotherapy has prompted some groups to recommend routine hematopoietic stem cell transplantation in first remission for these patients.[6] Others have suggested that the subtle myeloid-type genetic and immunophenotypic findings seen in ETP-ALL could argue for treatments more often considered in the context of myeloid neoplasms.[19,36] Novel and/or targeted

Table 4
Differential diagnosis in extramedullary sites

Neoplasm	Key Features/Comments
ETP-ALL	Indistinguishable from other blastic neoplasms with high nuclear-to-cytoplasmic ratio and blastic nuclear chromatin in tissue
ALL/MPAL	No morphologic features are useful in distinguishing tissue infiltrates of ETP-ALL from B-cell and other T-cell types of ALL and MPAL. Immunophenotyping is essential.
Thymoma	Lymphocyte-rich thymoma can mimic lymphoblastic lymphoma in tissue sections. Flow cytometry and immunohistochemical stain (especially keratin stain) are essential.
Other blastic neoplasms (BPDC, blastic neuroendocrine tumors, peripheral neuroectodermal tumor, etc.)	The suggestion of an organoid pattern in tissue sections should prompt comprehensive immunohistochemical assessment essential for the diagnosis of many nonleukemic childhood small blue cell tumors.

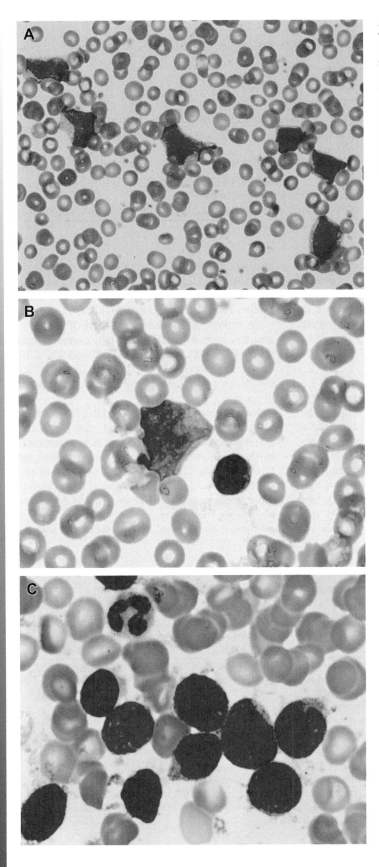

Fig. 5. (A) This blood smear in a patient with ETP-ALL shows a marked leukocytosis consisting of blasts with scant amounts of cytoplasm (Wright, 100×). (B) A side-by-side comparison of a small normal lymphocyte and an ETP-ALL blast is illustrated (Wright, 200×). (C) This bone marrow aspirate smear is from a patient with ETP-ALL show effacement by blasts with very scanty amounts of cytoplasm (Wright, 200×).

Fig. 5. (continued). (D) Bone marrow effacement by ETP-ALL is evident at low magnification in this core biopsy section (H&E, 10×). (E) On high magnification, ETP-ALL blasts exhibit dispersed chromatin and scant cytoplasm. Note rare myelocytes (H&E, 80×). (F) The leukemic cells in ETP-ALL are CD3 positive (CD3 immunohistochemistry, 80×).

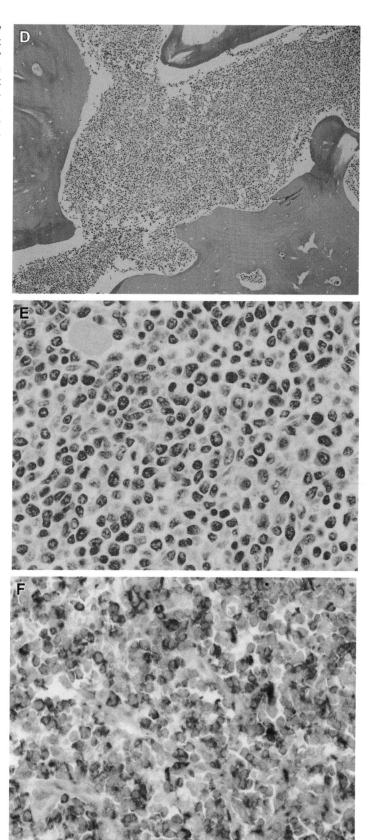

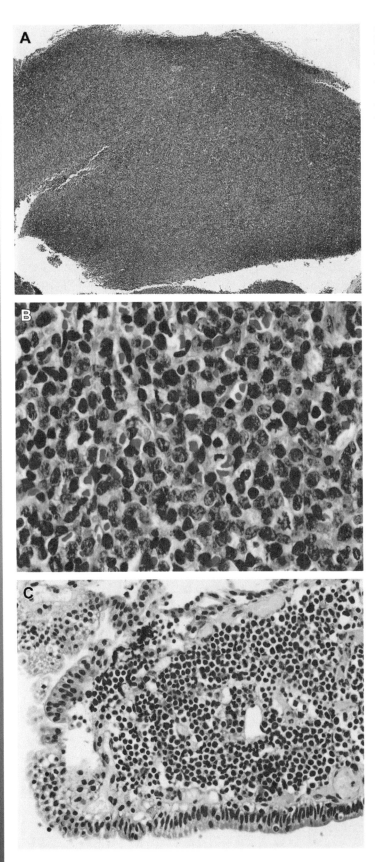

Fig. 6. (A) Lymph node effacement by ETP-ALL is shown at low magnification (H&E, 4×). (B) On high magnification, blasts with scant cytoplasm are evident. Note mitotic activity (H&E, 80×). (C) Infiltration of the duodenal mucosa is evident in this 11-year-old boy with ETP-ALL (H&E, 40×).

Fig. 6. (continued). (*D*) CD3 expression in ETP-ALL involving duodenum (CD3 immunohistochemistry, 40×). (*E*) CD45 expression in ETP-ALL involving duodenum (CD45 immunohistochemistry, 40×). (*F*) Simultaneous bone marrow infiltration by pleomorphic blasts in patient with ETP-ALL manifesting in duodenum (Wright, 120×).

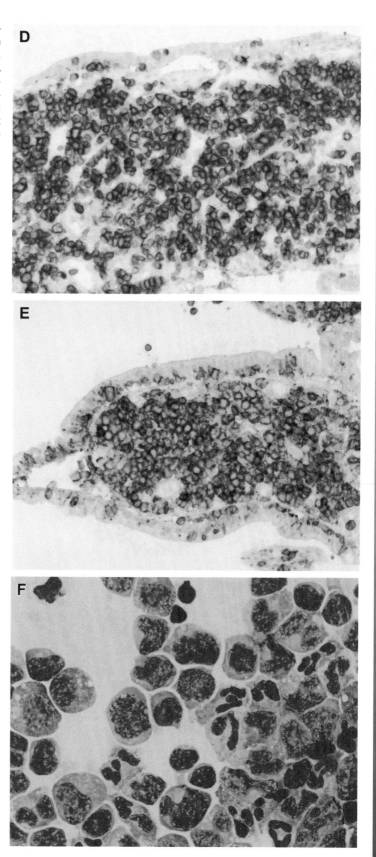

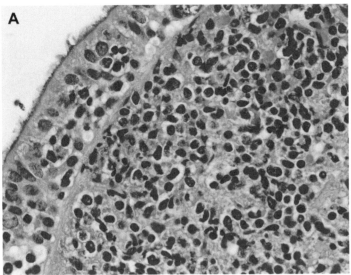

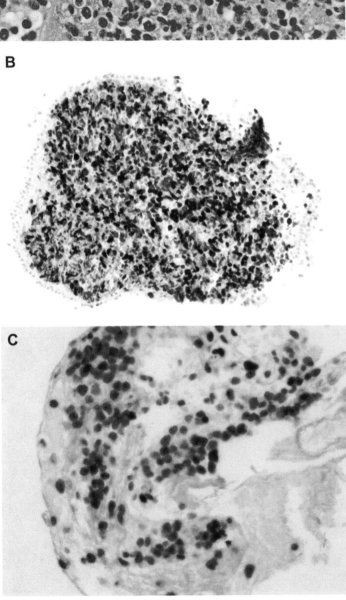

Fig. 7. (*A*) Infiltration into bronchial mucosa as a direct extension of mediastinal ETP-ALL is illustrated (H&E, 64×). (*B*) Increased proliferative rate in this case of ETP-ALL is evident by Ki67 (Ki67 immunohistochemistry, 40×). (*C*) Nuclear TdT is evident in this endobronchial biopsy of ETP-ALL of mediastinal origin (TdT immunohistochemistry, 50×).

therapies using tyrosine kinase inhibitors, epigenetic modifiers, γ-secretase inhibitors, and agents such as nelarabine may offer additional therapeutic approaches in this high-risk group of patients.[28,29,37] Identification of ETP-ALL in the routine diagnostic setting is imperative in light of these intensified and alternative treatment strategies.

REFERENCES

1. Kraszewska MD, Dawidowska M, Szczepanski T, et al. T-cell acute lymphoblastic leukaemia: recent molecular biology findings. Br J Haematol 2012; 156:303–15.

2. Borowitz MJ, Chan JK. T lymphoblastic leukemia/lymphoma. In: Swerdlow SH, Campo E, Harris NL, et al, editors. WHO classification of tumours of haematopoietic and lymphoid tissue. Lyon (France): International Agency for Research on Cancer; 2008. p. 176–8.

3. Acute lymphoblastic leukemia. 2013. Available at: nccn.org. Accessed April 12, 2013.

4. Onciu M. Acute lymphoblastic leukemia. Hematol Oncol Clin North Am 2009;23:655–74.

5. Streensma M, DeAngelo DJ. Looking under the hood of early T-Cell precursor acute lymphoblatic leukemia. The Hematologist 2012;9(3):12.

6. Coustan-Smith E, Mullighan CG, Onciu M, et al. Early T-cell precursor leukaemia: a subtype of very high-risk acute lymphoblastic leukaemia. Lancet Oncol 2009;10:147–56.

7. Schlenner SM, Rodewald HR. Early T cell development and the pitfalls of potential. Trends Immunol 2010;31:303–10.

8. Yang Q, Jeremiah Bell J, Bhandoola A. T-cell lineage determination. Immunol Rev 2010;238:12–22.

9. Ortolani C. Flow cytometry of hematological malignancies. West Sussex (United Kingdom): John Wiley & Sons; 2011.

10. Dunphy CH. Applications of flow cytometry and immunohistochemistry to diagnostic hematopathology. Arch Pathol Lab Med 2004;128:1004–22.

11. Awong G, Zuniga-Pflucker JC. Thymus-bound: the many features of T cell progenitors. Front Biosci (Schol Ed) 2011;3:961–9.

12. Rothenberg EV, Moore JE, Yui MA. Launching the T-cell-lineage developmental programme. Nat Rev Immunol 2008;8:9–21.

13. Wada H, Masuda K, Satoh R, et al. Adult T-cell progenitors retain myeloid potential. Nature 2008; 452:768–72.

14. Hao QL, George AA, Zhu J, et al. Human intrathymic lineage commitment is marked by differential CD7 expression: identification of CD7- lympho-myeloid thymic progenitors. Blood 2008;111:1318–26.

15. Weerkamp F, Baert MR, Brugman MH, et al. Human thymus contains multipotent progenitors with T/B lymphoid, myeloid, and erythroid lineage potential. Blood 2006;107:3131–7.

16. Bell JJ, Bhandoola A. The earliest thymic progenitors for T cells possess myeloid lineage potential. Nature 2008;452:764–7.

17. Czuczman MS, Dodge RK, Stewart CC, et al. Value of immunophenotype in intensively treated adult acute lymphoblastic leukemia: cancer and leukemia Group B study 8364. Blood 1999;93:3931–9.

18. Biagi C, Astolfi A, Masetti R, et al. Pediatric early T-cell precursor leukemia with NF1 deletion and high-sensitivity in vitro to tipifarnib. Leukemia 2010; 24:1230–3.

19. Zhang J, Ding L, Holmfeldt L, et al. The genetic basis of early T-cell precursor acute lymphoblastic leukaemia. Nature 2012;481:157–63.

20. Fielding AK, Banerjee L, Marks DI. Recent developments in the management of T-cell precursor acute lymphoblastic leukemia/lymphoma. Curr Hematol Malig Rep 2012;7:160–9.

21. Ma M, Wang X, Tang J, et al. Early T-cell precursor leukemia: a subtype of high risk childhood acute lymphoblastic leukemia. Front Med 2012; 6:416–20.

22. Inukai T, Kiyokawa N, Campana D, et al. Clinical significance of early T-cell precursor acute lymphoblastic leukaemia: results of the Tokyo Children's Cancer Study Group Study L99-15. Br J Haematol 2012;156:358–65.

23. Wood B, Winter S, Dunsmore K, et al. Patients with early T-Cell precursor (ETP) acute lymphoblastic leukemia (ALL) have high levels of minimal residual disease (MRD) at the end of induction–A Children's Oncology Group (COG) Study. ASH Annual Meeting Abstracts 2009;114:9.

24. Patel JL, Smith LM, Anderson J, et al. The immunophenotype of T-lymphoblastic lymphoma in children and adolescents: a Children's Oncology Group report. Br J Haematol 2012;159:454–61.

25. Neumann M, Heesch S, Gokbuget N, et al. Clinical and molecular characterization of early T-cell precursor leukemia: a high-risk subgroup in adult T-ALL with a high frequency of FLT3 mutations. Blood Cancer J 2012;2:e55.

26. Park S. Case study interpretation-Houston: case 3. Cytometry B Clin Cytom 2011;80B:261–3.

27. Yu S, Zhou X, Steinke FC, et al. The TCF-1 and LEF-1 transcription factors have cooperative and opposing roles in T cell development and malignancy. Immunity 2012;37:813–26.

28. Neumann M, Coskun E, Fransecky L, et al. FLT3 mutations in early T-cell precursor ALL characterize a stem cell like leukemia and imply the clinical use of tyrosine kinase inhibitors. PLoS One 2013;8: e53190.

29. Neumann M, Heesch S, Schlee C, et al. Whole-exome sequencing in adult ETP-ALL reveals

a high rate of DNMT3A mutations. Blood 2013;121: 4749–52.

30. Coskun E, Neumann M, Schlee C, et al. MicroRNA profiling reveals aberrant microRNA expression in adult ETP-ALL and functional studies implicate a role for miR-222 in acute leukemia. Leuk Res 2013; 37:647–56.

31. Dose M, Gounari F. Sleeping beauty: does ETP-ALL awaken later? Blood 2011;118:4500–1.

32. Gutierrez A, Dahlberg SE, Neuberg DS, et al. Absence of biallelic TCRgamma deletion predicts early treatment failure in pediatric T-cell acute lymphoblastic leukemia. J Clin Oncol 2010;28: 3816–23.

33. Hoehn D, Medeiros LJ, Chen SS, et al. CD117 expression is a sensitive but nonspecific predictor of FLT3 mutation in T acute lymphoblastic leukemia

and T/myeloid acute leukemia. Am J Clin Pathol 2012;137:213–9.

34. Zaremba CM, Oliver D, Cavalier M, et al. Distinct immunophenotype of early T-cell progenitors in T lymphoblastic leukemia/lymphoma may predict FMS-like tyrosine kinase 3 mutations. Ann Diagn Pathol 2012;16:16–20.

35. Borowitz MJ, Bene MC, Harris NL, et al. Acute leukaemias of ambiguous lineage. In: Swerdlow SH, Campo E, Harris NL, et al, editors. WHO classification of tumours of haematopoietic and lymphoid tissues. Lyon (France): IARC; 2008. p. 150–5.

36. Pui CH, Mullighan CG, Evans WE, et al. Pediatric acute lymphoblastic leukemia: where are we going and how do we get there? Blood 2012;120:1165–74.

37. Taub JW. Early T-cell precursor acute lymphoblastic leukaemia. Lancet Oncol 2009;10:105–6.

Myeloid Neoplasms with inv(3)(q21q26.2) or t(3;3)(q21;q26.2)

Heesun J. Rogers, MD, PhD*, Eric D. Hsi, MD

KEYWORDS

- Acute myeloid leukemia • Myelodysplastic syndrome • inv(3)(q21q26.2) • t(3;3)(q21;q26.2)
- Dysmegakaryopoiesis • Multilineage dysplasia • Dysregulated *EVI1*

KEY POINTS

- Acute myeloid leukemia (AML) with inv(3)(q21q26.2)/t(3;3)(q21;q26.2) [inv3/t(3;3)] is a distinct entity under the subgroup of AMLs with recurrent genetic abnormalities (RGAs) in the 2008 World Health Organization (WHO) classification.
- Myelodysplastic syndrome (MDS) with inv3/t(3;3) has a high risk of progression to AML.
- AML and MDS with inv3/t(3;3) have a similarly aggressive clinical course with short overall survival (OS) and are commonly refractory to therapy.
- Multilineage dysplasia is common.
- Characteristic small dysplastic megakaryocytes with nonlobated or bilobated nuclei are present in most inv3/t(3;3) patients.
- Dysregulation of *EVI1* plays an important role in stem cell self-renewal, leukemogenesis, and multilineage dysplasia and is associated with adverse prognosis.

ABSTRACT

Acute myeloid leukemia (AML) with inv(3)(q21q26.2)/t(3;3)(q21;q26.2) [inv3/t(3;3)] is a distinct entity under the subgroup of AMLs with recurrent genetic abnormalities in the 2008 World Health Organization classification. Myelodysplastic syndrome (MDS) with inv3/t(3;3) has a high risk of progression to AML. AML and MDS with inv3/t(3;3) have a similarly aggressive clinical course with short overall survival (OS) and are commonly refractory to therapy. In this article, clinical and pathologic features and prognosis in AML and MDS with inv3/t(3;3) are reviewed, and other myeloid neoplasms with similar dysplastic features to be differentiated from AML and MDS with inv3/t(3;3) are discussed.

OVERVIEW

Since 1976, rare cases of AML or preleukemia, with identical translocation of the long arm of chromosome 3 at band q26 and q21 have been reported. Those cases usually demonstrated thrombocytosis and atypical megakaryoctyes with small-size, monolobed or bilobed nuclei, and mature-appearing granular cytoplasm. These findings suggested a specific genetic alteration related to this translocation might play a role, at least in part, in the megakaryocytic proliferation or thrombocytosis.[1–4]

Today, AML with inv(3)(q21q26.2)/t(3;3)(q21;q26.2) [inv3/t(3;3)] is recognized as a rare aggressive myeloid neoplasm included as a distinct entity within AML with recurrent genetic

Conflict-of-Interest Disclosure: The authors declare no conflict of financial interests.

Robert J. Tomsich Pathology and Laboratory Medicine Institute, Cleveland Clinic, 9500 Euclid Avenue, Cleveland, OH 44195, USA

* Corresponding author. Robert J. Tomsich Pathology and Laboratory Medicine Institute, Cleveland Clinic, 9500 Euclid Avenue (L-11), Cleveland, OH 44195.

E-mail address: rogersj5@ccf.org

Surgical Pathology 6 (2013) 677–692
http://dx.doi.org/10.1016/j.path.2013.08.007
1875-9181/13/$ – see front matter © 2013 Elsevier Inc. All rights reserved.

Acronyms and Abbreviations: Myeloid neoplasms	
AML	Acute myeloid leukemia
APL	Acute promyelocytic leukemia
BM	Bone marrow
CML	Chronic myelogenous leukemia
EVI1	Ecotropic viral integration site 1
FISH	Fluorescence in situ hybridization
MDS	Myelodysplastic syndrome
MPNs	Myeloproliferative neoplasms
MRC	Myelodysplasia-related changes
OS	Overall survival
PB	Peripheral blood
RAEB	Refractory anemia with excess blasts
RCMD	Refractory cytopenia with multilineage dysplasia
RGA	Recurrent genetic abnormalities
RT-PCR	Reverse transcriptase–polymerase chain reaction
SNP	Single-nucleotide polymorphism

abnormalities (RGAs) in the 2008 WHO classification.[5] Although a subset of AML cases is recognized as AML regardless of the blast count, such as AML with t(8;21)(q22;q22), AML with inv(16) (p13.1q22) or t(16;16)(p13.1;q22) and acute promyelocytic leukemia (APL) with t(15;17) (q24.1;q21.1), inv3/t(3;3) is not considered this subtype.[5] MDS with inv3/t(3;3) is also recognized as aggressive disorder with a propensity to develop AML,[5–10] and this abnormality has been included as a high-risk genetic feature in a revision of a prognostic scoring system in MDS.[11,12]

Inv3/t(3;3) abnormalities result in aberrant expression of the oncogene ecotropic viral integration site 1 (EVI1). Chromosome 3q26.2 mapped for EVI1 and MDS1, and chromosome 3q21 mapped for ribophorin 1 (RPN1), GATA binding protein 2 (GATA2), and other genes.[7,8,13] EVI1/RPN1 fusion or a longer variant MDS1/EVI1 (also called MECOM) transcript by chimeric translocation leads to overexpression of EVI1 and/or GATA2. The breakpoint cluster regions of the RPN1 gene on chromosome 3q21 are known to play a role as an enhancer of EVI1 activation. The aberrant expression of the EVI1 gene is implicated in the pathogenesis of stem cell self-renewal leading to leukemogenesis, impairment of differentiation in erythroid and myeloid cells, and multilineage dysplasia.[6,8,14–17] The dysregulated EVI1 blocks endomitosis and impairs megakaryocytic differentiation, resulting in dysmegakaryopoiesis and characteristic small forms with mono/bilobated nuclei.[16,18] Clinically, it is associated with

an aggressive clinical course and poor therapeutic response in myeloid neoplasms.[19–21] This aberrant expression of EVI1 was noted in almost all inv3/t(3;3) AML and in 5% to 10% of de novo AML patients.[8,13,22]

The importance of EVI1 genetic alterations in leukemogensis has been shown in several transgenic mice experiments or implied in rare case reports after insertional activation of EVI1 during gene therapy.[14,23–28] Forced overexpression of EVI1 by transplantation or infection of bone marrow (BM) cells by an EVI1-containing retrovirus recapitulated myeloid hyperproliferation and down-regulation of genes related to myeloid differentiation, and resulted in features resembling MDS associated with progressive pancytopenia. Progression to AML is thought, however, to require additional genetic events by genomic instability. Recent murine models confirmed the concept of EVI1-induced leukemia with collaborating factors, such as CCAAT/enhancer-binding protein β, liver inhibitory protein, or mixed lineage leukemia. These mice showed dysplastic features in myeloid and erythroid cells, increased blasts, anemia, hepatosplenomegaly, and leukocytosis (in some of the mice) within 6 to 11 months after transplantation.[23–25]

Recent single-nucleotide polymorphism (SNP) microarray, sequencing, and fluorescence in situ hybridization (FISH) analyses have revealed

Pathology Key Features

1. Inv3/t(3;3) AML is a distinct entity under the group of AMLs with RGAs in the 2008 WHO classification.

2. Patients with inv3/t(3;3) MDS and AML have similarly aggressive clinical courses with poor OS.

3. The aberrant expression of the EVI1 gene is associated with leukemogenesis, impairment of differentiation in myeloid cells, and multilineage dysplasia.

4. Characteristic small dysplastic megakaryocytes with non/bilobated nuclei in almost all AML and MDS with inv3/t(3;3) is a useful clue.

5. Multilineage dysplasia is commonly present in inv3/t(3;3) AML and MDS.

6. Additional cytogenetic abnormalities including monosomy 7 are common in AML and MDS with inv3/t(3;3).

molecular heterogeneity of *EVI1* gene rearrangements.[13,15,19,20] In addition to several splicing variants of *EVI1*, other *EVI1* cryptic rearrangement, such as inv(3)(p24q26), t(3;21)(q26;q11) by *NRIP1-EVI1* fusion and der(7)t(3;7)(q26;q21) by *EVI1-CDK6* fusion, mediate a similar effect, leading to increased *EVI1* expression and adverse prognosis comparable to inv3/t(3;3).[13,20,21] Additional genetic abnormalities, such as *NRAS/KRAS*, *RUNX1*, *NF1*, or *FLT3*-ITD mutations, are identified in inv3/t(3;3) patients, more frequently in AML than MDS patients, and may associate with an even poorer outcome in this patient group.[29] In spite of molecular heterogeneity in inv3/t(3;3) and other *EVI1* rearrangements, however, a similarly poor survival in inv3/t(3;3) AML and MDS patients and progression to acute leukemia in more than half of inv3/t(3;3) MDS patients unifies these patients.[6,29]

CLINICAL FEATURES

According to earlier studies, the reported incidence of inv3/t(3;3) is approximately 1% to 2.5% of AML[5–7] and less than 1% in MDS.[11,12] The inv3/t(3;3) can occur rarely in other myeloid neoplasms, such as myeloproliferative neoplasms (MPNs), chronic myelomonocytic leukemia, and chronic or blast phase of chronic myelogenous leukemia (CML). This abnormality usually occurs in adults with no gender predilection. Their reported median ages are 48 to 56 years old in AML with inv3/t(3;3) patients and 62 to 67 years old in MDS with inv3/t(3;3) patients, which are slightly younger than the reported average age of adult AML (63 years old) and MDS (71 years old) in general.[5–8,11,12,30,31] It may present de novo, after therapy, or after history of MDS or other MPNs. Inv3/t(3;3) is extremely rare in childhood myeloid neoplasms.[32,33]

Inv3/t(3;3) patients typically present with anemia and normal or increased platelet counts. Thrombocytopenia can occur in less than 20% of inv3/t(3;3) patients, however. Some inv3/t(3;3) patients can develop hepatosplenomegaly, but lymphadenopathy is rare.[5] Leukocyte counts can be normal but can be slightly elevated. AML with inv3/t(3;3) patients with advanced age and high initial WBC counts are reported associated with poor clinical outcome.[7,34] MDS with inv3/t(3;3) share clinically similar features. Such cases have a poor prognosis with a short OS and high risk to progress to AML.[5–8]

DIAGNOSIS: MICROSCOPIC FEATURES

In addition to inv3/t(3;3) abnormality, the presence of 20% or more blasts in peripheral blood (PB) or BM is diagnostic of AML with inv3/t(3;3), and less than 20% blasts fell into the category of MDS with inv3/t(3;3). AML and MDS with inv3/t(3;3) share common morphologic features, however. Dysplastic features can be present in the PB smear and include dysgranulopoiesis with or without circulating blasts. Giant and/or hypogranular platelets are common. Rare circulating bare megakaryocyte nuclei can be present.[5]

Multilineage dysplasia is commonly present in the BM smear and can be present in more than half of AML and MDS with inv3/t(3;3) patients.[5,10,35] Megakaryocytes can be slightly increased in number and have atypical megakaryocytic morphology in almost all inv3/t(3;3) patients. Megakaryocytes demonstrate characteristically small forms with nonlobated or hypolobated nuclei, and other dysplastic features, such as multiple widely separated small nuclei or micromegakaryocytes, can be noted in the BM.[5,6,8,10] Examples of typical dysplastic megakaryocytes are shown in **Figs. 1** and **2**. Dyserythropoiesis and dysgranulopoiesis are also commonly present in inv3/t(3;3) patients[10,36] (shown in **Figs. 3** and **4**). Dyserythropoiesis includes irregular nuclearity, budding nuclei, multinuclearity, megaloblastoid changes, and ring sideroblasts. Dysgranulopoiesis includes nuclear hypolobation, hypersegmentation, cytoplasmic hypogranularity, and abnormal cytoplasmic granules. BM blasts can have morphologic features of any subtypes of AML except APL. BM blasts can show morphology of myeloblasts with or without differentiation, a mixture of myeloblasts and monoblasts, or megakaryoblasts. The BM cellularity is highly variable. Some cases may be hypocellular with myelofibrosis.[5,6,8] Megakaryocytes are normal to slightly increased in the BM core biopsy, and it may be difficult to recognize the characteristic small megakaryocytes with nonlobated or hypolobated nuclei on hematoxylin-eosin stain (**Fig. 5**A). Periodic acid–Schiff stain or immunohistochemistry specific for megakaryocytes, such as CD61, can often be helpful to recognize small megakaryocytes in the BM core biopsy (see **Fig. 5**B).

DIAGNOSIS: ANCILLARY STUDIES

Flow cytometry is an important diagnostic tool for characterizing the blasts in acute leukemia. Immunophenotypic analysis in AML with inv3/t(3;3), however, provides somewhat limited information. Blasts in inv3/t(3;3) demonstrate the immunophenotype of early myeloid cells, including CD13, CD33, CD117, and less commonly myeloperoxidase, and other uncommitted markers, such as

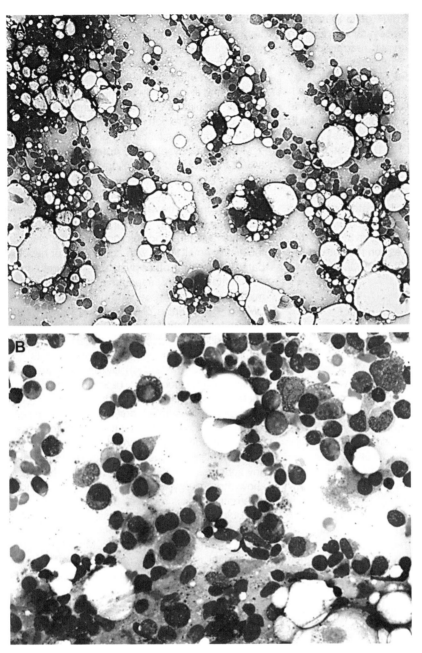

Fig. 1. Characteristic features of megakaryocytes in BM aspirate in inv3/t(3;3) patients. (*A;* Wright-Giemsa stain, ×20) MDS with inv3/t(3;3) and (*B;* Wright-Giemsa, ×40) AML with inv3/t(3;3) showing many small dysplastic megakaryocytes with nonlobated or bilobated nuclei in BM aspirate.

CD34, HLA-DR, CD38, and less commonly CD56. Some cases can have aberrant expression of CD7. Only a small subset expresses megakaryocytic markers, such as CD61 or CD41.[5,8,10,30]

Conventional cytogenetic evaluation of BM or PB is the gold standard for the diagnosis of inv3/t(3;3). Inv3/t(3;3) usually presents as the primary cytogenetic abnormality. Secondary cytogenetic abnormalities are reported, however, in 55% to 75% of inv3/t(3;3) patients.[7,8,22,37] The most common additional cytogenetic abnormality is monosomy 7, which is reported in 40% to 76% of AML with inv3/t(3;3) patients and associated with poor prognosis.[6,8,29,36] 5q Abnormalities or a complex karyotype can be identified in approximately one-third of the inv3/t(3;3) patients. Small numbers of inv3/t(3;3) patients may have t(9;22)(q34;q11.2)[t(9;22)]. CML patients may also

Fig. 2. Dysplastic mega-karyocytes in inv3/t(3;3) showing small megakaryocytes with nonlobated or bilobated nuclei and mature granular cytoplasm in BM aspirate at higher magnification (Wright-Giemsa stain, ×100).

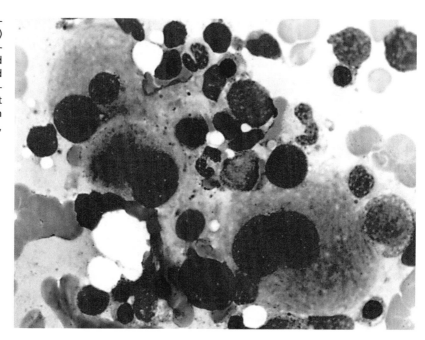

acquire the inv3/t(3;3) abnormality. Its clinical significance in CML is under evaluation; however, it is thought to be associated with progression to aggressive phase, such as accelerated or blast phase of the disease and worse prognosis.[36,38] Cases of t(9;22) and later acquiring inv3/t(3;3) abnormality are generally considered as aggressive phase of CML rather than AML with inv3/t(3;3). Inv3/t(3;3) patients can also have t(9;22) as secondary clonal evolution.[5] The late appearance of t(9;22) is very rare event in de novo or therapy-related AML and the appearance of t(9;22) has been closely associated with proliferation of leukemic blasts and an aggressive clinical course.[39] Although it is rare, the inv3/t(3;3) abnormality can occur as a secondary event as observed in a recent case report with MDS patients harboring monosomy 7.[6]

Fig. 3. Multilineage dysplasia in BM aspirate with MDS with inv3/t(3;3) showing significant dyserythropoiesis and dysgranulopoiesis (Wright-Giemsa stain, ×100).

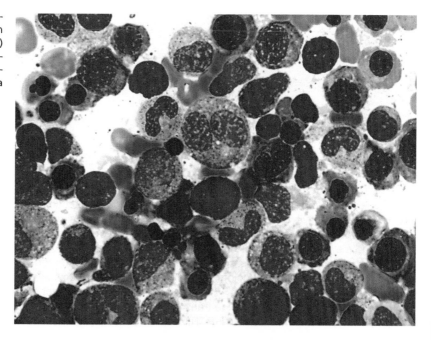

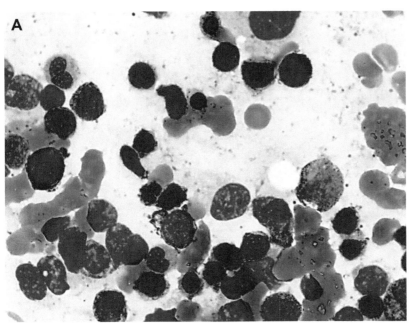

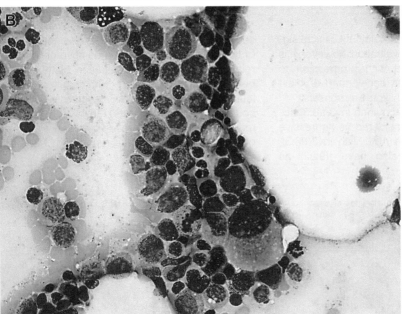

Fig. 4. (*A*; Wright-Giemsa stain, ×100) Prominent dyserythropoiesis, including irregular nuclei, multinucleation, and nuclear to cytoplasmic dyssynchrony, in BM aspirate of RAEB with inv3/t(3;3). (*B*; Wright-Giemsa stain, ×50) Prominent dysgranulopoiesis, including cytoplasmic hypogranularity and abnormal segmentation in BM aspirate of RAEB with inv3/t(3;3).

FISH analysis can be useful in the clinical laboratory with good sensitivity and specificity to detect the subtle appearance of inv3/t(3;3) and has rapid turnaround time without the need for cell culture. Interphase dual-color FISH allows coverage of a wide dispersion of 3q21 breakpoints, including *RPN1* locus, and 3q26, including *EVI1* locus involved in inv3/t(3;3). Although reverse transcriptase–polymerase chain reaction (RT-PCR) has difficulty detecting translocations due to the variability of breakpoints, FISH analysis has an advantage to detect wide heterogeneity of breakpoints, including cryptic rearrangements related to inv3/t(3;3).[40–42] Common additional cytogenetic abnormalities, which may suggest an additional negative prognostic impact, cannot be detected by FISH analysis. Molecular studies by RT-PCR or gene sequencing methods can detect overexpression

Fig. 5. BM core biopsy in AML with inv3/t(3;3). (*A*) Increased mononuclear cells with prominent nucleoli consistent with blasts and indistinct small megakaryocytes with hypolobated nuclei by hematoxylin-eosin stain (×20) and (*B*) numerous small megakaryocytes with non-lobated or hypolobated nuclei highlighted by CD61 immunohistochemistry (×20).

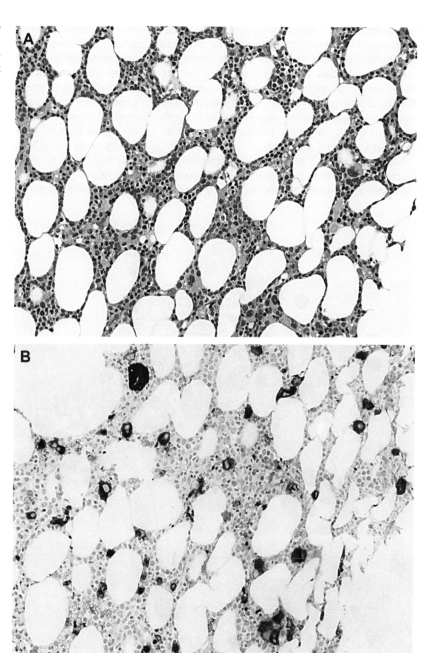

of EVI1 in this patient group; however, overexpression of EVI1 is not specific for inv3/t(3;3) because it can be identified in almost all inv3/t(3;3) AML and in 5% to 10% of de novo AML patients.[8,15,22]

SNP microarrays or comparative genomic hybridization arrays can be a potential complementary method with high-resolution to detect abnormalities that are not apparent by conventional karyotyping or cases that fail to culture subclones with the abnormalities. It can be useful to detect any additional cryptic deletions or duplication or

loss of alleles. Recent advance of technique shows an ability to detect balanced translocation in addition to unbalanced translocation.[38,43]

DIFFERENTIAL DIAGNOSIS

AML and MDS with inv3/t(3;3) have a similarly aggressive clinical course and share clinical and pathologic features. It is important to differentiate AML or MDS with inv3/t(3;3) patients, who have characteristically small dysplastic megakaryocytes, frequent multilineage dysplasia, and a dismal prognosis, from patients with similar pathologic features. The differential diagnosis includes MDS with isolated del(5q), AML with myelodysplasia-related changes (MRC), acute panmyelosis with myelofibrosis, acute megakaryoblastic leukemia, AML with t(1;22)(p13;q13), myeloid proliferations related to Down syndrome, and CML.

MDS with isolated del(5q) is characterized by macrocytic anemia and normal or increased platelets, commonly occurs in elderly women

and is known as an indolent disorder. The BM shows erythroid hypoplasia and megakaryocytic hyperplasia with small monolobated megakaryocytes that bear resemblance to those seen in the inv3/t(3;3) abnormality (Fig. 6). Dysgranulopoiesis is rare, however, in MDS with isolated del(5q) compared with common multilineage dysplasia in inv3/t(3;3).[44,45]

AML with inv3/t(3;3) abnormality and multilineage dysplasia is automatically included in AML with RGAs group in the 2008 WHO classification; however, AML with multilineage dysplasia and no

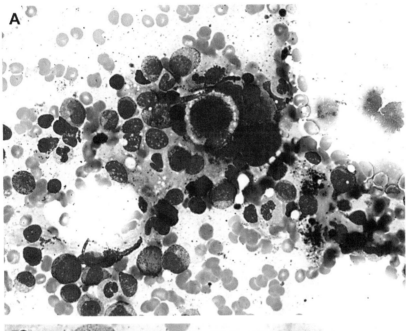

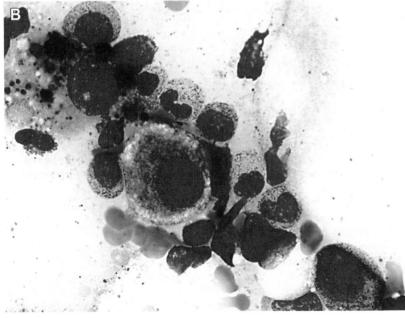

Fig. 6. (*A*; Wright-Giemsa stain, ×50, *B*; Wright-Giemsa stain, ×100) MDS with isolated del(5q) showing erythroid hypoplasia and megakaryocytic, hyperplasia with small megakaryocytes with nonlobated round nuclei in BM aspirate similar to the inv3/t(3;3) abnormality. Dysplasia in erythroid and granulocytic cells are rare, however, in MDS with isolated del(5q).

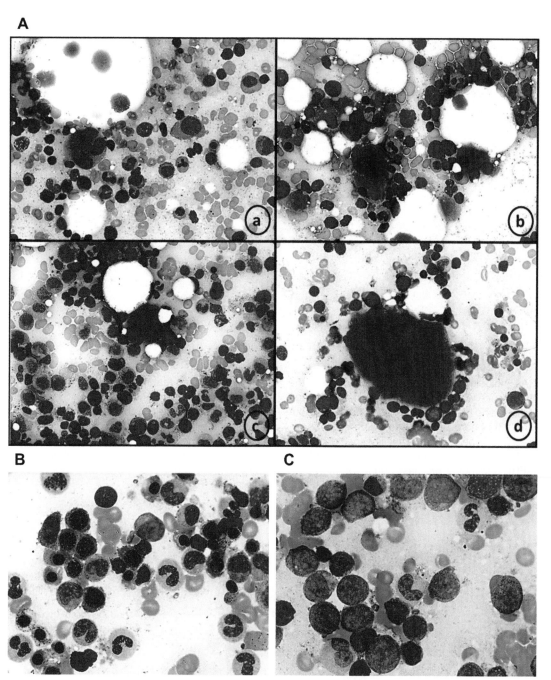

Fig. 7. (*A*; Wright-Giemsa stain, ×40) Various morphologic features of dysmegakaryopoiesis and multilineage dysplasia in BM aspirates. (a, b) RCMD showing small megakaryocytes with hypolobated nuclei or widely separate nuclei (pawn ball megakaryocytes) with dyserythropoiesis and dysgranulopoiesis. (c) RAEB showing small mega-karyocytes with hypolobated nuclei, dygranulopoiesis, and increased blasts. (d) AML-MRC showing large mega-karyocytes with abnormally lobated nuclei and increased blasts. (*B*; Wright-Giemsa stain, ×100) Significant dyserythropoiesis and dysgranulopoiesis in RCMD. (*C*) Increased myeloblasts and dysgranulopoiesis in AML-MRC (Wright-Giemsa stain, ×100).

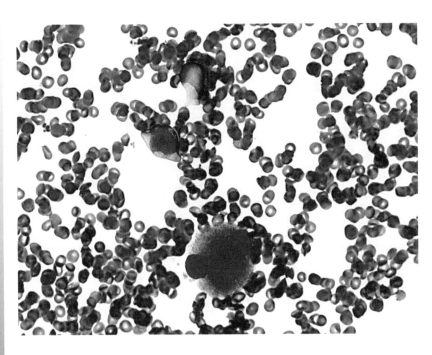

Fig. 8. Acute megakaryoblastic leukemia showing a small megakaryocyte with bilobated nuclei and megakaryoblasts in BM aspirate (Wright-Giemsa stain, ×100).

RGAs, including inv3/t(3;3) abnormality, falls in the category of AML-MRC. Also, cases of multilineage dysplasia and blasts less than 20% with or without inv3/t(3;3) abnormality fall into MDS, such as refractory cytopenia with multilineage dysplasia (RCMD) or refractory anemia with excess blasts (RAEB), depending on blast count. Small megakaryocytes with nonlobated or hypolobated nuclei are characteristic features in inv3/t(3;3) abnormality patients; however, AML-MRC, RCMD, or RAEB with other cytogenetic abnormalities can show significant bilineage or trilineage dysplasia with variable dysmegakaryocytic features, such as small to large megakaryocytes with hypolobated to hyperlobated nuclei or completely widely separate nuclei (**Fig. 7**).

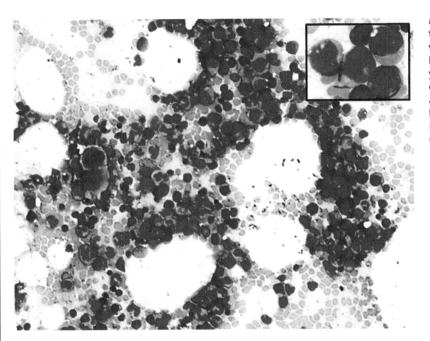

Fig. 9. Myeloproliferative disorder associated with Down syndrome. Dysplastic small megakaryocytes with nonlobated or hypolobated nuclei and increased megakaryoblasts (*highlighted in inset*) in BM aspirate (Wright-Giemsa stain, ×40).

Acute panmyelosis with myelofibrosis is an aggressive disorder with only a few months' survival and typically presents with abrupt fever, bone pain, and pancytopenia. The BM shows hypercellularity with acute panmyeloid proliferation, increased blasts (at least 20% by definition), and marked reticulin fibrosis. Megakaryocytes are typically dysplastic and show predominantly small forms with eosinophilic cytoplasm and nonlobated or hypolobated nuclei or micromegakaryocytes but are present with admixed immature granulocytic and erythroid elements (panmyelosis). Blasts are CD34 positive. Significant dysplasia in other cell lines is usually minimal and if prominent suggest AML-MRC. Acute megakaryoblastic leukemia show increased megakaryoblasts with cytoplasmic blebs (as opposed to CD34-positive myeloblasts), maturing dysplastic megakaryocytes, and fibrosis in BM (**Fig. 8**).[46,47]

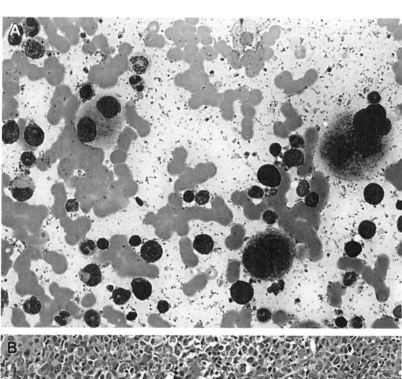
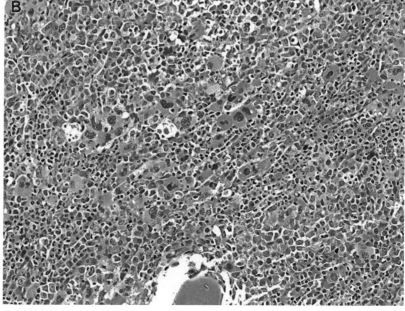

Fig. 10. CML in chronic phase. (*A*) Small megakaryocytes with hypolobated or nonlobated nuclei and left-shifted granulocytic hyperplasia in BM aspirate (Wright-Giemsa stain, ×50). (*B*) Hypercellular marrow with left-shifted granulocytic and megakaryocytic hyperplasia, and many small megakaryocytes with hypolobated or nonlobated nuclei in BM core biopsy (H&E stain, ×40).

AML with t(1;22)(p13;q13) is included in one of subtypes of AML with RGAs in the 2008 WHO classification. It typically occurs in infants or young children (younger than 3 years old) without Down syndrome. The BM shows similar morphologic findings to acute megakaryoblastic leukemia, including poorly differentiated blasts; megakaryoblasts; dysplastic megakaryocytes, such as atypical small to large megakaryocytes with nonlobated to hypolobated nuclei; and fibrosis. Dyserythropoiesis and dysgranulopoiesis are not typically present.[5]

Myeloid proliferations related to Down syndrome occur in young children with trisomy 21. They include various clinical entities, including transient abnormal myelopoiesis and AML, including acute megakaryoblastic leukemia in approximately half of AML patients in Down syndrome. In this entity, blasts with various stages of differentiation and dysmegakaryopoiesis, including small hypolobated or monolobated nuclei, are present (**Fig. 9**). Dyserythropoiesis and dysgranulopoiesis are rare, however.[5,48]

CML, *BCR-ABL1* positive, in chronic phase typically has hypercellularity, granulocytic hyperplasia, left shift in granulocytic maturation, and usually small megakaryocytes with hypolobated nuclei (dwarf megakaryocytes) in BM. Many of the CML patients have megakaryocytic proliferation and reticulin fibrosis. Small hypolobated megakaryocytes with myeloproliferative features, but no dysplastic features in erythroid or granulocytic features, in addition to presence of t(9;22), are diagnostic of CML (**Fig. 10**).

Differential Diagnosis

AML and MDS with inv3/t(3;3) Abnormality vs	Helpful Distinguishing Features
AML-MRC	Multilineage dysplasia with various morphology of dysplastic megakaryocytes, greater than 20% blasts, and no inv3/t(3;3) abnormality
RCMD or RAEB without inv3/t(3;3)	Similar morphology to AML-MRC but blasts less than 20%
MDS with isolated del(5q)	Macrocytic anemia in elderly women, erythroid hypoplasia, and megakaryocytic hyperplasia with small nonlobated megakaryocytes
Acute panmyelosis with myelofibrosis	Characteristic clinical features with abrupt fever, bone pain and pancytopenia, and hypercellular marrow with panmyeloid proliferation, increased blasts, reticulin fibrosis, and dysplastic megakaryocytes
Acute megakaryoblastic leukemia	Increased megakaryoblasts, dysmegakaryopoiesis, and fibrosis. Flow cytometry or immunohistochemistry with megakaryocytic markers is helpful
AML with t(1;22)(p13;q13)	Subtype of AMLs with RGAs in the WHO classification, typically young children without Down syndrome, and morphologically similar to acute megakaryoblastic leukemia
Myeloid proliferations related to Down syndrome	Young children with Down syndrome, various clinical entities and blasts with various stages of differentiation and dysmegakaryopoiesis, including small hypolobated or nonlobated nuclei
CML, *BCR-ABL1* positive	Hypercellular marrow with left-shifted granulocytic hyperplasia and small megakaryocytes, often megakaryocytic hyperplasia and t(9;22)(q34;q11.2)

PROGNOSIS

Inv3/t(3;3) is an aggressive disorder with short OS.[7–10] The revised International Prognostic Scoring System includes a comprehensive cytogenetic subgrouping to better define prognostic impact in MDS patients. In this system, inv3/t(3;3); monosomy 7; double abnormalities, including monosomy 7/del(7q); and complex karyotype with 3 abnormalities are automatically assigned as poor-risk cytogenetic subgroup with score 3, with an expected survival of 1.5 years and median time to 25% AML evolution of 1.7 years.[11,12] Approximately 55% to 65% of MDS with inv3/t(3;3) patients were reported to progress to AML.[6,7,10]

In AML with inv3/t(3;3), advanced age (older than 60 years) and high initial WBC are associated with poor clinical outcome.[34] Some studies report, however, that BM blast percentage or diagnosis as MDS or AML did not show significant differences in clinical outcome in inv3/t(3;3) patients.[6,11,34] In recent studies, the median OS was 13.0 to 17.5 months in MDS with inv3/t(3;3) patients and 9.6 to 13.8 months in AML with inv3/t(3;3) patients. Their OS was 33% at 1 year and 23% at 2 years and dropped to 3% at 5 years.[6,8,34] In a

multicenter study of 63 AML and 40 MDS with inv3/t(3;3) patients, the authors found a similarly short OS and no significant difference in OS between MDS and AML with inv3/t(3;3) (12.9 vs 7.9 months, $P = .149$ log rank) (Fig. 11). Greater than 80% of patients expired with a median follow-up of 7.9 months.[35] The similarly poor prognosis of AML and MDS patients from other studies suggests inv3/t(3;3) might be best considered as one of subtypes of AML with RGAs irrespective of blast count in the WHO classification.[6,29,35]

Some studies mention that inv3/t(3;3) alone predicts a dismal prognosis and OS seems not to be affected by additional cytogenetic abnormalities including monosomy 7 or complex karyotype.[6,10,12] Inv3/t(3;3) and additional monosomy 7 or complex karyotype are believed, however, to have an additional negative prognostic impact.[7,35,48] The authors have shown that complex karyotype or monosomal karyotype are independent prognostic risk factors, and inv3/t(3;3) patients with complex karyotype or monosomal karyotype had significantly shorter median OS than those without those karyotypic abnormalities (4.5 vs 11 months, $P<.001$ log rank, and 6 vs 11 months, $P = .002$ log rank, respectively).[35] Recent molecular studies in inv3/t(3;3) revealed *FLT3* internal tandem duplication,

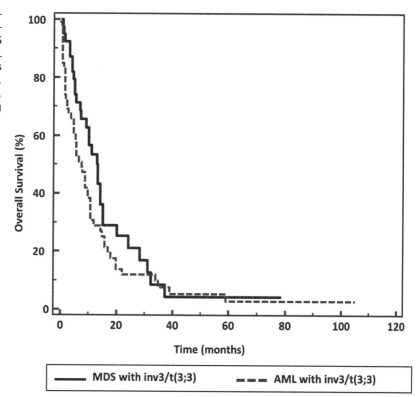

Fig. 11. Kaplan-Meier survival curve showing no significant difference in OS between MDS and AML with inv3/t(3;3) patients (N = 40, 12.9 months, and N = 63, 7.9 months, respectively; $P = .149$ log rank).

Pitfalls

! Establishing an accurate diagnosis is challenging in this rare disorder. Thorough morphologic evaluation, however, including characteristic dysmegakaryopoiesis and blast count and cytogenetic analysis, are required for the diagnosis.

! Small megakaryocytes with non/bilobated nuclei and multilineage dysplasia can be observed in other myeloid neoplasms. Cytogenetic abnormality confirms the diagnosis.

! AML with multilineage dysplasia and no inv3/ t(3;3) is diagnosed as AML-MRC, and MDS with inv3/t(3;3) is diagnosed as RCMD or RAEB, depending on the blast counts in the WHO classification.

! AML and MDS with inv3/t(3;3) need to be differentiated from other myeloid neoplasms with a similar dysplastic morphology because of their dismal prognosis with short survival and propensity to develop AML.

NRAS, EVI1 overexpression, or disproportionate EVI1 and MDS1/EVI1 expression is associated with unfavorable prognosis.[7,34] The clinical outcome related to these molecular findings needs to be confirmed, however. Inv3/t(3;3) is commonly refractory to conventional chemotherapy.[7,10,49] Inv3/t(3;3) patients who received allogeneic hematopoietic stem cell transplant showed, however, longer OS than patients who received chemotherapy alone in some studies.[8,34]

REFERENCES

1. Rowley JD, Potter D. Chromosomal banding patterns in acute leukemia. Blood 1976;47(5):705–22.

2. Golomb HM, Vardiman J, Rowley JD. Acute nonlymphocytic leukemia in adults: correlations with Q-banded chromosomes. Blood 1976;48(1):9–21.

3. Sweet DL, Golomb HM, Rowley JD, et al. Acute myelogenous leukemia and thrombocythemia associated with an abnormality of chromosome No. 3. Cancer Genet Cytogenet 1979;1:33–7.

4. Carroll AJ, Poon MC, Robinson NC, et al. Sideroblastic anemia associated with thrombocytosis and a chromosome 3 abnormality. Cancer Genet Cytogenet 1986;22:183–7.

5. Arber DA, Vardiman JW, Brunning RD, et al. Acute myeloid leukaemia with inv(3)(q21q26.2) or t(3;3)(q21;q26.2). In: Swerdlow SH, Campo E, Harris NL, et al, editors. WHO classification of tumours of haematopoietic and lymphoid tissues. 4th edition. Lyon (France): IARC Press; 2008. p. 110–8.

6. Cui W, Sun J, Cotta CV, et al. Myelodysplastic syndrome with inv(3)(q21q26.2) or t(3;3)(q21;q26.2) has a high risk for progression to acute myeoid leukemia. Am J Clin Pathol 2011;136(2):282–8.

7. Lugthart S, Groschel S, Beverloo HB, et al. Clinical, molecular, and prognostic significance of WHO type inv(3)(q21q26.2)/t(3;3)(q21;q26.2) and various other 3q abnormalities in acute myeloid leukemia. J Clin Oncol 2010;28(24):3890–8.

8. Sun J, Konoplev SN, Wang X, et al. De novo acute myeloid leukemia with inv(3)(q21q26.2) or t(3;3)(q21;q26.2): a clinicopathologic and cytogenetic study of an entity recently added to the WHO classification. Mod Pathol 2011;24(3):384–9.

9. Estey EH. Acute myeloid leukemia: 2012 update on diagnosis, risk stratification, and management. Am J Hematol 2012;87(1):89–99.

10. Shi G, Weh HJ, Diihrsen U, et al. Chromosomal abnormality inv(3)(q21q26) associated with multilineage hematopoietic progenitor cells in hematopoietic malignancies. Cancer Genet Cytogenet 1997; 96(1):58–63.

11. Schanz J, Tüchler H, Solé F, et al. New comprehensive cytogenetic scoring system for primary myelodysplastic syndromes (MDS) and oligoblastic acute myeloid leukemia after MDS derived from an international database merge. J Clin Oncol 2012; 30(8):820–9.

12. Greenberg PL, Tuechler H, Schanz J, et al. Revised international prognostic scoring system for myelodysplastic syndromes. Blood 2012;120(12): 2454–65.

13. Haferlach C, Bacher U, Grossmann V, et al. Three novel cytogenetically cryptic EVI1 rearrangements associated with increased EVI1 expression and poor prognosis identified in 27 acute myeloid leukemia cases. Genes Chromosomes Cancer 2012;51: 1079–85.

14. Kataoka K, Kurokawa M. Ecotropic viral integration site 1, stem cell self-renewal and leukemogenesis. Cancer Sci 2012;103(8):1371–7.

15. Martinelli G, Ottaviani E, Buonamici S, et al. Association of 3q21q26 syndrome with different RPN1/EVI1 fusion transcripts. Haematologica 2003;88(11): 1221–8.

16. Bitter MA, Neilly ME, Le Beau MM, et al. Rearrangements of chromosome 3 involving bands 3q21 and 3q26 are associated with normal or elevated platelet counts in acute nonlymphocytic leukemia. Blood 1985;66(6):1362–70.

17. Laricchia-Robbio L, Nucifora G. Significant increase of self-renewal in hematopoietic cells after forced expression of EVI1. Blood Cells Mol Dis 2008; 40(2):141–7.

18. Kilbey A, Alzuherri H, McColl J, et al. The EVI1 proto-oncoprotein blocks endomitosis in megakaryocytes by inhibiting sustained cyclin-dependent kinase 2 catalytic activity. Br J Haematol 2005;130(6):902–11.

19. Rockova V, Abbas S, Wouters BJ, et al. Risk stratification of intermediate-risk acute myeloid leukemia: integrative analysis of a multitude of gene mutation and gene expression markers. Blood 2011;118(4):1069–76.

20. Lahortiga I, Vázquez I, Agirre X, et al. Molecular heterogeneity in AML/MDS patients with 3q21q26 rearrangements. Genes Chromosomes Cancer 2004;40(3):179–89.

21. Wieser R. The oncogene and developmental regulator EVI1: expression, biochemical properties, and biological functions. Gene 2007;396(2):346–57.

22. Testoni N, Borsaru G, Martinelli G, et al. 3q21 and 3q26 cytogenetic abnormalities in acute myeloblastic leukemia: biological and clinical features. Haematologica 1999;84(8):690–4.

23. Watanabe-Okochi N, Yoshimi A, Sato I, et al. The shortest isoform of C/EBPβ, liver inhibitory protein (LIP), collaborates with Evi1 to induce AML in a mouse BMT model. Blood 2013;121(20):4142–55.

24. Goyama S, Kurokawa M. Evi-1 as a critical regulator of leukemic cells. Int J Hematol 2010;91(5):753–7.

25. Bindels EM, Havermans K, Lugthart S, et al. EVI1 is critical for the pathogenesis of a subset of MLL-AF9-rearranged AMLs. Blood 2012;119(24):5838–49.

26. Konrad TA, Karger A, Hackl H, et al. Inducible expression of EVI1 in human myeloid cells causes phenotypes consistent with its role in myelodysplastic syndromes. J Leukoc Biol 2009;86(4):813–22.

27. Buonamici S, Li D, Chi Y, et al. EVI1 induces myelodysplastic syndrome in mice. J Clin Invest 2004;114(5):713–9.

28. Stein S, Ott MG, Schultze-Strasser S, et al. Genomic instability and myelodysplasia with monosomy 7 consequent to EVI1 activation after gene therapy for chronic granulomatous disease. Nat Med 2010;16(2):198–204.

29. Haferlach C, Bacher U, Haferlach T, et al. The inv(3)(q21q26)/t(3;3)(q21;q26) is frequently accompanied by alterations of the RUNX1, KRAS and NRAS and NF1 genes and mediates adverse prognosis both in MDS and in AML: a study in 39 cases of MDS or AML. Leukemia 2011;25(5):874–7.

30. Medeiros BC, Kohrt HE, Arber DA. Immunophenotypic features of acute myeloid leukemia with inv(3)(q21q26.2)/t(3;3)(q21;q26.2). Leuk Res 2010;34(5):594–7.

31. Barxi A, Sekeres NA. Myelodysplastic syndromes: a practical approach to diagnosis and treatment. Cleve Clin J Med 2010;77:37–44.

32. Harrison CJ, Hills RK, Moorman AV, et al. Cytogenetics of childhood acute myeloid leukemia: United Kingdom Medical Research Council Treatment trials AML 10 and 12. J Clin Oncol 2010;28(16):2674–81.

33. Davis KL, Marina N, Arber DA, et al. Pediatric acute myeloid leukemia as classified using 2008 WHO Criteria: a single-center experience. Am J Clin Pathol 2013;139(6):818–25.

34. Weisser M, Haferlach C, Haferlach T, et al. Advanced age and high initial WBC influence the outcome of inv(3) (q21q26)/t(3;3) (q21;q26) positive AML. Leuk Lymphoma 2007;48(11):2145–51.

35. Rogers HJ, Vardiman JW, Anastasi J, et al. Complex karyotype but not blast percentage is associated with poor survival in acute myeloid leukemia and myelodysplastic syndrome with inv(3)(q21q26.2)/t(3;3)(q21;q26.2). Mod Pathol 2013;26(S2):358A.

36. Brunning RD, Orazi A, Germing U, et al. Myelodysplastic syndromes/neoplasms, overview. In: Swerdlow SH, Campo E, Harris NL, et al, editors. WHO classification of tumours of haematopoietic and lymphoid tissues. 4th edition. Lyon (France): IARC Press; 2008. p. 88–93.

37. Secker-Walker LM, Mehta A, Bain B. Abnormalities of 3q21 and 3q26 in myeloid malignancy: a United Kingdom Cancer Cytogenetic Group study. Br J Haematol 1995;91(2):490–501.

38. Toydemir R, Rowe L, Hibbard M, et al. Cytogenetic and molecular characterization of double inversion associated with a cryptic BCR-ABL1 rearrangement and additional genetic changes. Cancer Genet Cytogenet 2010;201(2):81–7.

39. Yagyu S, Morimoto A, Kakazu N, et al. Late appearance of a Philadelphia chromosome in a patient with therapy-related acute myeloid leukemia and high expression of EVI1. Cancer Genet Cytogenet 2008;180(2):115–20.

40. Braekeleer ED, Douet-Guilbert N, Basinko A, et al. Conventional cytogenetics and breakpoint distribution by fluorescent in situ hybridization in patients with malignant hemopathies associated with inv(3)(q21q26.2) or t(3;3)(q21;q26.2). Anticancer Res 2011;31:3441–8.

41. Shearer BM, Sukov WR, Flynn HC, et al. Development of a dual-color, double fusion FISH assay to detect RPN1/EVI1 gene fusion associated with inv(3), t(3;3), and ins(3;3) in patients with myelodysplasia and acute myeloid leukemia. Am J Hematol 2010;85(8):569–74.

42. Madrigal I, Carrió A, Gómez C, et al. Fluorescence in situ hybridization studies using BAC clones of the EVI1 locus in hematological malignancies with 3q rearrangements. Cancer Genet Cytogenet 2006;170(2):115–20.

43. Gruver AM, Rogers HJ, Cook JR, et al. Modified array-based comparative genomic hybridization detects cryptic and variant PML-RARA rearrangements in acute promyelocytic leukemia lacking

classic translocations. Diagn Mol Pathol 2013;22(1):10–21.

44. Hasserjuan RP, Le Beau MM, List AF, et al. Myelodysplastic syndrome with isolated del(5q). In: Swerdlow SH, Campo E, Harris NL, et al, editors. WHO classification of tumours of haematopoietic and lymphoid tissues. 4th edition. Lyon (France): IARC Press; 2008. p. 102.

45. Patnaik MM, Lasho TL, Finke CM. Isolated del(5q) in myeloid malignancies: clinicopathologic and molecular features in 143 consecutive patients. Am J Hematol 2011;86(5):393–8.

46. Grygalewicz B, Woroniecka R, pastwinska A, et al. Acute panmyelosis with myelofibrosis with EVI1 amplification. Cancer Genet 2012;205(5):255–60.

47. Arber DA, Brunning RD, Orazi A, et al. Acute myeloid leukaemia, not otherwise specified. In: Swerdlow SH, Campo E, Harris NL, et al, editors. WHO classification of tumours of haematopoietic and lymphoid tissues. 4th edition. Lyon (France): IARC Press; 2008. p. 130–9.

48. Hama A, Yagasaki H, Takahashi Y, et al. Acute megakaryoblastic leukaemia (AMKL) in children: a comparison of AMKL with and without Down syndrome. Br J Haematol 2008;140(5):552–61.

49. Reiter E, Greinix H, Rabitsch W, et al. Low curative potential of bone marrow transplantation for highly aggressive acute myelogenous leukemia with inversioin inv (3)(q21q26) or homologous translocation t(3;3) (q21;q26). Ann Hematol 2000;79(7):374–7.

Update on Myelodysplastic Syndromes Classification and Prognosis

Dita Gratzinger, MD, PhD[a],*, Peter L. Greenberg, MD[b]

KEYWORDS

- Myelodysplastic syndromes (MDS) • Cytogenetics • Dysplasia • Cytopenia
- Idiopathic cytopenia of uncertain significance (ICUS)

KEY POINTS

- MDS is a collection of cytogenetically heterogeneous clonal BM failure disorders derived from aberrant hematopoietic stem cells in the setting of an aberrant hematopoietic stem cell niche.
- The 2008 WHO classification of MDS incorporates peripheral blood and bone marrow morphologic findings, blast percentage, cytogenetics, and history of chemotherapy/radiation.
- Benign mimics of MDS include vitamin/micronutrient deficiencies, infections, drugs/toxins, autoimmune/rheumatologic disease and congenital syndromes.
- The Revised International Prognostic Scoring System (IPSS-R) incorporates a new blast count threshold of 2% in the marrow, necessitating careful quantification of blast counts below 5%.

ABSTRACT

Myelodysplastic syndromes (MDS) are a collection of cytogenetically heterogeneous clonal bone marrow (BM) failure disorders derived from aberrant hematopoietic stem cells in the setting of an aberrant hematopoietic stem cell niche. Patients suffer from variably progressive and symptomatic bone marrow failure with a risk of leukemic transformation. Diagnosis of MDS has long been based on morphologic assessment and blast percentage as in the original French-American-British classification. The recently developed Revised International Prognostic Scoring System provides improved prognostication using more refined cytogenetic, marrow blast, and cytopenia parameters. With the advent of deep sequencing technologies, dozens of molecular abnormalities have been identified in MDS.

OVERVIEW

MDS is an umbrella term for a clinically and cytogenetically heterogeneous collection of clonal BM failure disorders. The pathophysiology of MDS is shaped by its clonal origin from aberrant hematopoietic stem cells[1] in the setting of an aberrant hematopoietic stem cell niche.[2] Patients with MDS can have a relatively stable clinical course, may suffer from the complications of refractory cytopenias, or may develop acute myeloid leukemia. MDS is diagnosed in more than 10,000 patients a year in the United States and fewer than 50% of patients with MDS are alive 3 years from diagnosis. More than 80% of patients with MDS are over 60 years old at diagnosis, and their cytopenias and transfusion dependence interact with other age-related comorbidities to increase both patient morbidity and mortality[3] and at significant cost to the U.S. health care system.[4] Diagnosis of MDS has long been based on morphologic assessment and blast percentage as in the original French-American-British (FAB) classification.[5] More recently, refined histology and cytogenetic abnormalities have been added to the diagnostic algorithm in the world health organization (WHO) diagnostic schema,[6,7] although diagnosis remains problematic in patients with borderline morphologic abnormalities and normal

Disclosure Statement: The authors have nothing to disclose.
a Department of Pathology, Stanford University Medical Center, 300 Pasteur Drive, L235, Stanford, CA 94305, USA;
b Hematology Division, Stanford University Medical Center, 875 Blake Wilbur Drive, Stanford, CA 94305, USA
* Corresponding author.
E-mail address: ditag@stanford.edu

Surgical Pathology 6 (2013) 693–728
http://dx.doi.org/10.1016/j.path.2013.08.005
1875-9181/13/$ – see front matter © 2013 Elsevier Inc. All rights reserved.

surgpath.theclinics.com

Acronyms and Abbreviations for MDS

ALIP	Abnormal localization of immature precursors
AML	Acute myeloid leukemia
AML-MRC	AML with myelodysplasia-related changes
ANC	Absolute neutrophil count
BM	Bone marrow
CGH	Comparative genomic hybridization
CMML	Chronic myelomonocytic leukemia
del	Deletion
FAB	French-American-British (classification scheme preceding WHO)
FISH	Fluorescence in situ hybridization
G-CSF	Granulocyte colony stimulation factor
GM-CSF	Granulocyte-macrophage colony-stimulating factor
Hg	Hemoglobin
HHV	Human herpesvirus
HIV	Human immunodeficiency virus
ICUS	Idiopathic cytopenias of uncertain significance
IDUS	Idiopathic dysplasia of uncertain significance
IPSS	International Prognostic Scoring System
IPSS-R	Revised IPSS
IWG-PM	International Working Group for Prognosis in MDS
IWGM-MDS	International Working Group on Morphology of Myelodysplastic Syndrome
LDH	Lactate dehydrogenase
MDS	Myelodysplastic syndrome
MDS-U	MDS, unclassified
MMF	Mycophenolate mofetil
MonoMAC	Monocytopenia with Mycobacterium Avium Complex susceptibility
NCCN	National Comprehensive Cancer Network
NK	Natural killer
PB	Peripheral blood
RA	Refractory anemia
RAEB	RA with excess blasts
RAEB-T	RAEB in transformation
RARS	RA with ring sideroblasts
RCC	Refractory cytopenia of childhood
RN	Refractory neutropenia
RS	Ring sideroblasts
RT	Refractory thrombocytopenia
SM-AHNMD	Systemic mastocytosis with associated clonal hematologic non–mast cell lineage disease
SNP	Single-nucleotide polymorphism
WHO	World health organization

cytogenetics. With the advent of deep sequencing technologies, dozens of molecular abnormalities have been identified in MDS,[8] and a subset of these may soon become part of the standard clinicopathologic evaluation in known or suspected MDS.

GROSS FEATURES

MDS are diagnosed exclusively based on features of the peripheral blood (PB) and BM. Gross diagnosis is not applicable.

MICROSCOPIC FEATURES OF MDS

Examination of a high-quality PB smear and BM aspirate smear, iron stain, and core biopsy are crucial for accurate determination of blast count and morphologic dysplasi, as well as to identify or exclude alternate causes of cytopenias, such as hemolysis or lymphoproliferative disorders.

Red blood cell abnormalities include anemia, oval macrocytes, and poikilocytosis (Fig. 1A).

Fig. 1. Red blood cell findings in MDS. (*A*) Oval macrocytes, which can assume teardrop shapes, and bizarre poikilocytes (Wright-Giemsa stain, original magnification ×100). (*B*) Dimorphic red blood cells, including normochromic red cells admixed with hypochromic microcytes are often seen in sideroblastic anemias, including myelodysplastic syndromes with RS. In this case, hypogranular platelets are also present (Wright-Giemsa stain, original magnification ×100).

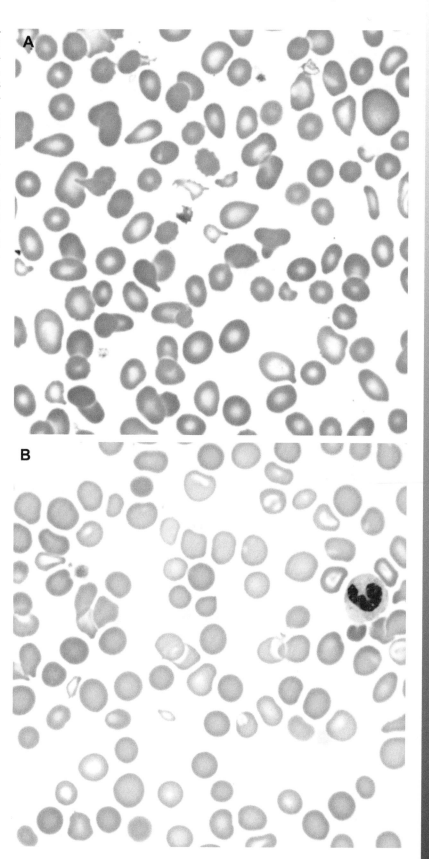

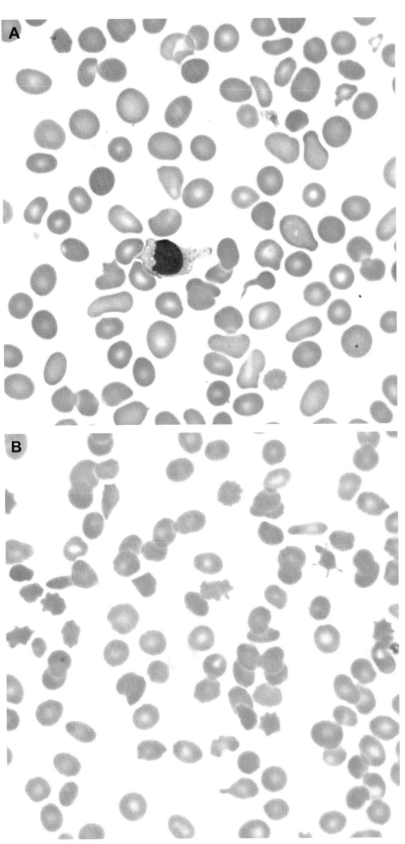

Fig. 2. Red blood cell findings in mimics of MDS. (*A*) The combination of spherocytes and polychromasia seen here should raise the possibility of autoimmune hemolysis; large granular lymphocytes may be seen in reactive settings as well as in association with MDS or other malignancy (Wright-Giemsa stain, original magnification ×100). (*B*) Alternate causes of red cell poikilocytosis should be considered, such as liver disease, in this case with numerous acanthocytes (Wright-Giemsa stain, original magnification ×100).

Fig. 3. Erythroid maturation abnormalities. (*A*)
Megaloblastoid erythroid
maturation is seen with
marked erythroid left-shift;
megalobastoid proerythro-
blasts are abnormally large
with immature chromatin
that can mimic myeloblasts
(Wright-Giemsa stain, original magnification ×100).
(*B*) The nuclear:cytoplasmic
dyssynchrony of megalo-
blastoid maturation is recognized by the combination
of hemoglobinized cyto-
plasm with uncondensed
blocky chromatin (Wright-
Giemsa stain, original magnification ×100).

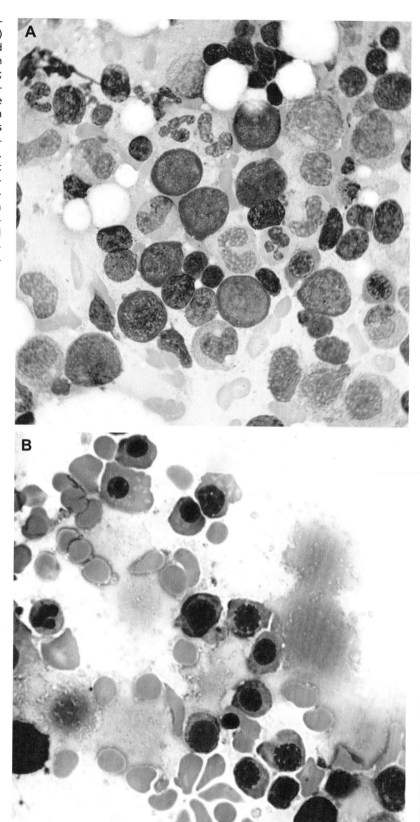

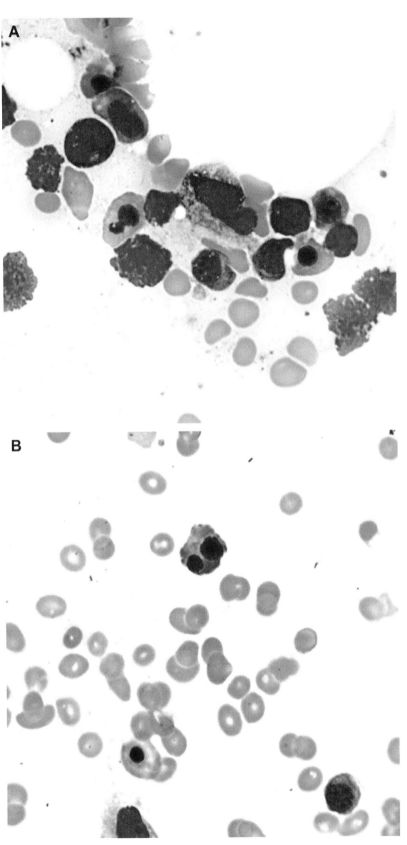

Fig. 4. Nuclear abnormalities in dyserythropoiesis. (A) Irregularities of nuclear shape, such as nuclear budding or fragmentation, are common features of dyserythropoiesis (Wright-Giemsa stain, original magnification ×100). (B) Although occasional binucleate forms can be seen in brisk erythropoiesis of any cause, unequal binucleation is seen in dyserythropoiesis (Wright-Giemsa stain, original magnification ×100).

Fig. 5. Iron staining to assess storage iron and RS. (A) Patients who are transfusion dependent or with ineffective erythropoiesis may show abundant stainable iron within marrow histiocytes (Perl's iron stain, original magnification ×40). (B) Perls iron stain also reveals numerous RS; erythroid nuclei are recognized by their dark red counterstain and perfectly round contour (×100).

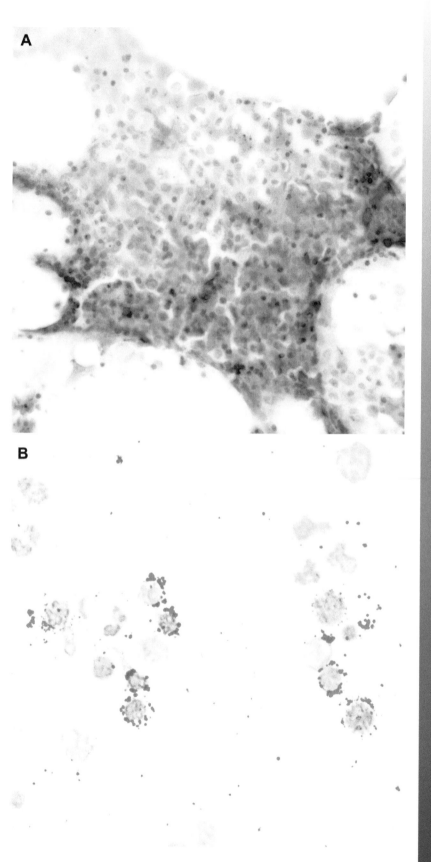

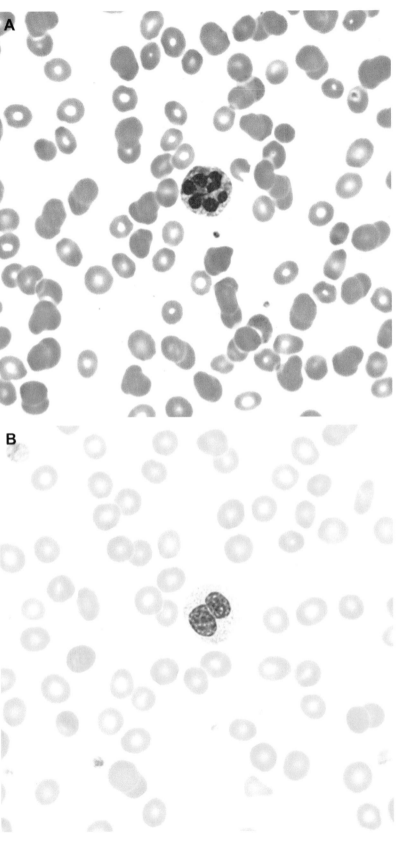

Fig. 6. Abnormalities of neutrophil segmentation. (A) Hypersegmented neutrophils (with 6 or more lobes) can be a sign of myelodysplasia or other causes of megaloblastic maturation (Wright-Giemsa stain, original magnification ×100). (B) Hypolobated, or pelgeroid, neutrophils are recognized not only by their nuclear shape but also by the exaggerated checkerboard pattern of their chromatin (Wright-Giemsa stain, original magnification ×100).

Fig. 7. Neutrophil cytoplasmic abnormalities. Hypogranular neutrophils can be a sign of dysplasia; it is good practice to find an internal positive control to exclude understaining as the cause (Wright-Giemsa stain, original magnification ×100).

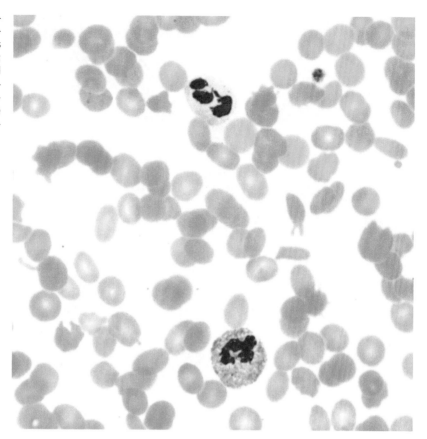

Dimorphic red blood cells, typically a mixture of normochromic normocytic or macrocytic forms and hypochromic microcytes, are seen in sideroblastic anemias (see **Fig. 1**B). Some red cell abnormalities may be clues to alternate etiologies of cytopenia, such as autoimmune hemolysis or liver disease (**Fig. 2**). BM erythroid lineage abnormalities commonly include erythroid hyperplasia with megaloblastoid maturation (**Fig. 3**); nuclear abnormalities, including binucleation, nuclear membrane irregularities, or budding; and cytoplasmic vacuolization (**Fig. 4**). Iron staining commonly reveals increased iron within histiocytes and on occasion also shows ring sideroblasts (RS), defined as 5 or more iron granules encircling one-third or more of the nucleus (**Fig. 5**).[9]

Dysgranulopoiesis may be most easily identified in the PB. Nuclear hypolobation (pseudo–Pelger-Huët anomaly, 1 to 2 round lobes with abnormally chunky chromatin) or hypersegmentation are frequent findings (**Fig. 6**). Cytoplasmic hypogranularity should be carefully distinguished from pale staining; usually a subset of neutrophils has normal cytoplasmic granularity as an internal positive control (**Fig. 7**). Similar findings may be seen in the marrow aspirate (**Fig. 8**). Cytoplasmic inclusions, such as Döhle bodies or abnormal granulation, may be present. Blasts generally have high nuclear/cytoplasmic ratios, visible nucleoli, fine nuclear chromatin, and lack a höf (**Figs. 9–11**).[9]

Evaluation for dysmegakaryopoiesis also begins in the PB, where giant (larger than a red blood cell) and bizarre, irregularly shaped platelets may be noted (**Fig. 12**). Whereas normal platelets are stippled with small purple granules, hypogranular platelets appear clear to pale blue and may be missed if not actively sought. BM megakaryocyte abnormalities include aberrant nucleation, often in the form of multiple round nuclei; nuclear hypolobation, typically in small megakaryocytes; and micromegakaryocytes, which should be sought at high power (**Fig. 13**).

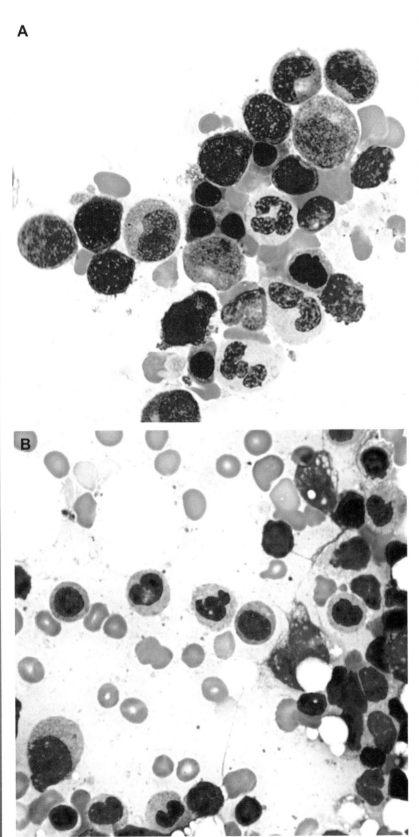

Fig. 8. Evaluation of the myeloid lineage in the BM aspirate. Dysplastic features of neutrophils easily seen in the PB may also be noted in the BM aspirate on careful inspection: (A; Wright-Giemsa stain, original magnification ×100) hypogranularity and (B; Wright-Giemsa stain, original magnification ×100) hyposegmentation/pelgeroid forms.

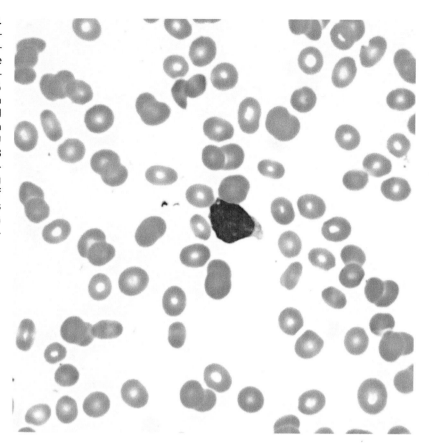

Fig. 9. Circulating blasts. The slide should be carefully scanned for circulating blasts; if any are present, careful enumeration is necessary—1% circulating blasts, even in the absence of increased BM blasts, necessitate a WHO diagnosis of MDS-U per the WHO 2008 criteria, and rare circulating blasts exceeding 1% merit a diagnosis of RA with excess blasts (RAEB) (Wright-Giemsa stain, original magnification ×100).

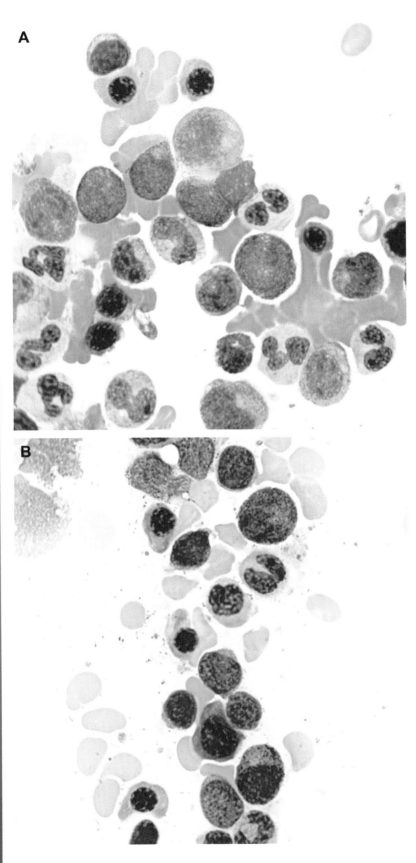

Fig. 10. Blast enumeration in the BM aspirate. (*A*; Wright-Giemsa stain, original magnification ×100) Enumeration of BM blasts should be performed in spiculate areas and only include intact forms. (*B*; Wright-Giemsa stain, original magnification ×100) Blasts in MDS may be small and ovoid; care must be taken not to pass over these as lymphocytes or hematogones (normal B-cell precursors).

Fig. 11. Pitfalls in blast enumeration in the BM. (*A*) In patients who have recently received G-CSF, there may be numerous promyelocytes, which can be distinguished from blasts by their granular cytoplasm and prominent höf (Wright-Giemsa stain, original magnification ×100). (*B*) Proerythroblasts have very round nuclei, dark cytoplasm, and small pale Golgi zones; the admixed blasts have slightly less round nuclei (Wright-Giemsa stain, original magnification ×100).

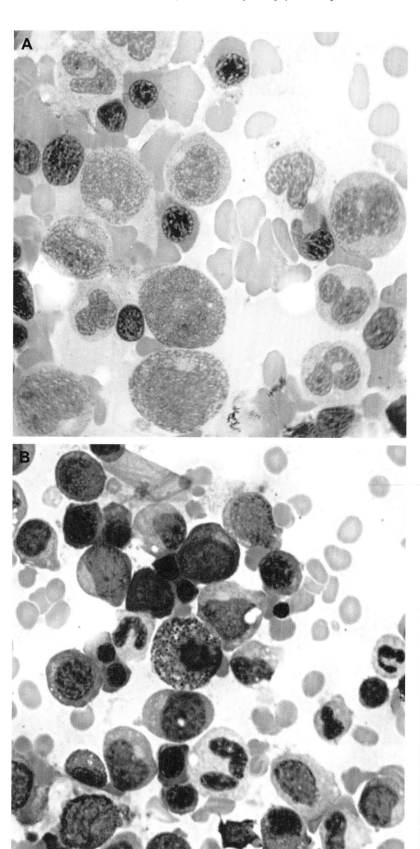

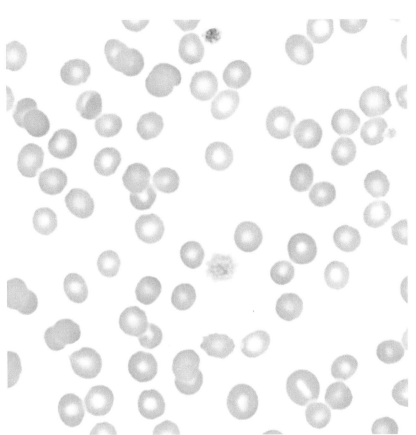

Fig. 12. Platelet abnormalities. Giant hypogranular platelets are as large or larger than red blood cells; their pale blue cytoplasm can blend in to the background of the slide so they should be actively sought (Wright-Giemsa stain, original magnification ×100).

Fig. 13. Megakaryocyte lineage abnormalities. (*A*) Multinucleated megakaryocytes are easily identified; their cytoplasm may share the hypogranular tinctorial quality of hypogranular platelets (Wright-Giemsa stain, original magnification ×100). (*B*) Monolobated micromegakaryocytes can be missed from low power (Wright-Giemsa stain, original magnification ×100).

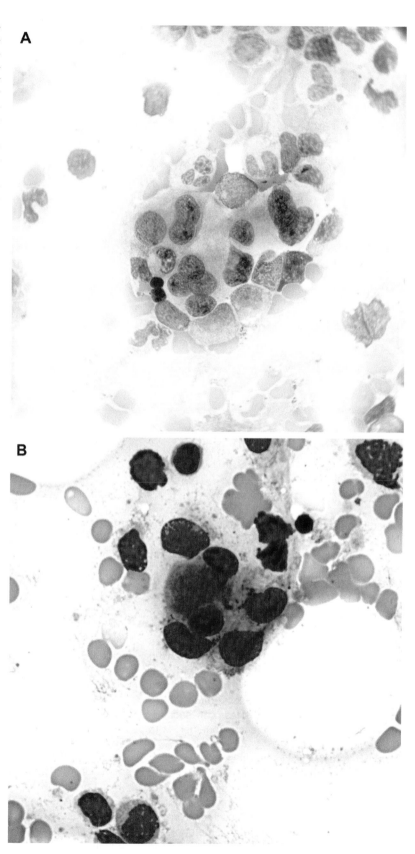

C

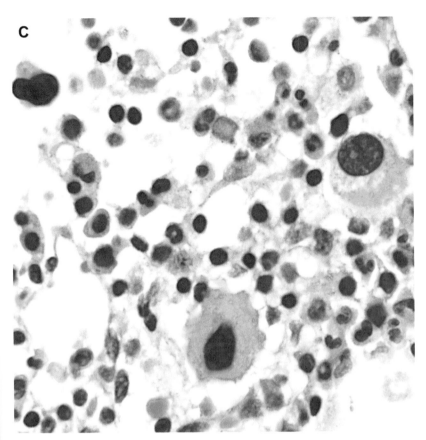

Fig. 13. (continued). Megakaryocyte lineage abnormalities. (C) The characteristic hypolobated megakaryocytes of MDS with isolated deletion of 5q can be appreciated on the core biopsy specimen (Haematoxylin & eosin stain, original magnification ×100).

DIFFERENTIAL DIAGNOSIS OF MDS

The differential diagnosis of MDS includes nutritional or infectious causes, drug or toxin effect, autoimmune/rheumatologic conditions, and congenital disorders (see **Differential Diagnosis box** and **Pitfalls box**).[10]

Vitamin B$_{12}$/folate deficiency induces megaloblastic maturation; in severe cases, sheets of megaloblastoid proerythroblasts can histologically mimic acute leukemia. Copper deficiency causes anemia and neutropenia with a characteristic constellation of vacuolization of erythroid and myeloid precursors, myeloid left shift, increased iron stores, and RS.[11] Zinc excess, often due to zinc-containing denture adhesives, can secondarily induce copper deficiency together with neurologic symptoms.[12]

Human immunodeficiency virus (HIV) infection can cause marked dysplasia,[13] including budding of erythroid nuclei and bizarre megakaryocyte nuclei (**Fig. 14**). Parvovirus B19 infects erythroid precursors, causing symptomatic anemia in patients with underlying inefficient hematopoiesis/ hemolysis. Occasionally, parvovirus B19 can cause bicytopenia or pancytopenia, associated with erythroid hypoplasia, giant pronormoblasts, and dyspoietic features.[14] Human herpesvirus (HHV)-6 can cause transient cytopenias and multilineage dysplasia in immunocompetent children.[15] Nonviral causes, such as visceral leishmaniasis, are also reported.[16]

Alcohol is a BM toxin that can induce megaloblastic erythroid maturation and RS.[17] The post-chemotherapy marrow frequently shows mild dyspoiesis, including megaloblastic maturation, mild erythroid nuclear budding, and occasional multinucleate megakaryocytes (**Fig. 15A**). GM-CSF can induce nuclear fragmentation or macro-polycytosis in neutrophils.[18] Several medications, most frequently mycophenolate mofetil,[19] produce a reversible pseudo–Pelger-Huët anomaly (see **Fig. 15B**). Valproic acid can cause cytopenias and megakaryocyte dysplasia in children,[20] mimicking the refractory cytopenia of childhood (RCC) type of MDS.

Systemic lupus erythematosus is well known to cause a reversible multilineage dysplasia (**Fig. 16**).[21] Autoimmune conditions, especially autoimmune hemolytic anemia and systemic

Differential Diagnosis
OF MYELODYSPLASTIC SYNDROMES

Differentials

Vitamin/micronutrient deficiencies	Vitamin B_{12}/folate, copper
Infections	HIV, parvovirus, visceral leishmaniasis
Toxins	Ethanol, heavy metals, zinc-induced copper deficiency
Drug effect	Chemotherapeutic agents/folate antagonists (megaloblastoid change), valproic acid, mycophenolate mofetil/ganciclovir (pelgeroid), isoniazid/chloramphenicol (RS)
Autoimmune/rheumatologic	Systemic lupus erythematosus, rheumatoid arthritis/felty syndrome
Congenital	Ineffective erythropoiesis or increased turnover due to thalassemias, hemoglobinopathies, glucose-6-phosphate dehydrogenase deficiency, hereditary spherocytosis

More frequent in children/young adults

Aplastic anemia	Must be differentiated from commonly hypocellular refractory cytopenia of childhood
Down syndrome	Myeloid proliferations related to Down syndrome
Inherited BM failure syndromes	Fanconi anemia, dyskeratosis congenita, Diamond-Blackfan anemia, Shwachman-Diamond syndrome, Pearson syndrome, congenital neutropenia/cyclic neutropenia, monocytopenia immunodeficiency (MonoMac) syndrome
Congenital anemias	Congenital dyserythropoietic anemias, congenital sideroblastic anemias
Infectious	HHV-6

Pitfalls
IN MDS

Non-neoplastic mimics of myelodysplasia

! Some ethnic groups, including several groups of African and Middle Eastern origin, may have absolute neutrophil count (ANC) <1.8 × 10^9/L under normal conditions[68]

! HIV dyspoiesis

! Megaloblastic anemia

! Copper deficiency

! Medication-induced pseudo–Pelger-Huët

Difficult-to-diagnose MDS

! MDS with fibrosis

! Hypoplastic MDS

Neoplastic mimics of MDS

! Oligoblastic acute myeloid leukemia (AML) with a recurring cytogenetic abnormality (eg, t[8;21] [q22;q22])

! Cytogenetic lesion due to separate hematolymphoid neoplasm (eg, deletion [del][13q] or del[11q] due to chronic lymphocytic leukemia)

! Morphologically subtle nonmyeloid neoplastic causes of cytopenia: hairy cell leukemia, T-cell large granular lymphocyte leukemia

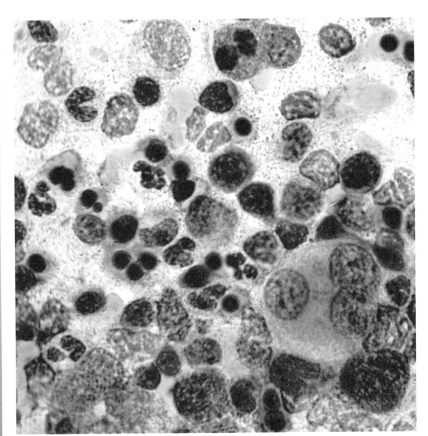

Fig. *14.* HIV-associated dysplasia. Marked multilineage dysplasia is present; multinucleated megakaryocytes dyserythropoiesis with nuclear budding are prominent (Wright-Giemsa stain, original magnification ×100).

vasculitis, are linked to an increased risk of myeloid neoplasia.[22] Brisk erythroid turnover of any cause— whether autoimmune, drug associated, or after chemotherapy—can be associated with dyserythropoiesis, such as binucleation or nuclear budding, so extreme care must be taken in rendering a diagnosis of myelodysplasia in this setting.

Congenital causes of cytopenias and dysplasia can present in adults as well as children. Inherited BM failure syndromes may involve a single lineage (Diamond-Blackfan anemia, severe congenital neutropenia, and congenital amegakaryocytic thrombocytopenia) or present with mixed cytopenias (Fanconi anemia [**Fig. 17**], dyskeratosis congenita, Shwachman-Diamond syndrome, or Pearson syndrome [**Fig. 18**]).[23] Fanconi anemia, dyskeratosis congenita,[24] and severe congenital neutropenia[25] carry a high risk of eventual MDS (**Fig. 19**) or AML. A more recently identified entity, monocytopenia immunodeficiency (MonoMac) syndrome (**Fig. 20**) presents with an unusual constellation of mycobacterial infections, monocytopenia, natural killer lymphocytopenia and B lymphocytopenia, and frequent progression to MDS/AML.[26] The MDS in these cases is frequently hypocellular with fibrosis.[27] Congenital sideroblastic anemias,[28] although rare, are important to recognize because some are responsive to dietary supplementation (pyridoxine or thiamine); younger age and microcytosis are diagnostic clues.[29] Congenital dyserythropoietic anemias present with marked erythroid hyperplasia and characteristic binucleated or multinucleated erythroblasts.[30]

Given the nonspecific nature of morphologic dyspoiesis, other neoplastic causes of chronic slowly evolving cytopenias must also be actively sought. Hairy cell leukemia and T-cell large granular lymphocyte leukemia (**Fig. 21**) are morphologically subtle neoplasms that are regularly discovered during BM evaluation for possible MDS.

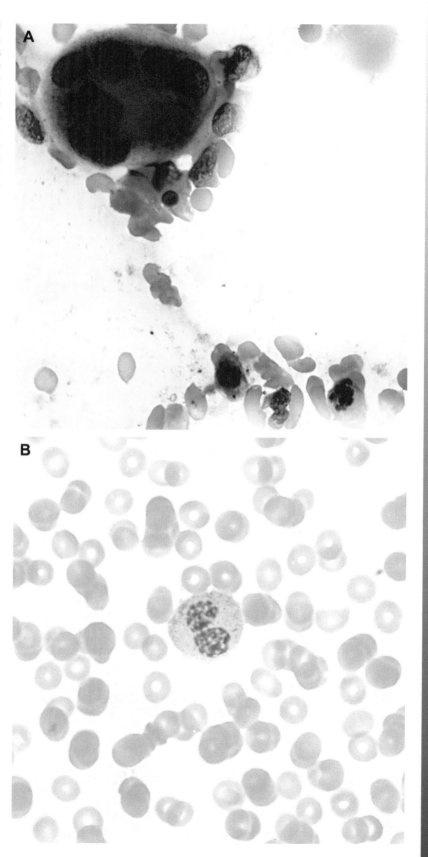

Fig. 15. Medication-induced dysplasia. (*A*) Common postchemotherapy changes include megakaryocyte multinucleation and dyserythropoiesis. (*B*) Pelgeroid change, characterized by hypolobation with an exaggerated chromatin clumping pattern, in neutrophils in a stem cell transplant patient treated with Mycophenolate mofetil (Wright-Giemsa stain, original magnification ×100).

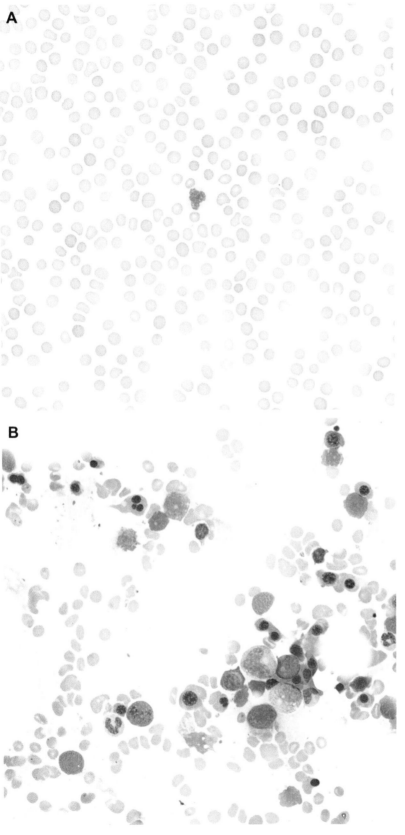

Fig. 16. Systemic lupus erythematosus-associated dysplasia. (*A*) Marked cytopenias with circulating hypogranular neutrophils (Wright-Giemsa stain, original magnification ×40). (*B*) The BM aspirate shows marked dyserythropoiesis with prominent nuclear budding (Wright-Giemsa stain, original magnification ×40).

Fig. 17. Fanconi anemia. (*A*) Mild nonspecific dyspoiesis may be seen in the BM aspirate (Wright-Giemsa stain, original magnification ×40). (*B*) The marrow is significantly hypocellular for age (Haematoxylin & eosin stain, original magnification ×40).

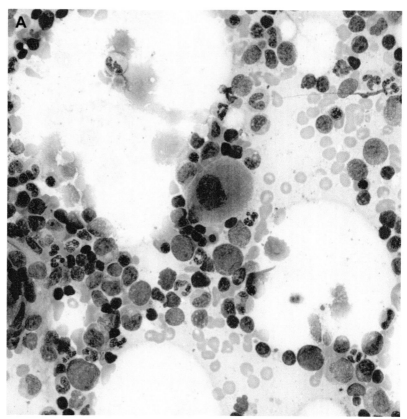

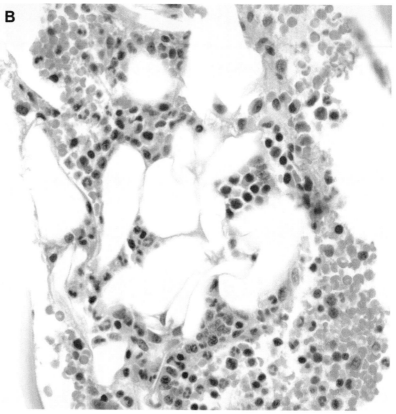

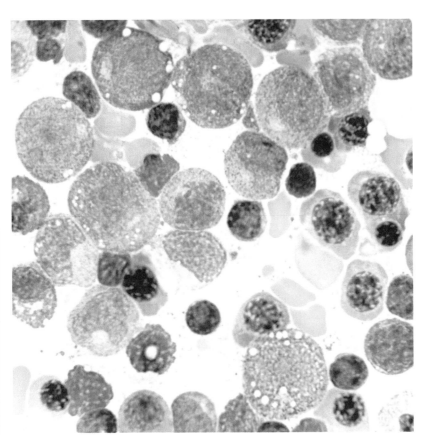

Fig. 18. Pearson syndrome. Cytoplasmic vacuolization is seen in both erythroid and myeloid precursors. Similar findings can also be seen in copper deficiency/zinc excess (Wright-Giemsa stain, original magnification ×100).

Fig. 19. Fanconi anemia with progression to a MDS. (*A*) In contrast to the mild nonspecific abnormalities seen at baseline, marked multilineage dysplasia is readily appreciated here. Note the monolobated micromegakaryocytes with hypogranular cytoplasm and numerous hypogranular neutrophils (Wright-Giemsa stain, original magnification ×40). (*B*) The marrow is now hypercellular rather than depleted as at baseline. The small dysplastic megakaryocytes are readily identified (Haematoxylin & eosin stain original magnification ×40).

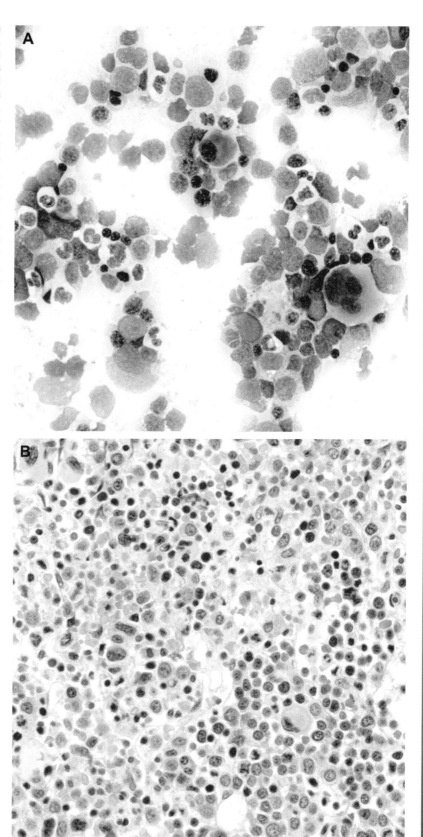

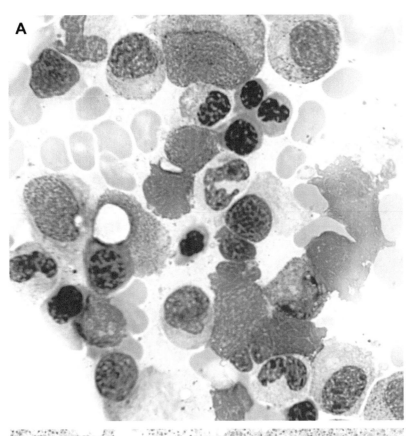

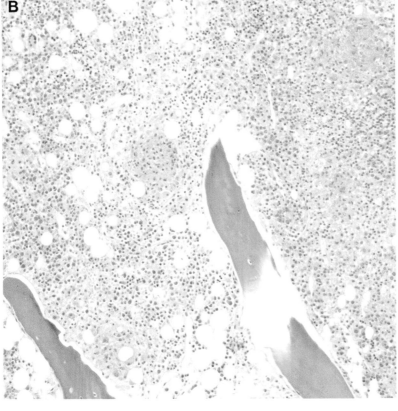

Fig. 20. MonoMac syndrome: this patient presented with monocytopenia, B lymphopenia and natural killer lymphopenia, and a mycobacterial infection. (*A*) Prominent dyserythropoiesis is present in the BM aspirate. Maturing myeloid precursors also show mildly aberrant segmentation (Wright-Giemsa stain, original magnification ×100). (*B*) Numerous granulomas seen on the BM core biopsy should prompt an evaluation for mycobacterial, fungal, or other infection (Haematoxylin & eosin stain, original magnification ×20).

Fig. 21. T cell large granular lymphocyte leukemia. T-cell large granular lymphocyte leukemia can be a morphologically subtle process presenting with cytopenias, particularly neutropenia. (*A*) Circulating large granular lymphocytes do not always have abundant cytoplasm, and granularity can be subtle as in this case (Wright-Giemsa stain, original magnification ×40). (*B*) On routine stains, bone marrow core biopsy involvement is very difficult to detect (Haematoxylin & eosin stain original magnification ×40).

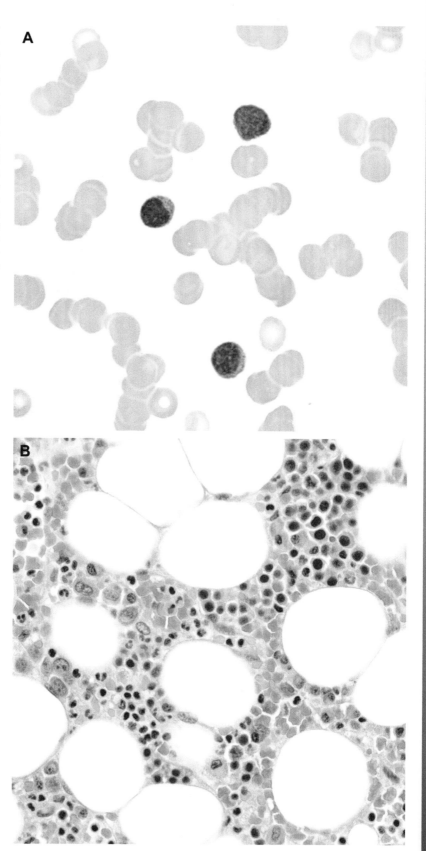

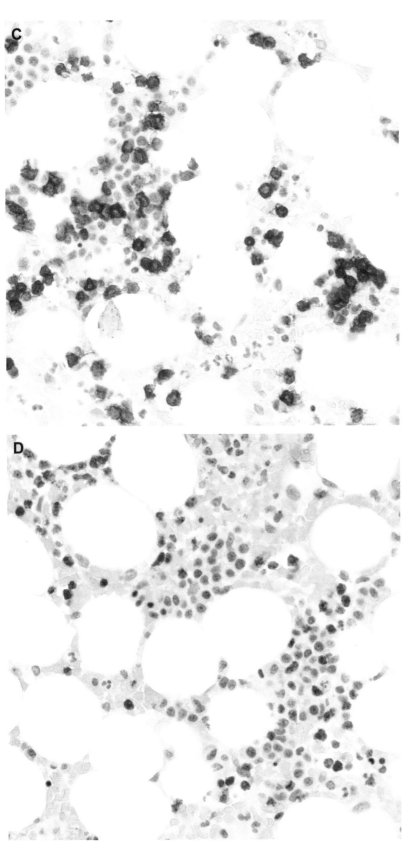

Fig. 21. (continued). T cell large granular lymphocyte leukemia. (*C* & *D*; Immunohistochemistry with diaminobenzidine chromogen and haematoxylin counterstain, ×40) Characteristic immunohistochemical findings of T-cell large granular lymphocyte leukemia[70] include clusters and linear arrays of CD8+ (*C*) granzyme+ (*D*) cytotoxic T cells.

DIAGNOSIS OF MDS

Minimal criteria for diagnosis of MDS were elucidated by the International Working Group on Morphology of Myelodysplastic Syndrome (IWGM-MDS) in 2006[31] and are largely reflected in the 2008 WHO criteria (**Table 1**).[6,7] These consist of a combination of clinical, morphologic, and cytogenetic findings (see **Pathologic Key Features Box**). Otherwise unexplained cytopenias must be present at least 6 months. Dysplasia is assessed in the erythroid, megakaryocytic, and myeloid lineages and must be present in at least 10% of that lineage. A marrow blast count of at least 500 cells, including at least 100 nonerythroid cells, has been proposed; in the PB, if any circulating blasts are seen on scan, a count of at least 500 nucleated cells is also recommended.[9] The presence of Auer rods automatically raises the category to RAEB-2 even at low blast counts.[32] Classical cytogenetics consists of the karyotypic analysis of at least 20 cultured BM mononuclear cells at metaphase for chromosomal abnormalities. Particular cytogenetic abnormalities, such as loss of the long arm of chromosome 7 or 5, are diagnostic of myelodysplastic syndromes even in cytopenic patients without overt morphologic dysplasia. In rare cases, cytogenetic studies may reveal a category-defining cytogenetic abnormality, such as t(8;21)(q22;q22) (**Fig. 22**). Fluorescence in situ hybridization (FISH) can identify selected abnormalities in a sensitive manner[33] (200 compared with 20 cells analyzed) but cannot identify nontargeted abnormalities. In patients for whom karyotyping is unsuccessful or suboptimal,

FISH for a panel of MDS-related abnormalities identifies unrecognized cytogenetic abnormalities in 14% to 20%.[34] If a BM aspirate is unavailable, PB is suitable for FISH for known cytogenetic abnormalities.[35]

Ancillary studies may be helpful in both rendering and accurately stratifying an MDS diagnosis. Blasts may be underrepresented in BM aspirates due to uneven distribution or fibrosis. Reticulin and trichrome stains should be graded using consensus criteria for fibrosis[36]; severe fibrosis may identify a clinically distinct subgroup of MDS.[37] In these cases, immunohistochemistry for CD34 may be helpful in estimating a blast count and identifying CD34+ blast cell clusters (**Fig. 23**).[38] Immunohistochemistry is also useful in the diagnosis of RCC; dysplastic micromegakaryocytes are highlighted by immunohistochemistry for a megakaryocyte marker, such as CD61 (**Fig. 24**).[39,40] Flow cytometry may be a helpful adjunct in MDS diagnosis thanks to abnormalities, such as decreased granulocyte side scatter, abnormal myeloid antigen acquisition, abnormal progenitor immunophenotype,[41] and decreased hematogones.[42] The complexity of flow cytometric criteria for dysplasia has limited their widespread use; simple reproducible criteria have been proposed.[43]

The WHO 2008 classification shows moderate reproducibility,[44] underlining the necessity of expert review.[45] Even among healthy stem cell donors, mild morphologic dysplasia is frequent.[46] Conversely, low-grade MDS can show subtle dyspoiesis and cannot be excluded on the basis of a normal karyotype, because more than half of cases of low-grade MDS show no abnormalities on standard cytogenetic analysis.[47] Recognizing the spectrum of unexplained cytopenias not meeting minimal morphologic/cytogenetic criteria for MDS, the IWGM-MDS has proposed a provisional category, idiopathic cytopenias of uncertain significance (ICUS),[48] for this group. Sophisticated approaches to identification of small genomic changes and uniparental disomy through array-based technologies, such as single-nucleotide polymorphism and comparative genomic hybridization arrays,[49] as well as deep sequencing approaches[8] may soon provide increased sensitivity and specificity in MDS diagnosis.

PROGNOSIS OF MDS

The clinical and biologic heterogeneity of MDS leads to difficulty in evaluating the prognosis of these patients. The International Prognostic Scoring System (IPSS) has been an important standard for assessing prognosis of primary

---

Pathologic Key Features

- Persistent cytopenias (usually hemoglobin [Hg] <10 g/dL, ANC <1.8 × 10^9/L, platelets <100 × 10^9/L)

- Overt dysplasia in ≥10% of one or more myeloid lineages AND/OR

- 5%–19% Marrow blasts AND/OR

- 1%–19% Circulating blasts AND/OR

- Defining cytogenetic lesion (eg, −7/del[7q]; −5/del[5q]; i[17q]; t[17p]; −13 or del[13q]; del[11q]; del[12p] or t[12p]; t[11;16][q23;p13.3]; t[3;21][q36.3;q21.2]; del[9q]; idic[X][q13]; t[1;3][p36.3;q21.2]; t[2;11] [p21;q23]; inv[3][q21q26.2]; t[6;9][p23q34])

Table 1
Diagnostic algorithm

	Cytopenias[a]	Dysplastic Lineages	MDS-defining Cytogenetics	PB Blasts	BM Blasts	RS
ICUS[48]	1, 2, or 3	None	—	0%	<5%	0%
IDUS[48]	None	≥10% of 1, 2, or 3	±	0%	<5%	±
MDS-U (cytogenetic)[6]	1, 2, or 3	≤10%	+	<1%	<5%	<15%
RCUD (RA, RT, or RN)[6]	1 or 2	≥10% of 1 lineage	±	<1%	<5%	<15%
RARS[6]	1 or 2	≥10% of erythroids	±	0%	<5%	≥15%
RCMD[6]	1 or 2	≥10% of 2 or 3 lineages	±	<1%	<5%	±
MDS-U (pancytopenia)[6]	3	≥10% of 1 lineage	±	<1%	<5%	<15%
MDS-U (PB blasts)[6]	1, 2, or 3	1 or more	±	1%	<5%	±
RAEB-1[6]	1, 2, or 3	1 or more	±	2%–4% AND/OR	5%–9%	±
RAEB-2[6]	1, 2, or 3	1 or more	±	5%–19% OR Auer rods	10%–19% OR Auer rods	±
AML-MRC/FAB RAEB-T[6,b]	1, 2, or 3	≥50% of 2 lineages	±	20%–29%	20%–29%	±
MDS with isolated del(5q)[6]	Usually 1 (anemia)	Hypolobated small megakaryocytes	Isolated del(5q)	<1%	<5%	±
RCC (children)[6]	1, 2, or 3	≥10% of 1, or ≤10% of 2 or 3	±	<2%	<5%	±

Abbreviations: AML-MRC, AML with myelodysplasia-related changes; IDUS, idiopathic dysplasia of uncertain significance; MDS-U, MDS, unclassified; RA, refractory anemia; RAEB-T, RAEB in transformation; RARS, RA with ring sideroblasts; RN, refractory neutropenia; RT, refractory thrombocytopenia.

If monocytes >1 × 10^9/L, classify as chronic myelomonocytic leukemia.

If prior chemotherapy or radiation therapy, classify as therapy-related myeloid neoplasm.

If associated systemic mastocytosis, classify as systemic mastocytosis with associated clonal hematologic non–mast cell lineage disease and classify the AHNMD.

Separate criteria apply to childhood MDS.[40]

[a] Specific levels of cytopenias required by the WHO are Hg <10 g/dL; ANC <1.8 × 10^9/L; and platelets <100 × 10^9/L. Thresholds for cytopenias in ICUS/IDUS are Hg <11 g/dL; ANC <1.0 × 10^9/L; and platelets <100 × 10^9/L.

[b] Current National Comprehensive Cancer Network (NCCN) guidelines reaffirm the clinical utility of the FAB RAEB-T category (including clinical stability for at least 2 months) in combination with the WHO 2008 schema (2014 NCCN guidelines[69]).

Data from Greenberg PL, Attar E, Bennett JM, et al. Myelodysplastic syndromes: clinical practice guidelines in oncology. J Natl Compr Canc Netw 2013;11:838–74.

untreated adult MDS patients since 1997, combining critical clinical and biologic features: marrow blast percentage, cytogenetics, and number of cytopenias.[50] Both modification of existing parameters and additional prognostic systems have since been proposed to provide additional meaningful differences in clinical outcomes.[51–55] Importantly, newer cytogenetic groupings have been shown prognostically valuable and have refined features used in the IPSS.[56] Other variables suggested as providing prognostic information in MDS include BM core biopsy features, such as marrow fibrosis[38,57]; abnormal localization of immature precursors[58]; and patient features, including serum LDH,[59] ferritin,[60] β$_2$-microglobulin,[61,62] patient comorbidities, and performance status.[54,63,64]

Fig. 22. Oligoblastic AML with t(8;21)(q22q22). A cytogenetic finding of t(8;21)(q22q22) is definitional of AML, even with a low blast count. (*A*) The PB shows anemia, thrombocytopenia, granulocytic dysplasia, and rare blasts (Wright-Giemsa stain, original magnification ×40). (*B*) The BM aspirate shows dyserythropoiesis with no increase in blasts. Nevertheless, the diagnosis of acute leukemia is rendered based on the cytogenetic findings (Wright-Giemsa stain, original magnification ×100).

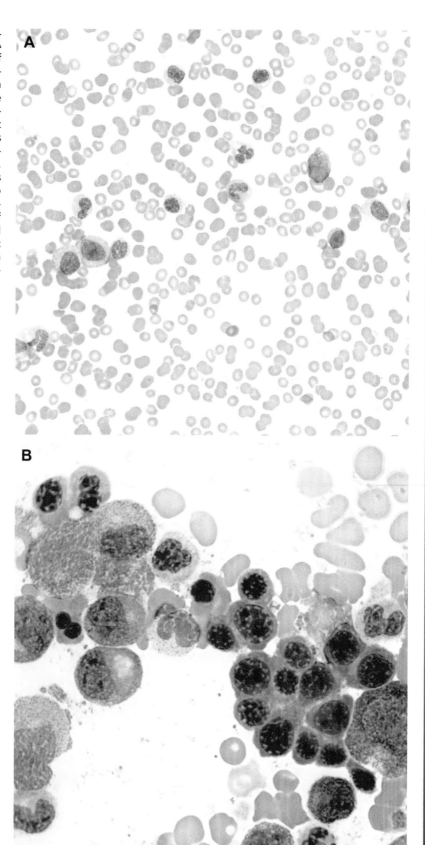

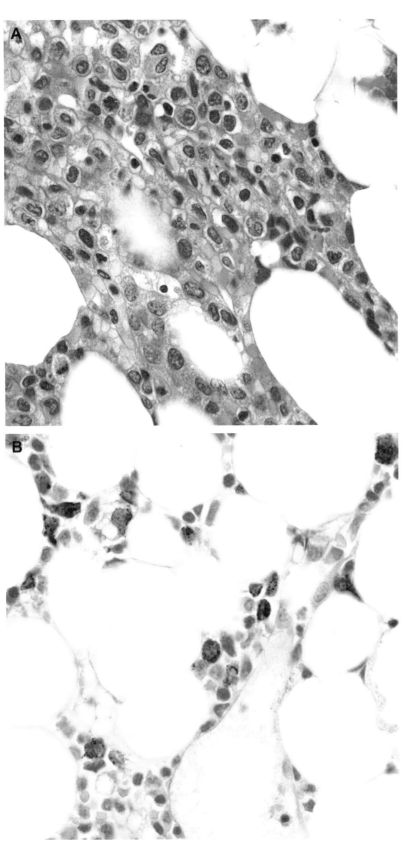

Fig. 23. Identification of blast clusters by CD34 immunohistochemistry. (*A*) Clusters of immature cells seen on the BM core biopsy should prompt immunohistochemical evaluation (Haematoxylin & eosin stain original magnification ×40). (*B*) CD34 immunohistochemistry reveals small clusters of blasts and an increased overall CD34+ blast percentage exceeding 20%. CD34+ blasts must be distinguished from capillaries seen end-on; endothelial staining is bright and linear, whereas CD34+ blast staining is often weaker and more diffuse or speckled (Immunohistochemistry with diaminobenzidine chromogen and haematoxylin counterstain, original magnification ×40).

Fig. 24. RCC and CD61 immunohistochemistry. (*A*) Review of the BM aspirate shows erythroid predominance with an increased proportion of proerythroblasts and mild dyspoiesis (Wright-Giemsa stain, original magnification ×100). (*B*) The BM core biopsy is often hypocellular for age, showing prominent erythroid islands. Myelopoiesis is decreased and megakaryocytes are difficult to identify (Haematoxylin & eosin stain, original magnification ×20).

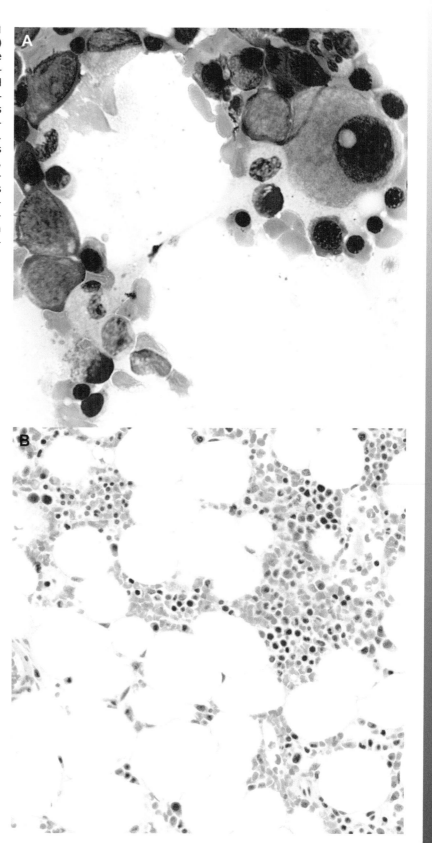

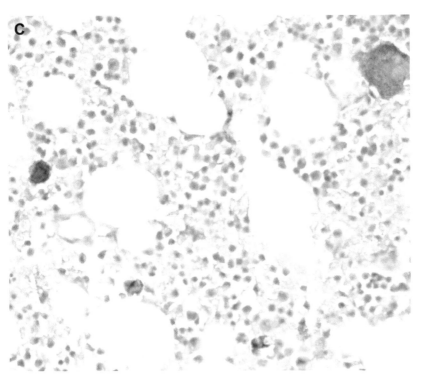

Fig. 24. (*continued*). RCC and CD61 immunohisto-chemistry. (*C*) Immunohisto-chemistry for CD61 reveals characteristic dysplastic micromegakaryocytes (Immunohistochemistry with diaminobenzidine chromogen and haematoxylin counterstain, original magnification ×20).

The International Working Group for Prognosis in MDS recently published the new revised IPSS (IPSS-R) based on a much larger group of primary untreated MDS patients (IPSS-R, n = 7012; IPSS, n = 816)[65] from multiple international institutions. The IPSS-R improves on the IPSS, albeit marrow cytogenetics, marrow blast percentage, and cytopenias remain the major basis of its predictive capability. Novel components of this system include 5 rather than 3 cytogenetic prognostic subgroups with specific and new classifications of several less common cytogenetic subsets (Table 2),[56] splitting the low marrow blast percentage value (yielding 2 groups of 2% or less and greater than 2 to less than 5%), and assessing the depth (rather than merely the number) of cytopenias (Table 3).[65] This model defines 5 rather than 4 major prognostic categories for both survival and risk of AML progression (Table 4). Patient age, performance status, serum ferritin, and lactate dehydrogenase were significant additive minor features for survival but not for AML transformation. The utility of this prognostic system has recently been confirmed for untreated patients[66] and in preliminary fashion for those who have been treated with disease-altering therapy.[67] As such, the IPSS-R

is proving beneficial for predicting the clinical outcomes of untreated MDS patients and aiding design and analysis of clinical trials in this disease. Further investigations to determine the

Table 2
IPSS-R cytogenetic risk groups

	Cytogenetic Abnormalities
Very good	−Y, del(11q)
Good	Normal, del(5q), del(12p), del(20q), double including del(5q)
Intermediate	del(7q), +8, +19, i(17q), Any other single or double independent clones
Poor	−7, inv(3)/t(3q)/del(3q), Double including −7/del(7q), complex: 3 abnormalities
Very poor	Complex: >3 abnormalities

The data were derived from Schanz and colleagues.[56]
Data from Greenberg PL, Tuechler H, Schanz J, et al. Revised International Prognostic Scoring System (IPSS-R) for myelodysplastic syndromes. Blood 2012;120:2454–65. © The American Society of Hematology.

Table 3
IPSS-R prognostic score values

	0	0.5	1	1.5	2	3	4
Cytogenetics	Very good	—	Good	—	Intermediate	Poor	Very poor
BM blast (%)	≤2	—	>2–<5	—	5–10	>10	—
Hemoglobin	≥10	—	8–<10	<8	—	—	—
Platelets	≥100	50–<100	<50	—	—	—	—
ANC	≥0.8	<0.8	—	—	—	—	—

Data from Greenberg PL, Tuechler H, Schanz J, et al. Revised International Prognostic Scoring System (IPSS-R) for myelodysplastic syndromes. Blood 2012;120:2454–65. © The American Society of Hematology.

Table 4
IPSS-R: prognostic risk scores and categories: clinical outcomes

	No. Patients	Very Low	Low	Intermediate	High	Very High
Risk score	—	≤1.5	>1.5–3	>3–4.5	>4.5–6	>6
Patients (%)	—	19	38	20	13	10
Survival[a]	7012	8.8	5.3	3.0	1.6	0.8
AML/25%[a,b]	6485	NR	10.8	3.2	1.4	0.7

Web sites for IPSS-R calculator tool: http://www.ipss-r.com and http://mds-foundation.org/calculator/index.php.
[a] Medians, years.
[b] Median time to 25% AML evolution.
Data from Greenberg PL, Tuechler H, Schanz J, et al. Revised International Prognostic Scoring System (IPSS-R) for myelodysplastic syndromes. Blood 2012;120:2454–65. © The American Society of Hematology.

impact of molecular and flow cytometric technologies on the IPSS-R are warranted and ongoing.

REFERENCES

1. Pang WW, Pluvinage JV, Price EA, et al. Hematopoietic stem cell and progenitor cell mechanisms in myelodysplastic syndromes. Proc Natl Acad Sci U S A 2013;110:3011–6.
2. Raaijmakers MH. Myelodysplastic syndromes: revisiting the role of the bone marrow microenvironment in disease pathogenesis. Int J Hematol 2012;95:17–25.
3. Ma X. Epidemiology of myelodysplastic syndromes. Am J Med 2012;125:S2–5.
4. Goldberg SL, Chen E, Sasane M, et al. Economic impact on US Medicare of a new diagnosis of myelodysplastic syndromes and the incremental costs associated with blood transfusion need. Transfusion 2012. http://dx.doi.org/10.1111/j.1537-2995.2012.03626.x.
5. Bennett JM, Catovsky D, Daniel MT, et al. Proposals for the classification of the myelodysplastic syndromes. Br J Haematol 1982;51:189–99.
6. Swerdlow S, International Agency for Research on Cancer, World Health Organization. WHO classification of tumours of haematopoietic and lymphoid tissues. Lyon: International Agency for Research on Cancer; 2008.
7. Vardiman JW, Thiele J, Arber DA, et al. The 2008 revision of the World Health Organization (WHO) classification of myeloid neoplasms and acute leukemia: rationale and important changes. Blood 2009;114:937–51.
8. Tothova Z, Steensma DP, Ebert BL. New strategies in myelodysplastic syndromes: application of molecular diagnostics to clinical practice. Clin Cancer Res 2013. http://dx.doi.org/10.1158/1078-0432.CCR-12-1251.
9. Mufti GJ, Bennett JM, Goasguen J, et al. Diagnosis and classification of myelodysplastic syndrome: International Working Group on Morphology of myelodysplastic syndrome (IWGM-MDS) consensus proposals for the definition and enumeration of myeloblasts and ring sideroblasts. Haematologica 2008;93:1712–7.
10. Steensma DP. Dysplasia has A differential diagnosis: distinguishing genuine myelodysplastic syndromes (MDS) from mimics, imitators, copycats and impostors. Curr Hematol Malig Rep 2012;7:310–20.
11. Lazarchick J. Update on anemia and neutropenia in copper deficiency. Curr Opin Hematol 2012;19:58–60.
12. Gabreyes AA, Abbasi HN, Forbes KP, et al. Hypocupremia associated cytopenia and myelopathy: a

national retrospective review. Eur J Haematol 2013; 90:1–9.

13. Karcher DS, Frost AR. The bone marrow in human immunodeficiency virus (HIV)-related disease. Morphology and clinical correlation. Am J Clin Pathol 1991;95:63–71.

14. Yarali N, Duru F, Sipahi T, et al. Parvovirus B19 infection reminiscent of myelodysplastic syndrome in three children with chronic hemolytic anemia. Pediatr Hematol Oncol 2000;17:475–82.

15. Kagialis-Girard S, Durand B, Mialou V, et al. Human herpesvirus 6 infection and transient acquired myelodysplasia in children. Pediatr Blood Cancer 2006; 47:543–8.

16. Sheikha A. Dyserythropoiesis in 105 patients with visceral leishmaniasis. Lab Hematol 2004;10:206–11.

17. Budde R, Hellerich U. Alcoholic dyshaematopoiesis: morphological features of alcohol-induced bone marrow damage in biopsy sections compared with aspiration smears. Acta Haematol 1995;94:74–7.

18. Bain BJ, Nam D. Neutrophil dysplasia induced by granulocyte colony-stimulating factor. Am J Hematol 2010;85:354.

19. Wang E, Boswell E, Siddiqi I, et al. Pseudo-Pelger-Huët anomaly induced by medications: a clinicopathologic study in comparison with myelodysplastic syndrome-related pseudo-Pelger-Huët anomaly. Am J Clin Pathol 2011;135: 291–303.

20. Benjamin B, Gesundheit B, Kirby M, et al. Thrombocytopenia and megakaryocyte dysplasia: an adverse effect of valproic acid treatment. J Pediatr Hematol Oncol 2002;24(7):589–90.

21. Oka Y, Kameoka J, Hirabayashi Y, et al. Reversible bone marrow dysplasia in patients with systemic lupus erythematosus. Intern Med 2008;47:737–42.

22. Anderson LA, Pfeiffer RM, Landgren O, et al. Risks of myeloid malignancies in patients with autoimmune conditions. Br J Cancer 2009;100:822–8.

23. Dokal I, Vulliamy T. Inherited aplastic anaemias/ bone marrow failure syndromes. Blood Rev 2008; 22:141–53.

24. Alter BP, Giri N, Savage SA, et al. Malignancies and survival patterns in the National Cancer Institute inherited bone marrow failure syndromes cohort study. Br J Haematol 2010;150:179–88.

25. Carlsson G, Fasth A, Berglöf E, et al. Incidence of severe congenital neutropenia in Sweden and risk of evolution to myelodysplastic syndrome/ leukaemia. Br J Haematol 2012;158:363–9.

26. Hsu AP, Sampaio EP, Khan J, et al. Mutations in GATA2 are associated with the autosomal dominant and sporadic monocytopenia and mycobacterial infection (MonoMAC) syndrome. Blood 2011;118: 2653–5.

27. Calvo KR, Vinh DC, Maric I, et al. Myelodysplasia in autosomal dominant and sporadic monocytopenia

immunodeficiency syndrome: diagnostic features and clinical implications. Haematologica 2011;96: 1221–5.

28. Harigae H, Furuyama K. Hereditary sideroblastic anemia: pathophysiology and gene mutations. Int J Hematol 2010;92:425–31.

29. Ohba R, Furuyama K, Yoshida K, et al. Clinical and genetic characteristics of congenital sideroblastic anemia: comparison with myelodysplastic syndrome with ring sideroblast (MDS-RS). Ann Hematol 2013;92:1–9.

30. Iolascon A, Esposito MR, Russo R. Clinical aspects and pathogenesis of congenital dyserythropoietic anemias: from morphology to molecular approach. Haematologica 2012;97:1786–94.

31. Valent P, Horny HP, Bennett JM, et al. Definitions and standards in the diagnosis and treatment of the myelodysplastic syndromes: consensus statements and report from a working conference. Leuk Res 2007;31:727–36.

32. Willis MS, McKenna RW, Peterson LC, et al. Low blast count myeloid disorders with auer rods: a clinicopathologic analysis of 9 cases. Am J Clin Pathol 2005;124:191–8.

33. Cherry AM, Brockman SR, Paternoster SF, et al. Comparison of interphase FISH and metaphase cytogenetics to study myelodysplastic syndrome: an Eastern Cooperative Oncology Group (ECOG) study. Leuk Res 2003;27:1085–90.

34. Coleman JF, Theil KS, Tubbs RR, et al. Diagnostic yield of bone marrow and peripheral blood FISH panel testing in clinically suspected myelodysplastic syndromes and/or acute myeloid leukemia a prospective analysis of 433 cases. Am J Clin Pathol 2011;135:915–20.

35. Cherry AM, Slovak ML, Campbell LJ, et al. Will a peripheral blood (PB) sample yield the same diagnostic and prognostic cytogenetic data as the concomitant bone marrow (BM) in myelodysplasia? Leuk Res 2012;36:832–40.

36. Thiele J, Kvasnicka HM, Facchetti F, et al. European consensus on grading bone marrow fibrosis and assessment of cellularity. Haematologica 2005;90:1128–32.

37. Kröger N, Zabelina T, Biezen A van, et al. Allogeneic stem cell transplantation for myelodysplastic syndromes with bone marrow fibrosis. Haematologica 2011;96:291–7.

38. Della Porta MG, Malcovati L, Boveri E, et al. Clinical relevance of bone marrow fibrosis and CD34-positive cell clusters in primary myelodysplastic syndromes. J Clin Oncol 2009;27:754–62.

39. Baumann I, Führer M, Behrendt S, et al. Morphological differentiation of severe aplastic anaemia from hypocellular refractory cytopenia of childhood: reproducibility of histopathological diagnostic criteria. Histopathology 2012;61:10–7.

40. Niemeyer CM, Baumann I. Classification of childhood aplastic anemia and myelodysplastic syndrome. Hematology Am Soc Hematol Educ Program 2011;2011:84–9.

41. Wood BL. Myeloid malignancies: myelodysplastic syndromes, myeloproliferative disorders, and acute myeloid leukemia. Clin Lab Med 2007;27:551–75.

42. Maftoun-Banankhah S, Maleki A, Karandikar NJ, et al. Multiparameter flow cytometric analysis reveals low percentage of bone marrow hematogones in myelodysplastic syndromes. Am J Clin Pathol 2008;129:300–8.

43. Della Porta MG, Picone C, Pascutto C, et al. Multicenter validation of a reproducible flow cytometric score for the diagnosis of low-grade myelodysplastic syndromes: results of a European LeukemiaNET study. Haematologica 2012;97:1209–17.

44. Senent L, Arenillas L, Luño E, et al. Reproducibility of the World Health Organization 2008 criteria for myelodysplastic syndromes. Haematologica 2013; 98:568–75.

45. Naqvi K, Jabbour E, Bueso-Ramos C, et al. Implications of discrepancy in morphologic diagnosis of myelodysplastic syndrome between referral and tertiary care centers. Blood 2011;118:4690–3.

46. Parmentier S, Schetelig J, Lorenz K, et al. Assessment of dysplastic hematopoiesis: lessons from healthy bone marrow donors. Haematologica 2012;97:723–30.

47. Haase D, Germing U, Schanz J, et al. New insights into the prognostic impact of the karyotype in MDS and correlation with subtypes: evidence from a core dataset of 2124 patients. Blood 2007;110: 4385–95.

48. Valent P, Bain BJ, Bennett JM, et al. Idiopathic cytopenia of undetermined significance (ICUS) and idiopathic dysplasia of uncertain significance (IDUS), and their distinction from low risk MDS. Leuk Res 2012;36:1–5.

49. Shaffer LG, Ballif BC, Schultz RA. In: Banerjee D, Shah SP, editors. Array comparative genomic hybridization. Humana Press; 2013. p. 69–85. Available at: <http://link.springer.com.laneproxy.stanford.edu/protocol/10.1007/978-1-62703-281-0_5>; 2013.

50. Greenberg P, Cox C, LeBeau MM, et al. International scoring system for evaluating prognosis in myelodysplastic syndromes. Blood 1997;89:2079–88.

51. Malcovati L, Porta MGD, Pascutto C, et al. Prognostic factors and life expectancy in myelodysplastic syndromes classified according to WHO criteria: a basis for clinical decision making. J Clin Oncol 2005;23:7594–603.

52. Malcovati L, Germing U, Kuendgen A, et al. Time-dependent prognostic scoring system for predicting survival and leukemic evolution in myelodysplastic syndromes. J Clin Oncol 2007;25: 3503–10.

53. Kantarjian H, O'Brien S, Ravandi F, et al. Proposal for a new risk model in myelodysplastic syndrome that accounts for events not considered in the original International Prognostic Scoring System. Cancer 2008;113:1351–61.

54. Della Porta MG, Malcovati L, Strupp C, et al. Risk stratification based on both disease status and extra-hematologic comorbidities in patients with myelodysplastic syndrome. Haematologica 2011; 96:441–9.

55. Nösslinger T, Tüchler H, Germing U, et al. Prognostic impact of age and gender in 897 untreated patients with primary myelodysplastic syndromes. Ann Oncol 2010;21:120–5.

56. Schanz J, Tüchler H, Solé F, et al. New comprehensive cytogenetic scoring system for primary myelodysplastic syndromes (MDS) and oligoblastic acute myeloid leukemia after MDS derived from an international database merge. J Clin Oncol 2012;30:820–9.

57. Buesche G, Teoman H, Wilczak W, et al. Marrow fibrosis predicts early fatal marrow failure in patients with myelodysplastic syndromes. Leukemia 2008;22:313–22.

58. Verburgh E, Achten R, Maes B, et al. Additional prognostic value of bone marrow histology in patients subclassified according to the International Prognostic Scoring System for myelodysplastic syndromes. J Clin Oncol 2003;21: 273–82.

59. Germing U, Hildebrandt B, Pfeilstöcker M, et al. Refinement of the international prognostic scoring system (IPSS) by including LDH as an additional prognostic variable to improve risk assessment in patients with primary myelodysplastic syndromes (MDS). Leukemia 2005;19:2223–31.

60. Sanz G, Nomdedeu B, Such E, et al. Independent impact of iron overload and transfusion dependency on survival and leukemic evolution in patients with myelodysplastic syndrome. Blood 2008;112:238–9.

61. Gatto S, Ball G, Onida F, et al. Contribution of beta-2 microglobulin levels to the prognostic stratification of survival in patients with myelodysplastic syndrome (MDS). Blood 2003;102:1622–5.

62. Neumann F, Gattermann N, Barthelmes HU, et al. Levels of beta 2 microglobulin have a prognostic relevance for patients with myelodysplastic syndrome with regard to survival and the risk of transformation into acute myelogenous leukemia. Leuk Res 2009;33:232–6.

63. Wang R, Gross CP, Halene S, et al. Comorbidities and survival in a large cohort of patients with newly diagnosed myelodysplastic syndromes. Leuk Res 2009;33:1594–8.

64. Naqvi K, Garcia-Manero G, Sardesai S, et al. Association of comorbidities with overall survival

in myelodysplastic syndrome: development of a prognostic model. J Clin Oncol 2011;29:2240–6.

65. Greenberg PL, Tuechler H, Schanz J, et al. Revised International Prognostic Scoring System (IPSS-R) for myelodysplastic syndromes. Blood 2012;120: 2454–65. http://dx.doi.org/10.1182/blood-2012-03-420489.

66. Lamarque M, Raynaud S, Itzykson R, et al. The revised IPSS is a powerful tool to evaluate the outcome of MDS patients treated with azacitidine: the GFM experience. Blood 2012;120:5084–5.

67. Sekeres M, Adès L, Tüchler H. Revised International Prognostic Scoring System (IPSS-R) for primary treated MDS patients: a report from the IWG-PM. Proc Int'l Symposium on MDS. Leuk Res 2013;37:S74.

68. Haddy TB, Rana SR, Castro O. Benign ethnic neutropenia: what is a normal absolute neutrophil count? J Lab Clin Med 1999;133:15–22.

69. Greenberg PL, Attar E, Bennett JM, et al. NCCN clinical practice guidelines in oncology: myelodysplastic syndromes. J Natl Compr Canc Netw 2013; 11:838–74 Version 1.2014.

70. Morice WG, Kurtin PJ, Tefferi A, et al. Distinct bone marrow findings in T-cell granular lymphocytic leukemia revealed by paraffin section immunoperoxidase stains for CD8, TIA-1, and granzyme B. Blood 2002;99:268–74.

Atypical Phenotypes in Classical Hodgkin Lymphoma

Lawrence M. Weiss, MD

KEYWORDS

- Immunohistochemistry • CD30 • CD15 • PAX-5 • CD45 • CD20 • CD79a • OCT-2 • BOB.1

KEY POINTS

- Most cases of classical Hodgkin lymphoma have a characteristic phenotype, with expression of CD30, CD15, and PAX-5, and absence of CD45 and most B-lineage markers.
- A significant subset of cases of classical Hodgkin lymphoma has atypical phenotypes, usually absence of CD15 or expression of one or more B-lineage markers, such as CD20, CD79a, OCT-2, and BOB.1.
- The most common problems in the immunodiagnosis of classical Hodgkin lymphoma involve the misidentification of other cells types, such as immunoblasts or histiocytes, as Hodgkin cells, or the inability to assess multiple antigens in small tissue biopsies.
- Cases expressing the full B-cell program may represent a borderline lymphoma intermediate between classical Hodgkin lymphoma and diffuse large B-cell lymphoma.
- Novel multiplexing technologies may help provide better assessment of antigen expression on Hodgkin cells.

ABSTRACT

Classical Hodgkin lymphoma has a characteristic immunophenotype in most cases, with expression of CD30, CD15, and PAX-5, and absence of CD45 and T-lineage markers. However, in a significant subset of cases, atypical staining patterns may be seen for one or more antigens, particularly negative staining for CD15 or staining for one or more B-lineage markers, such as CD20, CD79a, OCT-2, or BOB.1. The greatest pitfall is in the misinterpretation of other cells, such as immunoblasts or histiocytes, as Hodgkin cells.

OVERVIEW

Classical Hodgkin lymphoma is diagnosed by the identification of Reed-Sternberg cells and variants (collectively Hodgkin cells) in the appropriate cellular milieu. This was previously accomplished using solely morphologic criteria.

The development of effective immunohistochemical studies that can be performed in formalin-fixed and paraffin-embedded sections, along with the availability of antibodies reactive on formalin-resistant epitopes, has allowed a more accurate immunohistochemical recognition of Hodgkin cells, with the realization that many cases previously regarded as classical Hodgkin lymphoma actually represented other entities, such as T-cell/histiocyte-rich large B-cell lymphoma. The purpose of this article was to review the immunophenotypes that may be observed in classical Hodgkin lymphoma.

The typical phenotype observed in Hodgkin lymphoma is shown in **Table 1**. CD30 is the most consistent of the major diagnostic markers of Hodgkin cells, expressed in virtually 100% of cases. The older literature suggested a lower incidence of CD30 expression, on the order of 90% of cases, probably as a reflection of the results obtained before the current era of optimal antigen retrieval.[1] The staining pattern for CD30

Dr Weiss is affiliated with Clarient, a GE Healthcare Company, which is the developer of the Hodgkin lymphoma MultiOmyx laboratory developed test.
Clarient Diagnostic Services, Inc, 31 Columbia, Aliso Viejo, CA 92656, USA
E-mail address: lweiss@clarientinc.com

Surgical Pathology 6 (2013) 729–742
http://dx.doi.org/10.1016/j.path.2013.08.011
1875-9181/13/$ – see front matter © 2013 Elsevier Inc. All rights reserved.

Table 1
Immunophenotype of Hodgkin cells in classical Hodgkin lymphoma

CD30	100%
CD15	70%
PAX-5	95%
CD45	5%
CD20	25%
CD79a	15%
BOB.1	15%–25%
OCT-2	15%–50%
MUM-1	100%
Fascin	100%
EMA	5%
EBER/EBV-LMP-1	30%
BCL2	25%
BCL6	15%
CD138	40%
CD10	0%
CD3, other T-lineage	0%

is membranous and/or paranuclear, as well as weaker diffuse cytoplasmic; however, diffuse cytoplasmic staining alone is nonspecific (**Fig. 1**). It is controversial whether Hodgkin cells are truly ever CD30-negative or whether the negativity is a technical artifact, although I believe that I have rarely seen cases of classical Hodgkin lymphoma that were truly CD30-negative. CD30 remains expressed, even after anti-CD30 therapy.[2] CD15 is a less-consistent marker of Hodgkin cells, expressed in the literature in about 85% of cases.[3] Again, the staining is membranous and/or paranuclear, with a nonspecific diffuse granular cytoplasmic staining (the latter may frequently be seen in peripheral T-cell lymphoma) (**Fig. 2**). In my recent personal experience, the percentage of CD15 positivity is much lower than 85%, probably less than 50%. Although much of that difference can be explained by referral pattern, specifically the tendency of pathologists to refer CD15-negative cases for expert consultation, I still believe that the true percentage of CD15 positivity in classical Hodgkin lymphoma is well below 85% and probably closer to 70%. I attribute most of the lower positivity (even in the advent of more effective immunohistochemical technology) to the greater recognition of CD15 positivity in histiocytes and other cell types that can mimic CD15 expression in Hodgkin cells. It is now well recognized that histiocytes may show a granular cytoplasmic positivity for CD15 that is concentrated in the paranuclear region, and that neoplastic T cells may also show a granular pattern of cytoplasmic CD15 reactivity.

PAX-5 is another consistent marker of Hodgkin cells, evidence of the derivation of Hodgkin cells from the B-cell lineage. The most comprehensive studies have reported PAX-5 expression in approximately 95% of cases.[4] In addition, the expression is consistently weak to moderate in intensity, in contrast to the consistently strong

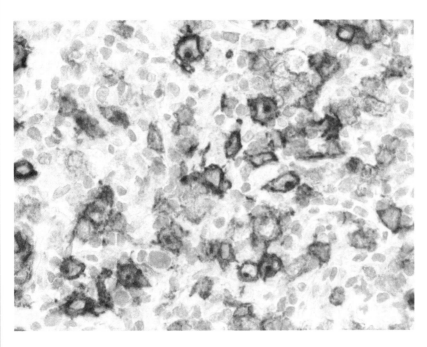

Fig. 1. CD30 in classical Hodgkin lymphoma. Membrane and/or paranuclear staining is evidence of true CD30 staining. Cytoplasmic staining alone lacks specificity.

Fig. 2. CD15 staining. (*A*) Classical Hodgkin lymphoma. Note the relatively specific membrane and/or paranuclear staining pattern. (*B, C*) CD15 staining in histiocytes can vary from weak to strong, is typically granular cytoplasmic; the latter may show a paranuclear localization.

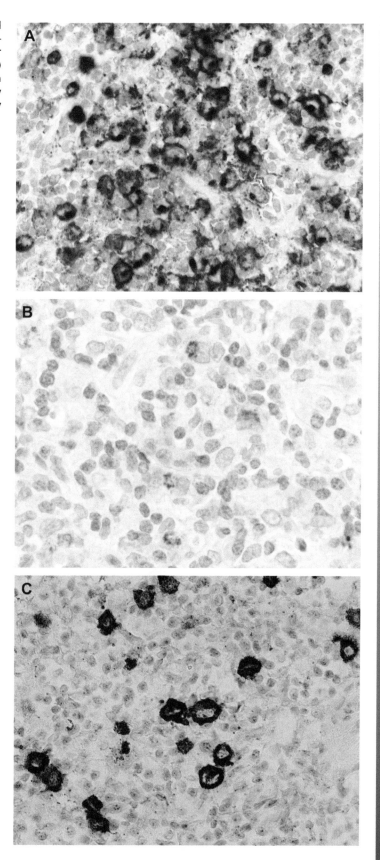

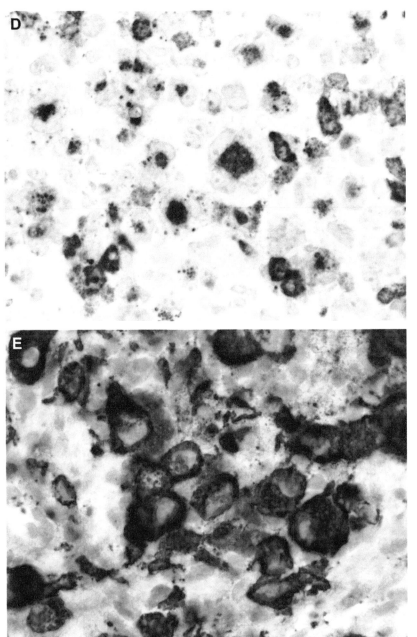

Fig. 2. (continued). CD15 staining. (D, E) CD15 staining in T-cell lymphoma. A coarse granular staining pattern is typical, which may on occasion show a paranuclear localization.

staining seen in small B-lymphocytes (Fig. 3). It is my experience that PAX-5 is even more consistently expressed in Hodgkin cells than the early literature suggests. Although there are undoubted cases of classical Hodgkin lymphoma in which the PAX-5 is negative on the Hodgkin cells, I would be very cautious in diagnosing a case of classical Hodgkin lymphoma in the face of negativity for PAX-5. One caveat about using the weak to moderate intensity of PAX-5 staining as a clue to the diagnosis of classical Hodgkin lymphoma is that the large B cells of diffuse large B-cell lymphoma may also show moderate staining for PAX-5.

CD45 is another potentially useful marker for the diagnosis of classical Hodgkin lymphoma, but must be interpreted very carefully. In the earlier literature, it is stated that about 10% of cases of

Fig. 3. PAX-5 staining in classical Hodgkin lymphoma. The staining is almost always weak to moderate in intensity. Note the strongly staining small B-lymphocytes.

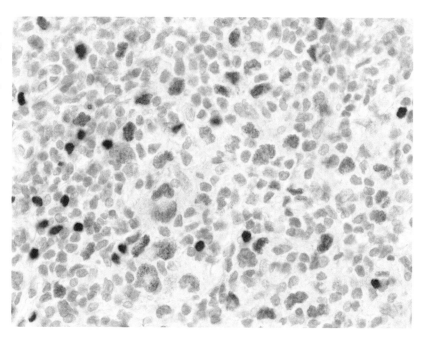

classical Hodgkin lymphoma are positive for CD45, but my experience is that the proportion of CD45-positive cases is much lower, and probably closer to 5% of cases or even less.[5] The key issue is that it is very difficult to assess CD45 positivity in Hodgkin cells, for several reasons. First, Hodgkin cells are generally disposed singly and are found in close apposition to small T-cell lymphocytes. Even when T-lymphocytes are not seen adjacent to Hodgkin cells, they still may have been present either above or below the plane of a 5-μm to 10-μm section, and their membranes may be still present adherent to the Hodgkin cells. Therefore, for a Hodgkin cell to be regarded as CD45-positive, there must be a ring of membrane positivity extending completely around the Hodgkin cells, staining at an intensity that is as great or greater than the adjacent small lymphoid cells. It is most helpful to assess staining when Hodgkin cells abut other Hodgkin cells (**Fig. 4**). The second pitfall in the assessment of CD45 staining is staining of CD45-positive histiocytes that can be confused with Hodgkin cells, particularly when the nuclear counterstain is weak, as most immunostains omit an eosin counterstain that would highlight the more prominent nucleoli of Hodgkin cells. In some lymphocyte-rich cases, it is not possible to assess the Hodgkin cells for CD45, but in cases that can be assessed, CD45 remains a very helpful negative marker.

Although Hodgkin cells have been definitively shown to derive from the B-lymphoid lineage,

part of the molecular deficit of classical Hodgkin lymphoma includes loss of the B-lineage program, with consequent absence of surface immunoglobulin and relative loss of pan B-cell antigens. CD20 is expressed in about 15% to 40% of cases of classical Hodgkin lymphoma in various series, and, in my experience, is expressed in about 25% of cases.[6] The staining is usually variable in the positive cases, with some Hodgkin cells strongly positive, other cells moderately to weakly positive, and a variable proportion negative (**Fig. 5**). Expression of CD20 in cases of Hodgkin lymphoma has been associated with adverse prognosis in some but not other studies.[7,8] Focal CD20 staining of Hodgkin cells must be distinguished from CD20 staining of scattered immunoblasts, which may be present in cases of classical Hodgkin lymphoma. This can be a very difficult exercise, given the variable CD20 staining that may be seen in immunoblasts. Similarly, CD79a reactivity is also seen in only a minority of cases of classical Hodgkin lymphoma, lower than the incidence seen with CD20, and in my experience approximately 15% of cases.[9] Similar to CD20, it is most unusual for most Hodgkin cells to be CD79a-positive, and in most positive cases, only a small subpopulation of Hodgkin cells shows expression of the antigen. Again, this staining must be distinguished from staining of immunoblasts, usually an even more difficult exercise with CD79a than with CD20, given the smaller proportion of positive Hodgkin cells

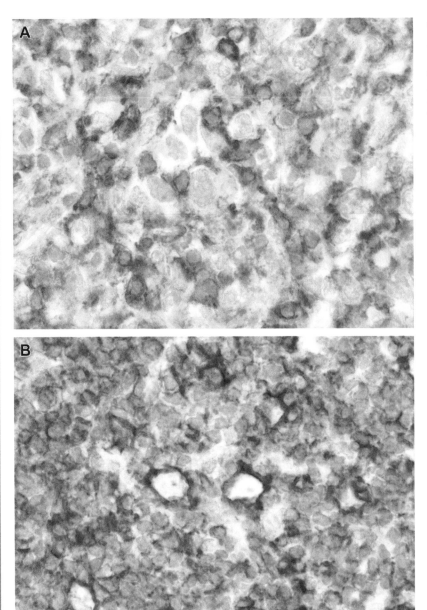

Fig. 4. CD45 staining in Hodgkin lymphoma. (*A*) Classical Hodgkin lymphoma. The staining pattern is best assessed when atypical cells abut each other, after eliminating the possibility of histiocytes. (*B*) Nodular lymphocyte predominance in Hodgkin lymphoma, showing positive staining of lymphocyte-predominant cells for contrast.

usually present in a positive case and the generally weak staining of CD79a in both Hodgkin cells and immunoblasts. Surface or cytoplasmic immunoglobulin light chain restriction is never seen, although Hodgkin cells may show diffuse nonspecific cytoplasmic uptake of immunoglobulin light and heavy chains.

The loss of surface immunoglobulin and pan B-cell antigens may be due to the loss of B-cell transcription factors in a subset of cases, and this loss has also been used in the diagnosis of Hodgkin lymphoma. For example, the B-cell transcription factors BOB.1 and OCT-2 are often aberrantly absent in Hodgkin cells, and are detectable in only about 15% to 25% and 15% to 50% of cases, respectively (**Fig. 6**).[10,11] The variation in the percentages of positive cases between different series, is probably due to inclusion or exclusion of cases with weak staining, but strong staining for one or both antigens is unusual in

Fig. 5. CD20 staining in classical Hodgkin lymphoma. Staining may be seen in about 25% of cases, usually staining a subset of the Hodgkin cells, with variable intensity.

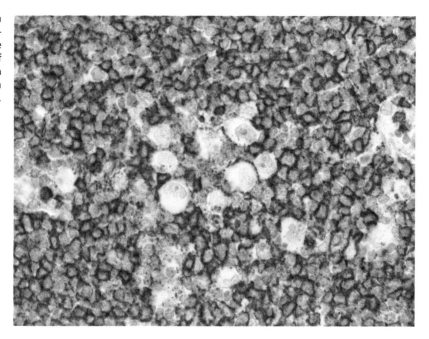

cases of classical Hodgkin lymphoma, whereas moderate to strong staining for both markers is typical of B-cell lymphoma or nodular lymphocyte predominance Hodgkin lymphoma.

Multiple myeoloma oncogene 1 (MUM-1) and fascin are consistent markers of Hodgkin cells.[12,13] Both are absent in nodular lymphocyte predominant Hodgkin lymphoma, and are thus important in this differential diagnosis; however, both MUM-1 and fascin are often positive in cases of diffuse large B-cell lymphoma. In addition, MUM-1 is usually expressed on reactive immunoblasts and fascin is expressed on normal dendritic cells in the lymph node, limiting their value in differential diagnosis in other settings. EMA expression is unusual in Hodgkin lymphoma,

Fig. 6. OCT-2 staining in classical Hodgkin lymphoma. When positive, the staining is usually of weak to moderate intensity.

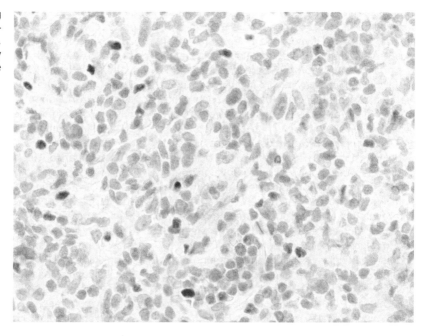

but has been reported in a small subset of cases, probably with an incidence of expression of about 5%.[14] Epstein-Barr virus (EBV) infection, as detected by either EBV-encoded RNA (EBER) or EBV latent membrane protein 1 (LMP-1), is detected in a varying proportion of cases, depending on the geographic region studied.[15] In Western countries, it averages about 30% to 40% of cases, being most common in children and older adults, particularly in cases of mixed cellularity and the rare lymphocyte depletion.

BCL2, BCL6, and CD138 are expressed in a significant subset of cases of classical Hodgkin lymphoma, whereas CD10 and BLIMP-1 are consistently negative.[16] In about 60% of cases, the Hodgkin cells are negative for BCL6 and CD138, which, in concert with expression of MUM-1 and negativity for CD10 and BLIMP-1, suggests a later germinal center or early post–germinal center immunophenotype. In about 25% of cases, BCL6 is negative but CD138 is positive, consistent with a post–germinal center phenotype, whereas in about 15% of cases, both BCL6 and CD138 are expressed in the Hodgkin cells, showing an indeterminate phenotype.

The incidence of expression of T-cell markers in Hodgkin lymphoma is still somewhat controversial. Early studies suggested that expression of T-lineage antigens could be seen on Hodgkin cells. For example, expression of CD3, particularly with a cytoplasmic distribution, was reported in approximately 25% to 33% of cases, and membrane or cytoplasmic expression of T-cell-receptor beta was reported in about 20% of cases.[17,18] More recent studies have suggested that, if specific T-lineage antigen expression is seen at all in cases of classical Hodgkin lymphoma, however, it must be a very rare event; these results fit well with near uniform absence of clonal T-cell receptor gene rearrangements in Hodgkin lymphoma, even with microdissection of the atypical cells. I prefer to regard such cases with CD3 expression as probably representing a peripheral T-cell lymphoma, noting that rare cases of T-cell lymphoma may closely mimic classical Hodgkin lymphoma. This is particularly true when cutaneous T-cell lymphoma involves lymph nodes, and probably explains some if not most of the previously reported association between cutaneous T-cell lymphoma and Hodgkin lymphoma.

Recent studies have focused on the presence of Hodgkinlike cells in peripheral T-cell lymphomas, particularly cases of angioimmunoblastic T-cell lymphoma, thus simulating Hodgkin lymphoma.[19] The Hodgkinlike cells show expression of CD30 and CD15, with variable positivity for CD20, and are also positive for EBV (Fig. 7).

Molecular studies have demonstrated that these cells represent oligoclonal B cells rather than part of the neoplastic T-cell clone, possibly arising as a result of local immunosuppression caused by the underlying T-cell lymphoma. Similar Hodgkinlike cells have been found in association with cases of follicular T-cell lymphoma, although many of these cases are negative for EBV infection, and show a peculiar rosetting of PD-1–positive neoplastic T cells around the Reed-Sternberg–like cells.[20,21] The expression of CD43 and other T-related antigens must also be rare in true cases of classical Hodgkin lymphoma,[22] and probably represents cases of peripheral T-cell lymphoma mimicking Hodgkin lymphoma. Nonetheless, expression of cytotoxic molecules have been reported in a very small subset of cases of true Hodgkin lymphoma, and has been associated with a poor prognosis.[23]

Similar Reed-Sternberg–like cells have also been reported in a variety of B-cell lymphomas, most commonly in the settings of chronic lymphocytic leukemia and follicular lymphoma. In chronic lymphocytic leukemia, the Hodgkin cells are found in the context of a background of chronic lymphocytic leukemia, and express CD30, and usually also CD15 and CD20.[24] These cells are usually also EBV-positive. This phenomenon may be responsible for cases of Hodgkinlike Richter's transformation, in which true Hodgkin lymphoma is seen composite with separate areas of chronic lymphocytic leukemia. In contrast, the Hodgkinlike cells present in Hodgkinlike lymphoproliferations occurring in immunosuppressed individuals usually possess an immunophenotype closer to B cells.[25] Although CD30 is uniformly expressed, these cells are typically positive for CD20 and other B-lineage markers, but negative for CD15. Although EBV is uniformly positive, a type III latency pattern is usually seen, in contrast to the type II latency pattern seen in classical Hodgkin lymphoma. Similarly, Hodgkinlike cells with an identical phenotype may be observed in EBV-positive diffuse large B-cell lymphoma of the elderly.

To summarize, Hodgkin cells in cases of classical Hodgkin lymphoma show consistent expression of CD30, often with CD15, but without CD45, and, at best, only abortive evidence of B-cell antigen expression, typically weak to moderate PAX-5 expression. However, rare cases may show expression of CD30, and usually CD15, in Hodgkinlike cells in concert with a B-cell program that includes at least several B-lineage markers.[26] Such cases had been designated as gray zone lymphomas, and are referred to in the 2008 World Health Organization classification as

Fig. 7. Hodgkinlike cells in angioim-
munoblastic T-cell lymphoma. (*A*)
Hematoxylin and eosin. (*B*) CD30.
(*C*) CD15.

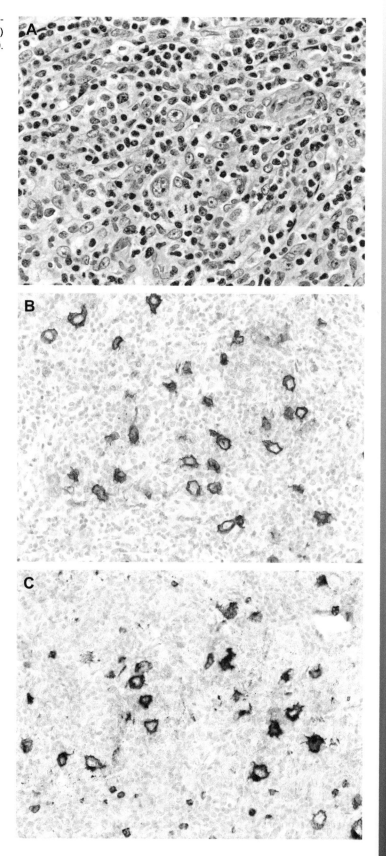

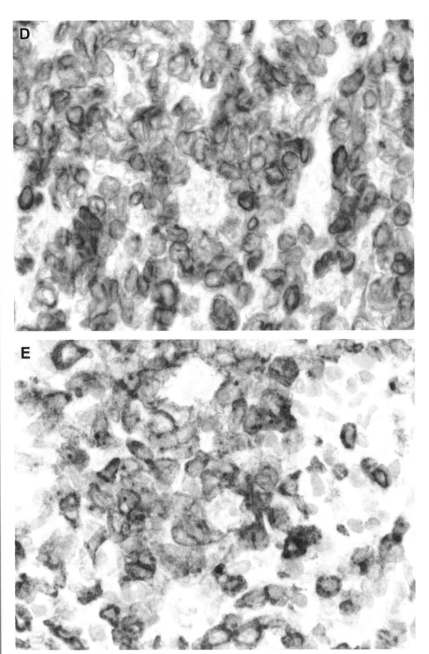

Fig. 7. (continued). Hodgkinlike cells in angioimmunoblastic T-cell lymphoma. (*D*) CD3. (*E*) CD10. The phenotype is indistinguishable from true classical Hodgkin cells.

B-cell lymphoma, unclassifiable, with features intermediate between diffuse large B-cell lymphoma and classical Hodgkin lymphoma. These cases usually, but not exclusively, occur in the mediastinum, and may be intermediate forms in a biologic continuum between mediastinal (thymic) large B-cell lymphoma and classical Hodgkin lymphoma.

In the final analysis, the major difficulty in the immunophenotypic diagnosis of classical Hodgkin lymphoma is probably not the variable expression of different markers on Hodgkin cells, but the difficulty in assessing true antigen expression on the rare Hodgkin cells in a sea of reactive lymphoid cells in a given case. This is particularly difficult in small-needle core biopsy specimens, such as are commonly obtained in the mediastinum. This is no doubt reflected in the conflicting studies reporting widely differing incidences of various antigens in Hodgkin lymphoma, particularly of antigens expressed in directly adjacent cells (eg, CD45 and CD3) or

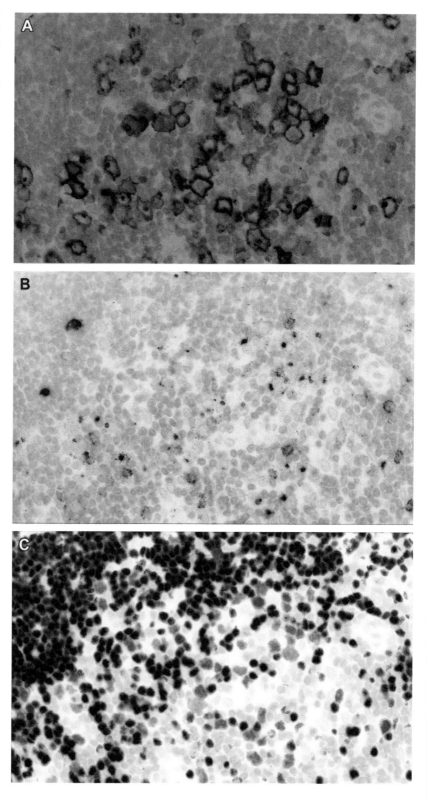

Fig. 8. Classical Hodgkin lymphoma, showing staining of 9 antibodies in a single section, by Multi-Omyx, ensuring the CD30-positive cells are the ones evaluated in the other sections. (*A*) CD30. (*B*) CD15. (*C*) PAX-5.

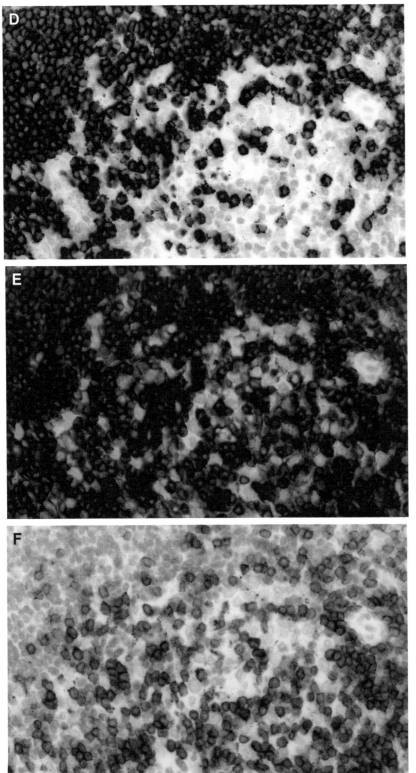

Fig. 8. (continued). Classical Hodgkin lymphoma, showing staining of 9 antibodies in a single section, by Multi-Omyx, ensuring the CD30-positive cells are the ones evaluated in the other sections. (D) CD20. (E) CD45. (F) CD3.

Fig. 8. (continued). Classical Hodgkin lymphoma, showing staining of 9 antibodies in a single section, by Multi-Omyx, ensuring the CD30-positive cells are the ones evaluated in the other sections (*G*) CD79a. (*H*) BOB.1. (*I*) OCT-2.

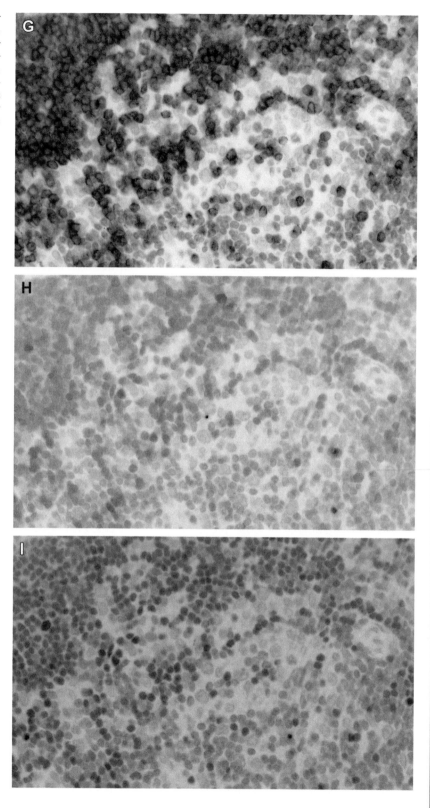

antigens expressed in CD30+ immunoblasts (eg, CD20 and other B-lineage markers) or histiocytes (eg, CD15). This problem may be potentially addressed in the near future, with the development of multiplex staining protocols that allow assessment of multiple markers at the same time.[27] In one such platform, MultiOmyx (Clarient Diagnostic Services, Inc., Aliso Viejo, CA), 9 common Hodgkin markers can be assessed either serially or in combination on a single section (**Fig. 8**).

REFERENCES

1. Chang KL, Arber DA, Weiss LM. CD30: a review. Appl Immunohistochem 1993;1:244–55.
2. Nathwani BN, Krishnan AY, Huang Q, et al. Persistence of CD30 expression in Hodgkin lymphoma following brentuximab vedotin (SGN-35) treatment failure. Leuk Lymphoma 2012;53:2051–3.
3. Arber DA, Weiss LM. CD15: a review. Appl Immunohistochem 1993;1:17–30.
4. Torlakovic E, Torlakovic G, Nguyen PL, et al. The value of anti-pax-5 immunostaining in routinely fixed and paraffin-embedded sections: a novel pan pre-B and B-cell marker. Am J Surg Pathol 2002;26:104–14.
5. Weiss LM, Arber DA, Chang KL. CD45: a review. Appl Immunohistochem 1993;1:166–81.
6. Chang KL, Arber DA, Weiss LM. CD20: a review. Appl Immunohistochem 1996;4:1–15.
7. Rassidakis GZ, Medeiros LJ, Viviani S, et al. CD20 expression in Hodgkin and Reed-Sternberg cells of classical Hodgkin's disease: associations with presenting features and clinical outcome. J Clin Oncol 2002;20:1278–87.
8. Portlock CS, Donnelly GB, Qin J, et al. Adverse prognostic significance of CD20 positive Reed-Sternberg cells in classical Hodgkin's disease. Br J Haematol 2004;125:701–8.
9. Korkolopoulou P, Cordell J, Jones M, et al. The expression of the B-cell marker mb-1 (CD79a) in Hodgkin's disease. Histopathology 1994;24:511–5.
10. Stein H, Marafioti T, Foss HD, et al. Down-regulation of BOB.1/OBF.1 and Oct2 in classical Hodgkin disease but not in lymphocyte predominant Hodgkin disease correlates with immunoglobulin transcription. Blood 2001;97:496–501.
11. Garcia-Cosio M, Santon A, Martin P, et al. Analysis of transcription factor OCT.1, OCT.2 and BOB.1 expression using tissue arrays in classical Hodgkin's lymphoma. Mod Pathol 2004;17:1531–8.
12. Carbone A, Gloghini A, Aldinucci D, et al. Expression pattern of MUM1/IRF4 in the spectrum of pathology of Hodgkin's disease. Br J Haematol 2002;117:366–72.
13. Pinkus GS, Pinkus JL, Langhoff E, et al. Fascin, a sensitive new marker for Reed-Sternberg cells of Hodgkin's disease. Evidence for a dendritic or B cell derivation? Am J Surg Pathol 1997;150:543–62.
14. Carbone A, Gloghini A, Volpe R. Paraffin section immunohistochemistry in the diagnosis of Hodgkin's disease and anaplastic large cell (CD30+) lymphomas. Virchows Arch A Pathol Anat Histopathol 1992;420:527–32.
15. Rezk SA, Weiss LM. Epstein-Barr virus-associated lymphoproliferative disorders. Hum Pathol 2007;38:1293–304.
16. Bai M, Panoulas V, Papoudou-Bai A, et al. B-cell differentiation immunophenotypes in classical Hodgkin lymphomas. Leuk Lymphoma 2006;47:495–501.
17. Cibull ML, Stein H, Gatter KC, et al. The expression of the CD3 antigen in Hodgkin's disease. Histopathology 1989;15:599–605.
18. Dallenbach FE, Stein H. Expression of T-cell-receptor Â·chain in Reed-Sternberg cells. Lancet 1989;2:828–30.
19. Quintanilla-Martinez L, Fend F, Moguel LR, et al. Peripheral T-cell lymphoma with Reed-Sternberg-like cells of B-cell phenotype and genotype associated with Epstein-Barr virus infection. Am J Surg Pathol 1999;23:1233–40.
20. Nicolae A, Pittaluga S, Venkataraman G, et al. Peripheral T-cell lymphomas of follicular T-helper cell derivation with Hodgkin/Reed-Sternberg cells of B-cell lineage: both EBV-positive and EBV-negative variants exist. Am J Surg Pathol 2013;37:816–26.
21. Moroch J, Copie-Bergman C, de LL, et al. Follicular peripheral T-cell lymphoma expands the spectrum of classical Hodgkin lymphoma mimics. Am J Surg Pathol 2012;36:1636–46.
22. Arber DA, Weiss LM. CD43: a review. Appl Immunohistochem 1993;1:88–96.
23. Asano N, Kinoshita T, Tamaru J, et al. Cytotoxic molecule-positive classical Hodgkin's lymphoma: a clinicopathological comparison with cytotoxic molecule-positive peripheral T-cell lymphoma of not otherwise specified type. Haematologica 2011;96:1636–43.
24. Momose H, Jaffe ES, Shin SS, et al. Chronic lymphocytic leukemia/small lymphocytic lymphoma with Reed-Sternberg-like cells and possible transformation to Hodgkin's disease. Mediation by Epstein-Barr virus. Am J Surg Pathol 1992;16:859–67.
25. Pitman S, Huang Q, Zuppan C, et al. Hodgkin lymphoma-like posttransplant lymphoproliferative disorder (HL-like PTLD) simulates monomorphic B-cell PTLD both clinically and pathologically. Am J Surg Pathol 2006;30:470–6.
26. Traverse-Glehen A, Pittaluga S, Gaulard P, et al. Mediastinal gray zone lymphoma: the missing link between classic Hodgkin's lymphoma and mediastinal large B-cell lymphoma. Am J Surg Pathol 2005;29:1411–21.
27. Gerdes MJ, Sevinsky CJ, Sood A, et al. High-order, multiplexed, quantitative, in situ, single cell analysis of cancer tissue. Proc Natl Acad Sci U S A 2013;110(29):11982–7.

Blastic Plasmacytoid Dendritic Cell Neoplasm
How do You Distinguish It from Acute Myeloid Leukemia?

Kaaren K. Reichard, MD

KEYWORDS

• Blastic • Plasmacytoid • Dendritic • CD123 • Leukemia • Myeloid • Cutis • Monocytic

ABSTRACT

BPDCN is a recently elucidated clinicopathologic entity. This disease typically involves the skin, with 30% to 40% of patients showing an additional concurrent leukemic component. Although BPDCN often exhibits cytologic features akin to acute lymphoblastic leukemia, the main differential diagnostic challenge, in the skin and in the bone marrow, is distinction from AML, in particular AML with monocytic differentiation.

Abbreviations: Blastic Plasmacytoid Dendritic Cell Neoplasm	
AML	Acute myeloid leukemia
BPDCN	Blastic plasmacytoid dendritic cell neoplasm
EBER	Epstein-Barr virus RNA-encoded molecules
MPO	Myeloperoxidase
NK	Natural killer
pDC	Plasmacytoid dendritic cell
TdT	Terminal deoxynucleotidyl transferase
T-LL	T-cell lymphoblastic leukemia/lymphoma

OVERVIEW

Blastic plasmacytoid dendritic cell neoplasm (BPDCN) is a recently elucidated clinicopathologic entity, heretofore known as CD4+ CD56+ hematodermic neoplasm and blastic NK-cell lymphoma.[1–6] The designation BPDCN stems from functional studies that demonstrated biologic similarities of the constituent cells of BPDCN with plasmacytoid dendritic cell (pDC) precursors.[1,6–10] This disease typically involves the skin, with 30% to 40% of patients showing an additional concurrent leukemic component. BPDCN behaves in a clinically aggressive fashion in adults and has been classified in the category of acute myeloid leukemia (AML) and related precursor neoplasms by the World Health Organization.[1] Although BPDCN often exhibits cytologic features akin to acute lymphoblastic leukemia, the main differential diagnostic challenge, in the skin and in the bone marrow, is distinction from AML, in particular, AML with monocytic differentiation. This distinction is critical because conventional chemotherapy is typically inadequate for the treatment of BPDCN in adults.[2,4,5,11] Recent studies suggest that stem cell transplantation may be indicated to provide a more durable response.[12–16] In contrast,

Disclosure: The author has no relevant financial or other conflicts to disclose.
Division of Hematopathology, Mayo Clinic, 200 1st Street Southwest, Hilton Building 8th Floor, Rochester, MN 55902, USA
E-mail address: reichard.kaaren@mayo.edu

Surgical Pathology 6 (2013) 743–765
http://dx.doi.org/10.1016/j.path.2013.08.010
1875-9181/13/$ – see front matter © 2013 Elsevier Inc. All rights reserved.

surgpath.theclinics.com

Pathologic Key Features
OF BPDCN

Clinical presentation

- Asymptomatic, single or multiple cutaneous nodules, patches/plaques, and/or bruise-like lesions
- 20% Involvement of regional lymph nodes
- Variable involvement of peripheral blood and bone marrow at diagnosis; >90% leukemic involvement at relapse

Cytology

- Intermediate cells with blastic chromatin, inconspicuous nucleoli, and scant cytoplasm (lymphoblast-like)
- Occasional myeloblast-like: larger size, 1 or more prominent nucleoli, abundant cytoplasm
- Circumferential nuclear rimming by vacuoles (pearl necklace appearance)
- Pseudopod cytoplasmic extensions

Morphology

- Skin: if minimal involvement, periadnexal and perivascular infiltrate; if dense involvement, diffuse dermal infiltrate with minimal epidermal component
- Bone marrow: interstitial, nodular, or diffuse infiltrate
- Lymph node: paracortical expansion

Immunophenotypic profile

- Positivity for CD4, CD56, CD45RA, CD123, HLA-DR, BDCA-2, TCL1, BDCA-4, CD2AP, terminal deoxynucleotidyl transferase (TdT) (50% of cases)
- Negative for myeloperoxidase (MPO) and nonspecific esterase/butyrate esterase cytochemical stains
- Negative for lysozyme and CD11c; associated with monocytic differentiation
- Negative CD34/CD117 (immature markers)
- Negative for CD3 (excludes T-cell lineage)
- Negative for CD19, CD20, and cytoplasmic CD79a (excludes B-cell lineage)
- Negative for Epstein-Barr virus (excludes NK/T-cell malignancy)

Genetics

- Nonspecific abnormalities
- Large genomic losses, including 5q, 12p, 13q, 6q, and chromosome 9
- Loss of *CDKN1B* and *CDKN2A*
- *TET2* and *TP53* mutations

long-term successful eradication of the disease in children may be more readily achieved with high-risk combination cytotoxic therapies.[17]

CLINICAL FEATURES

The clinical features of BPDCN are largely attributable to the manifestations of cutaneous involvement.[18–20] The skin lesions in BPDCN consist of bruise-like patches and tumor nodules that may be single or multiple. Affected regions of the body often include the face and scalp followed by the trunk and limbs. A subset of patients presents with more diffuse disease composed of a combination of nodules and patches.[18,19] The diffuse presentation is typically what alerts an examining physician to the possibility of BPDCN. Disseminated cutaneous disease is most likely to correlate with concurrent leukemic involvement.[19]

MICROSCOPIC FEATURES

BPDCN, also known as hematodermic neoplasm, characteristically shows involvement of the skin and/or peripheral blood and bone marrow. Any tissue type may be infiltrated, however, ranging from sites, such as lymph nodes and spleen, to rarer tissues, like the nasopharynx, uterus, and ovaries.

In the skin, BPDCN often shows a diffuse dermal infiltrate with rare involvement of the epidermis. With less advanced lesions, the infiltrates are sparsely cellular and may exhibit a perivascular and periadnexal pattern (**Figs. 1** and **2**). Regardless of the infiltrative pattern, the tumor cells are predominantly medium in size with dispersed chromatin, irregular nuclear contours, variably prominent nucleoli, and inconspicuous mitoses. When the infiltrates are sparse, the initial identification of the neoplastic cells and/or a neoplastic process in general may be problematic and result in a delay in diagnosis.

In the peripheral blood and bone marrow, the tumor cells of BPDCN often demonstrate lymphoblast-like cytology: medium-sized cells with round to slightly irregular nuclei, inconspicuous nucleoli, and scant cytoplasm lacking granules or Auer rods (**Figs. 3–5**). Less frequently, BPDCN cells exhibit features akin to myeloid blasts, such as larger overall cell size, 1 or more prominent nucleoli, and more abundant cytoplasm (**Figs. 6** and **7**). On occasion, the cells of BPDCN show a tadpole-like appearance with a unipolar extension of cytoplasm (see **Fig. 5**). This finding is, however, nonspecific and may be seen in a variety of acute leukemias. The neoplastic cells may also show a unique feature characterized by a circumferential ring of evenly sized vacuoles around the nucleus, the so-called pearl necklace. The extent of bone marrow involvement by BPDCN varies, ranging from morphologically occult and subtle interstitial infiltrates requiring ancillary techniques for identification to overt nodular collections of tumor cells and marrow effacement (**Fig. 8**).[21]

When BPDCN involves lymph nodes, the cytologic features are similar to those described for the skin and bone marrow. BPDCN commonly demonstrates a paracortical infiltration pattern (**Figs. 9–12**). Splenic involvement by BPDCN shows prominent red pulp and sinusoidal infiltrates (**Figs. 13** and **14**).

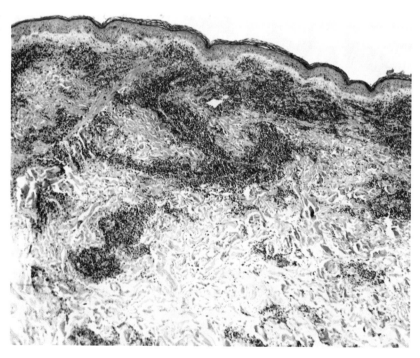

Fig. 1. Cutaneous involvement by BPDCN exhibiting a periadnexal and perivascular infiltration pattern. This corresponds clinically to a patch-like lesion (skin, hematoxylin-eosin, original magnification ×20).

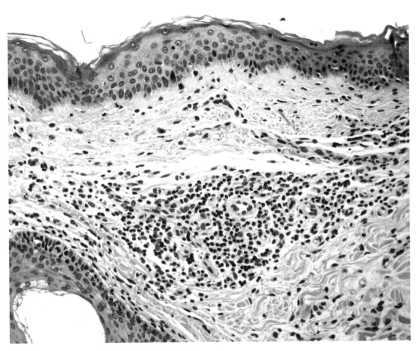

Fig. 2. Early cutaneous involvement by BPDCN demonstrates a histologically bland, mature lymphocyte-like infiltrate that can be easily missed initially. Clinically, this may appear as a bruise-like lesion in the skin. A high index of clinical suspicion is often the first clue to the diagnosis (skin, hematoxylin-eosin, original magnification ×100).

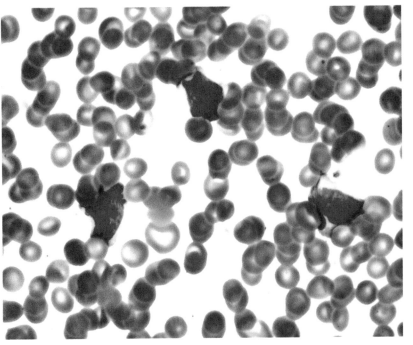

Fig. 3. Leukemic involvement by BPDCN often demonstrates a lymphoblast-like cytology. The cells are small to intermediate with inconspicuous nucleoli and scant cytoplasm (peripheral blood, Wright-Giemsa, original magnification ×100).

Fig. 4. The cytologic appearance of BDPCN is often lymphoblast-like characterized by small to medium-sized cells with blastic chromatin, inconspicuous nucleoli, and scant cytoplasm, which is devoid of granules (bone marrow aspirate, Wright-Giemsa, ×100 oil).

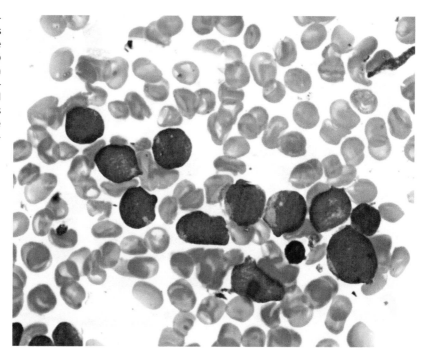

Fig. 5. In this case of BPDCN involving the bone marrow, not only do the cells exhibit the typical lymphoblast-like cytology (small to medium-sized cells with blastic chromatin, inconspicuous nucleoli, and scant cytoplasm, which is devoid of granules) but also they show pseudopod cytoplasmic extensions (bone marrow aspirate, Wright-Giemsa, ×100).

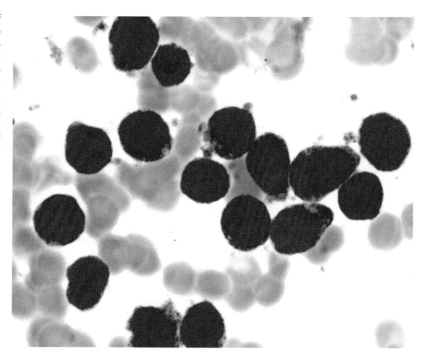

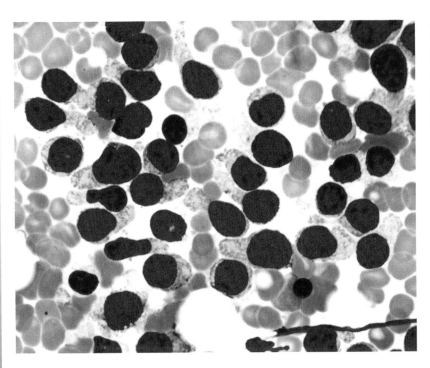

Fig. 6. The cells of BDPCN may show cytologic features more akin to immature myeloid cells as in this case with overall slightly larger cell size and more abundant cytoplasm (bone marrow aspirate, Wright-Giemsa, ×100 oil).

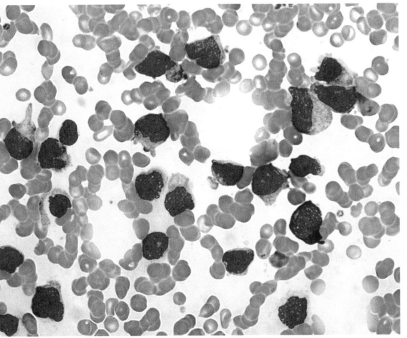

Fig. 7. The cells of BPDCN exhibit a striking resemblance to monocytic cells in this example with large cell size, an occasional prominent nucleolus, abundant lightly basophilic cytoplasm, and variably indented nuclear contours (bone marrow aspirate, Wright-Giemsa, ×100 oil).

Fig. 8. BPDCN may involve the bone marrow in a subtle, nodular, interstitial, or diffuse pattern. In this example, the cells diffusely involve the bone marrow clot section with only an occasional megakaryocyte remaining. The cells of BPDCN are lymphoid-like with small to intermediate in size with scant cytoplasm and open chromatin (bone marrow clot section, hematoxylin-eosin, original magnification ×100).

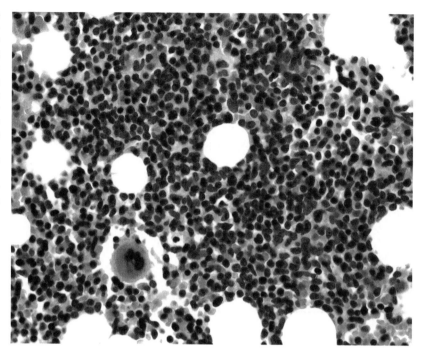

Fig. 9. BPDCN involves lymph nodes in a paracortical distribution pattern and shows a monotonous proliferation of blastic cells with scattered tangible-body macrophages (lymph node, hematoxylin-eosin, original magnification ×10).

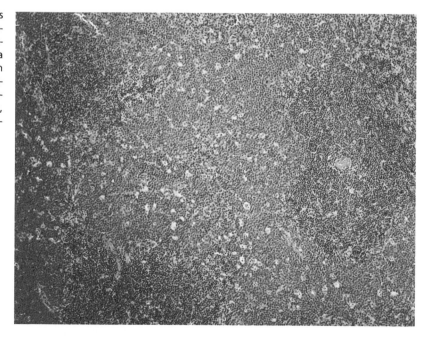

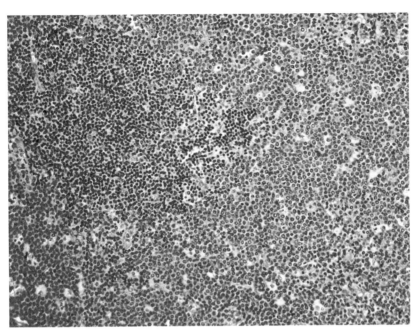

Fig. 10. Paracortical expansion of a lymph node involved by BPDCN. The cells of BPDCN are intermediate in size, with round to slightly indented nuclear contours, open chromatin, inconspicuous nucleoli, and scant cytoplasm in contrast to typical small, mature lymphocytes (*upper left*) (lymph node, hematoxylin-eosin, original magnification ×20).

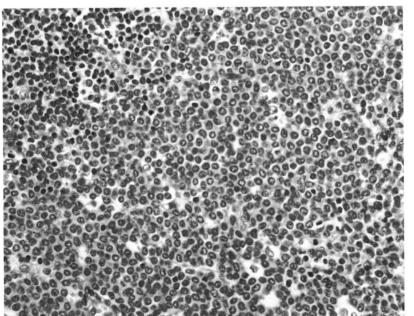

Fig. 11. The cells of BPDCN are intermediate in size, with round to slightly indented nuclear contours, open chromatin, inconspicuous nucleoli, and scant cytoplasm in contrast to typical small, mature lymphocytes (*upper left*) (lymph node, hematoxylin-eosin, original magnification ×60).

Fig. 12. The cells of BPDCN are intermediate in size, with round to slightly indented nuclear contours, open chromatin, inconspicuous nucleoli and scant cytoplasm (*upper left*) (lymph node, hematoxylin-eosin, original magnification ×100).

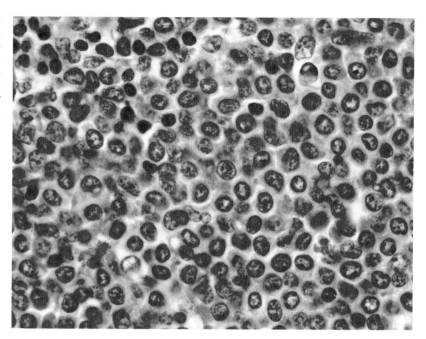

Fig. 13. Splenic red pulp infiltration by BPDCN in this case of a patient presenting with cytopenias and splenomegaly (spleen, hematoxylin-eosin, original magnification ×20).

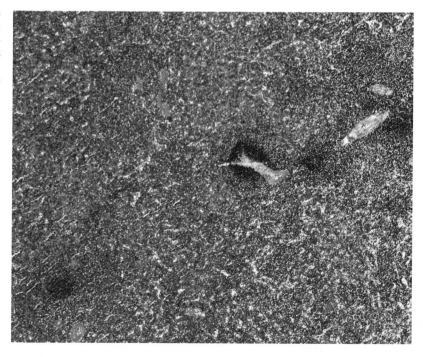

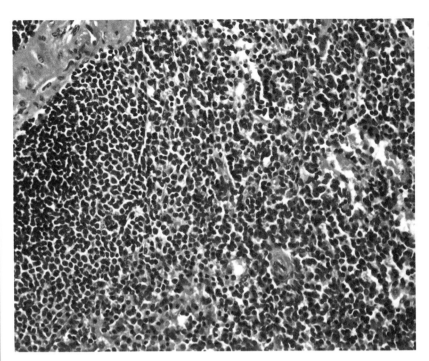

Fig. 14. The cells of BPDCN bear somewhat of a resemblance to lymphocytes (*upper left*) although they are slightly larger in size with more open chromatin (spleen, hematoxylin-eosin, original magnification ×60).

DIAGNOSIS

Establishing a diagnosis of BPDCN requires a multifaceted approach, including histopathologic examination and a thorough immunophenotypic and cytochemical assessment. Given that a majority of cases of BPDCN do not present with a leukemic component (which yields tumor cells readily amenable for multiparametric flow cytometric evaluation), a broad repertoire of immunohistochemical antibodies is available for use in paraffin-embedded tissue specimens. An extensive immunophenotypic panel is needed to diagnose BPDCN for at least 3 reasons: it is a rare entity, it is a diagnosis of exclusion, and many of the markers positive in BPDCN are not individually specific for this entity (see **Pitfalls box**).

The classic immunophenotypic profile for BPDCN is CD4+, CD56+, lineage negative, CD43+, HLA-DR+, CD45RA+, TCL1+, CD123+, BDCA2+, and CD2AP+ (**Figs. 15–22**B).[1,3,5,11,22–27] Many of these markers may be assessed by both immunohistochemical and flow cytometric methods. *Lineage negative* refers to absence of markers diagnostic of B-cell, T-cell, natural killer (NK)-cell, or myeloid derivation (for a list of typical lineage-associated antigens, see **Pathologic Key Features of BPDCN box**). Aside from TdT, markers of immaturity/blasts (eg, CD34 and CD117) are absent. TdT expression is seen in

approximately 50% of cases of BPDCN but shows a unique staining pattern compared with classic acute lymphoblastic leukemia in that it is patchy with weak and variable nuclear positivity (**Fig. 23**). Cytochemical stains for MPO and nonspecific esterase/butyrate esterase are negative, and cytoplasmic nucleophosmin is absent.[28] The intracytoplasmic detection of TCL1 by flow cytometry may be a helpful diagnostic criterion.[29]

Other recently described markers of potential diagnostic significance in BPDCN include SP1B, BDCA-4, CD2AP, and BAD-LAMP.[24,25,30–33] SP1B is expressed among a variety of B-cell and T-cell lymphomas but seems absent in cutaneous mimickers of BPDCN.[32] CD2AP seems exclusively expressed in pDCs. BDCA-4 (also known as neuropilin 1) is expressed on normal pDCs and BPDCN.

Expression of myeloid (eg, CD33) or T-cell (CD2 and CD7)–associated markers is not uncommon in BPDCN and should not result in a misdiagnosis of AML or T lymphoblastic leukemia (T-LL) given that the remainder of the immunohistochemical profile is in keeping with BPDCN.[1,3,34,35] CD22 expression (antibody S-HCL 1) has been documented on normal pDCs and their neoplasms.[36] In addition, other deviations from the typical BPDCN immunophenotypic profile of BPDCN, such as lack of CD56 expression, are well documented in the literature.

Fig. 15. BPDCN cells are uniformly positive for CD4 as part of the typical immunophenotypical profile for BPDCN (bone marrow clot section, CD4 immunohistochemistry ×100).

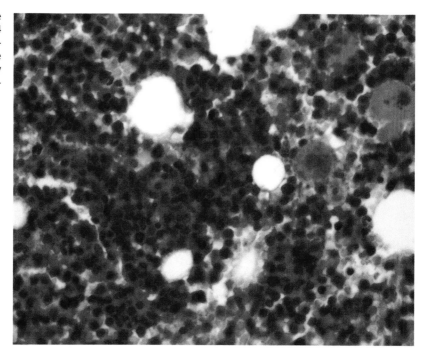

Fig. 16. BPDCN cells are positive for CD56 as part of the typical immunophenotypical profile for BPDCN (bone marrow clot section, CD56 immunohistochemistry ×100).

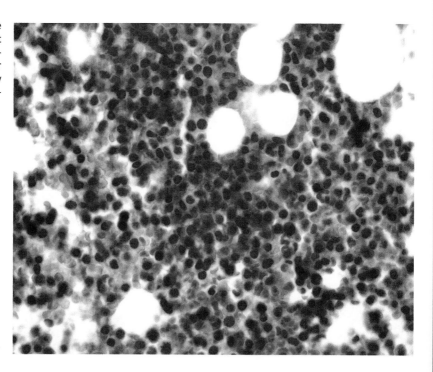

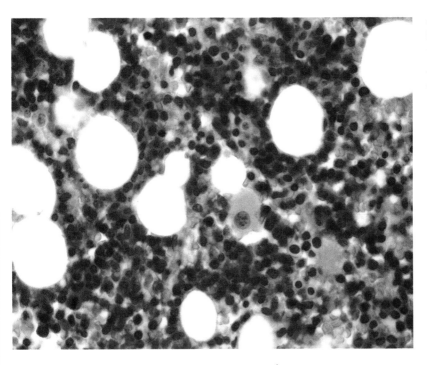

Fig. 17. BPDCN cells are positive for CD123 as part of the typical immunophenotypical profile for BPDCN (bone marrow clot section, CD123 immunohistochemistry ×100).

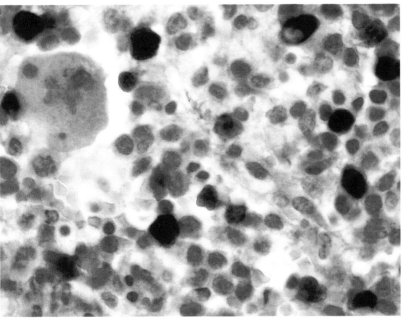

Fig. 18. This clot section involved by BPDCN illustrates a lack of expression of the myeloid-associated marker MPO in the tumor cells. A few positively staining background granulocytes are noted (bone marrow clot section, MPO immunohistochemistry ×100).

Fig. 19. This clot section involved by BPDCN illustrates a lack of expression of the monocytic-associated marker lysozyme in the tumor cells. A few positively staining background monocytes are noted (bone marrow clot section, lysozyme immunohistochemistry ×100).

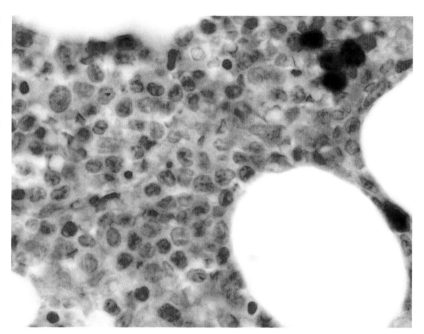

Fig. 20. CD123 highlights the tumor cells of BPDCN in the spleen. Although CD123 is not specific for BPDCN, the remaining immunophenotypic features (not shown) of positivity for CD4, CD56, TCL1, and negative for markers of B-cell, T-cell, NK-cell, and myeloid/monocytic leukemia confirm the diagnosis (spleen, CD123 immunohistochemistry ×100).

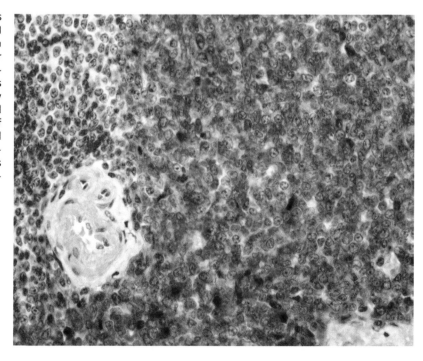

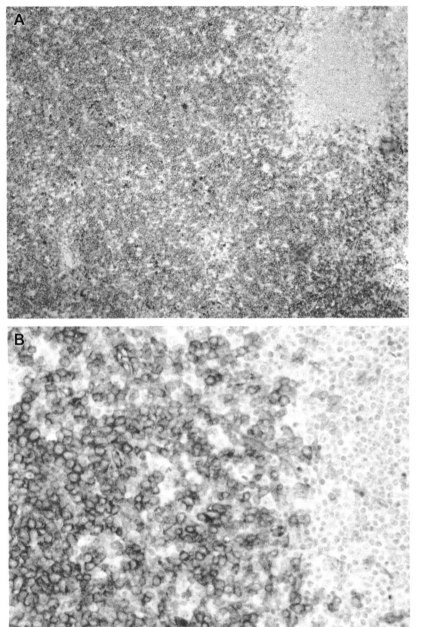

Fig. 21. (*A*; lymph node, CD123 immunohisto- chemistry, original magni- fication ×10, *B*; lymph node, CD123 immuno- histochemistry, original magnification ×40) The cells of BPDCN demon- strate membrane positiv- ity for CD123.

Fig. 22. (*A, B*) The cells of BPDCN demonstrate uniform nuclear and cytoplasmic positivity for TCL1 (lymph node, TCL1 immunohistochemistry, original magnification ×10 and ×40).

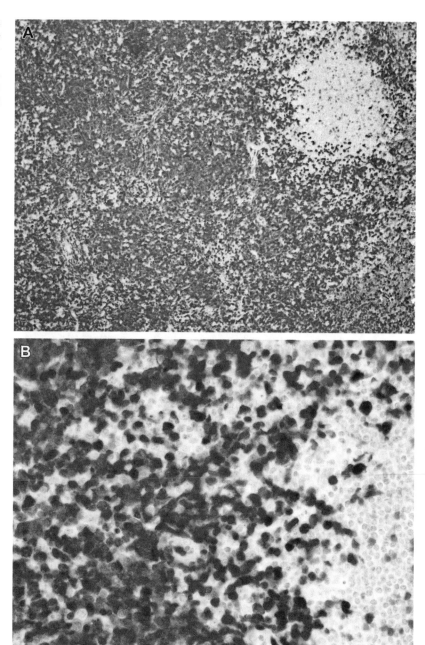

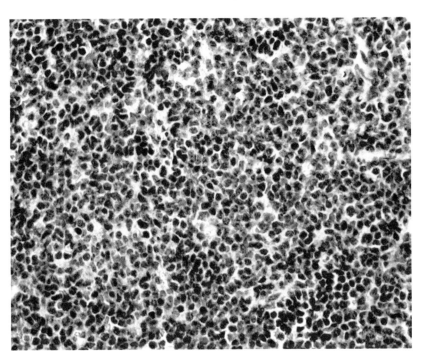

Fig. 23. BPDCN shows variable weak nuclear positivity for TdT in approximately 50% of cases. This pattern contrasts with that of acute lymphoblastic leukemia, which shows uniform TdT positivity (lymph node, TdT immunohistochemistry, original magnification ×100).

These potential antigenic pitfalls should not result in a misdiagnosis if the complete immunophenotypic and cytochemical panel is performed. Ultimately, this panel excludes myeloid/monocytic and T-cell malignancy.

The genetic alterations in BPDCN are thus far nonspecific, with a diagnostic recurring abnormality yet to be identified.[37–41] BPDCN cytogenetic aberrations tend to manifest as large losses of genomic material affecting 5q, 12p, 13q, 6q, and chromosome 9.[38] Using array-based comparative genomic hybridization techniques, loss of *RB1* and *LATS2* genes were noted.[37] Losses of *CDKN1B, CDKN2A, TET2*, and *TP53* mutations have been reported.[42] Biallelic deletions of the 9p21.3 loci involving *CDKN2A/CDKN2B* affect the G1/S segment of the cell cycle and may play a significant role in the pathogenesis of this disease.[39] The *MYD88* L265P mutation, commonly associated with lymphoplasmacytic lymphoma, seems absent in BPDCN.[43,44]

DIFFERENTIAL DIAGNOSIS

The differential diagnostic considerations for BPDCN range from acute leukemia, myeloid and lymphoid types, and myeloid sarcoma/leukemia cutis to NK/T-cell lymphoma/leukemia, blastic mantle cell lymphoma and other high-grade lymphomas, to collections of pDCs in association with a chronic myeloid malignancy or reactive

conditions. This differential diagnosis is based on cytologic and/or immunophenotypic similarity to BPDCN (discussed later). Distinguishing these various entities from BPDCN is important for therapeutic management and prognostic reasons. Recognition of the immunophenotypic overlap of many of the markers seen in BPDCN with non-BPDCN entities is critical such that 1 or 2 positive antigens or a small panel of markers do not result in a misdiagnosis.

Almost certainly the most challenging entity to distinguish from BPDCN is AML/monocytic leukemia and myeloid sarcoma/myeloid leukemia cutis (**Figs. 24–26**). Several independent research studies have shown, however, that a panel of immunohistochemical antibodies, in conjunction with cytochemical stains, may serve as a reliable discriminator of BPDCN from its mimics.[3,5,22,45–47] The immunophenotypic overlap between BPDCN and monocytic leukemia and MPO-negative myeloid sarcoma in particular is well-known because both entities may express CD33, CD4, CD56, and HLA-DR and lack expression of CD34 and CD117. The cytochemical detection of nonspecific esterase and/or monocyte-associated markers (CD36/CD64 coexpression, lysozyme, and CD14) is helpful in the identification of monocytic leukemia. A panel showing tumor cells positive for CD4, CD56, CD123, and TCL1 seems indicative of a diagnosis of BPDCN in this scenario. CD123 as an isolated marker is not

Fig. 24. A low-power view of myeloid leukemia cutis demonstrates morphologic overlap with BPDCN given its nodular and perivascular pattern (hematoxylin-eosin, ×10 magnification).

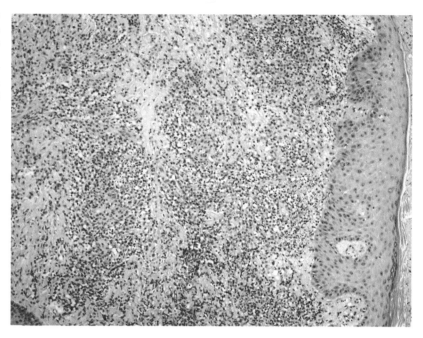

helpful in distinguishing AML from BPDCN because it is expressed on a significant number of AMLs.[48,49] Although many phenotypic markers may need to be performed, the final immunohistochemical panel, when BPDCN remains a diagnostic consideration, should include at least MPO, lysozyme, CD4, CD56, CD123, and TCL1. B-cell, T-cell, NK-cell, and cytochemical studies for MPO and nonspecific esterase and immature markers should be performed.

Differentiation of B-cell lymphoblastic leukemia/lymphoma and T-cell lymphoblastic

Fig. 25. A medium-power view of myeloid leukemia cutis may resemble BPDCN with intermediate-sized cells, blastic chromatin, and variably prominent nucleoli (hematoxylin-eosin, magnification ×40).

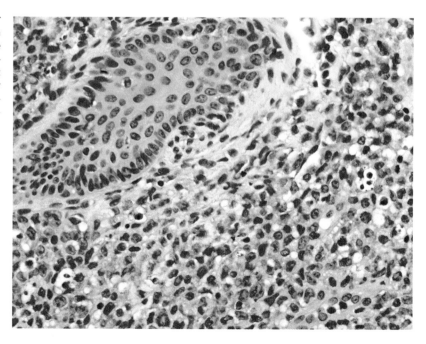

leukemia/lymphoma (T-LL) from BPDCN is generally straightforward with a typical immunophenotypic assessment (**Fig. 27**). BPDCN does not express B-lineage–associated markers, such as CD19 and CD20. Cytoplasmic CD22 has been described in one case of BPDCN.[36] Although T-LL may share some phenotypic similarities with BPDCN, such as expression of CD4, CD2, and TdT, expression of CD3 and a more complete repertoire of T-cell markers is absent. The pattern of TdT expression in BPDCN is different from T-LL in that it is patchy and weak rather than of uniform intensity.

Nonacute clinicopathologic entities that may exhibit a blastic appearance (eg, high-grade lymphoma and myeloma) are generally readily distinguished from BPDCN based on their antigen expression pattern indicating B-cell, T-cell or plasma cell lineage. Furthermore, these blastic mimickers are not expected to show positivity for all of the BPDCN markers, CD4, CD56, CD123, and TCL1. B-cell lymphomas express several B-cell markers (eg, CD19, CD20, and PAX5) and often show surface or cytoplasmic light chain restriction. T-cell lymphomas express a various admixture of T-cell markers, including CD3; typically, a clonal T-cell receptor gene rearrangement is detectable. Blastic mantle cell lymphoma expresses cyclin D1. Plasma cell myeloma, which is often CD56 positive and rarely CD4 positive, may potentially mimic BPDCN. The neoplastic tumor cells, however, demonstrate CD138 and bright CD38 positivity and cytoplasmic light chain restriction, unlike BPDCN. The author has seen one case of myeloma that not only expressed CD123 in a subset of the tumor cells but also showed tadpole-like cytology (**Fig. 28**). NK/T-cell lymphomas/leukemias express Epstein-Barr virus RNA-encoded molecules (EBER).

Collections of pDCs may pose a diagnostic challenge with BPDCN. Nodules of pDCs occur in a variety of neoplastic and non-neoplastic scenarios, perhaps the most well regarded are chronic myelomonocytic leukemia and Kikuchi-Fujimoto lymphadenitis.[9,50–54] These pDC aggregates show a similar immunophenotypic expression profile to BPDCN; however, less often they show CD56 positivity. Distinction of pDC nodules from BPDCN does not generally pose a significant diagnostic dilemma due to the known associated pathologic conditions, lack of architectural effacement, and absence of a typical hematodermic clinical presentation.

ΔΔ
Differential Diagnosis
BPDCN DIFFERENTIAL DIAGNOSTIC CONSIDERATIONS

Differential Diagnosis	Possible Overlap With BPDCN	Features Helpful to Distinguish from BPDCN
AML with monocytic differentiation/myeloid sarcoma	CD4+, CD56+, CD123+, CD33+, CD2+, CD3−	CD36/CD64+, lysozyme+, cytochemical butyrate esterase+ in monocytic leukemias, TdT−, TCL1−
Myeloid leukemia cutis	CD4+, CD56+, CD123+, CD33+	MPO+, uniform CD4+/CD56+/CD123+/TCL1+ not seen, CD34+
pDC nodules in chronic myelomonocytic leukemia, other conditions	CD4+, CD68+	Lack of blastic cytology, lack of tissue effacement often CD56− and TdT−
B lymphoblastic leukemia	Cytology, TdT+	Expression of B-cell markers, CD34+, CD10+, B-cell receptor gene rearrangement+
T lymphoblastic leukemia	CD2+, CD7+, TdT+, and cytology	Expression of cytoplasmic/surface CD3, T-cell receptor gene rearrangement+, generally strong expression of CD2, CD5, and/or CD7, CD1A+
Aggressive NK/T-cell lymphoma	CD56+, CD2+	EBER+
Plasma cell myeloma	CD56+, CD4+, CD34−	CD138+, CD38 bright+, and cytoplasmic immunoglobulin restriction

Data from Refs.[3,10,18,26,35,45–47,50,53,54]

Fig. 26. A high-power view of myeloid leukemia cutis reveals morphologic similarity to some cases of BPDCN with inter-mediate-sized cells, blastic chromatin, and variably prominent nucleoli. A stra-tegic immunohistochem-ical assessment is most useful in distinguishing the two entities (hematox-ylin-eosin, magnification ×100).

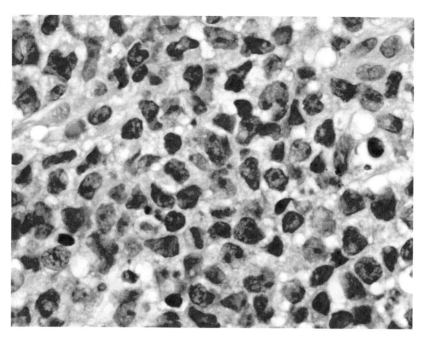

PROGNOSIS

The overall prognosis in BPDCN treated with conventional chemotherapeutic regimens is poor. In the adult population, there is often an initial adequate tumor response to acute leukemia–like therapy, but relapse is inevitable, resulting in a median survival of approximately 12 to 14 months.[1,12,55–58] Because of the rarity of BPDCN, no optimal standardized therapeutic approach

Fig. 27. B lymphoblastic leukemia/lymphoma cutis is morphologically indis-tinguishable from other cutaneous infiltrative blas-tic processes. Immunophe-notypic studies, including positivity for CD19, CD34, and CD10, are useful in arriving at the diagnosis (hematoxylin-eosin, mag-nification ×100).

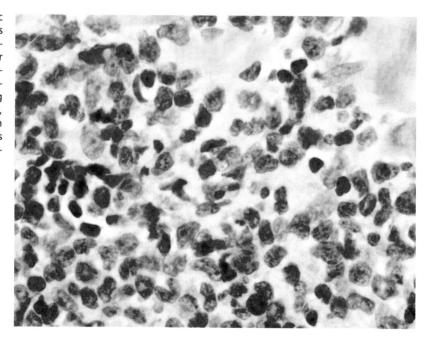

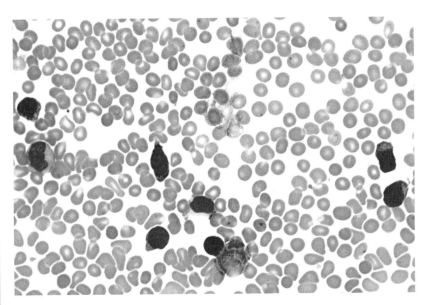

Fig. 28. This bone marrow aspirate shows intermediate-sized cells with reticulated chromatin, scant cytoplasm, and pseudopod cytology in a case of myeloma, which morphologically mimics BPDCN. Additionally, the cells immunophenotypically mimicked BPDCN by expressing CD4, CD56, and CD123 (subset). Further investigation demonstrated uniform CD138 positivity and cytoplasmic κ light chain restriction (bone marrow aspirate, Wright-Giemsa, original magnification ×60).

has yet been realized. Both high-risk acute lymphoblastic leukemia and AML regimens seem incapable of inducing long-term remissions. Recently, it has been shown that high-dose chemotherapy followed by allogeneic stem cell transplantation may induce long-term durable disease control.[12,13,15,59,60]

BPDCN seems less clinically aggressive in the pediatric population compared with in adults.[17] It has been suggested that stem cell transplantation in childhood may be reserved for those patients who relapse and subsequently obtain a second remission. Although it is only a few reported cases, those children with BPDCN who underwent stem cell transplantation achieved an overall survival similar to those who received chemotherapy only. Therefore, to date, there is no significant advantageous benefit to children undergoing initial stem cell transplantation.

Pitfalls

! None of the antigens that constitute the typical BPDCN immunophenotypic profile may be used individually as a diagnostic tool for BPDCN. Many of these markers are normally or abnormally in other cell types and diseases (eg, CD4, T cells, monocytes-macrophages; TCL1A, T-PLL, hairy cell leukemia; CD123, a variety of AMLs, B lymphoblastic leukemia/lymphoma; CD56, NK cells, plasma cell myeloma, aberrant monocytes, subset of AMLs, neuroendocrine/small cell carcinoma; and BDCA-2, normal pDCs).

! Early cutaneous involvement by BPDCN may be clinically nonspecific and histologically sparsely cellular. A subtle perivascular and/or periadnexal pattern by BPDCN associated with an admixed small lymphocyte population may result in a heterogeneous-appearing infiltrate leading to initial diagnostic difficulty.

! Rare cases of BPDCN are CD56 negative.

! Low-level bone marrow involvement by BPDCN may be morphologically undetectable requiring the use of ancillary techniques (eg, immunohistochemistry or flow cytometry) for identification.

! BPDCN is rare and a diagnosis of exclusion. A thorough cytologic and immunophenotypic evaluation is required to exclude more common mimickers.

Data from Refs.[3,5,21,22,48,49,61]

REFERENCES

1. Facchetti F, Jones D, Petrella T. Blastic plasmacytoid dendritic cell neoplasm. In: Swerdlow SH, Ellias C, Harris NL, et al, editors. WHO classification of tumours of haematopoietic and lymphoid tissues. 4th edition. Lyon (France): IARC Press; 2008. p. 145–7.

2. Feuillard J, Jacob MC, Valensi F, et al. Clinical and biologic features of CD4(+)CD56(+) malignancies. Blood 2002;99(5):1556–63.

3. Herling M, Jones D. CD4+/CD56+ hematodermic tumor: the features of an evolving entity and its relationship to dendritic cells. Am J Clin Pathol 2007; 127(5):687–700.

4. Jacob MC, Chaperot L, Mossuz P, et al. CD4+ CD56+ lineage negative malignancies: a new entity developed from malignant early plasmacytoid dendritic cells. Haematologica 2003;88(8):941–55.

5. Petrella T, Bagot M, Willemze R, et al. Blastic NK-cell lymphomas (agranular CD4+CD56+ hematodermic neoplasms): a review. Am J Clin Pathol 2005;123(5):662–75.

6. Petrella T, Comeau MR, Maynadié M, et al. 'Agranular CD4+ CD56+ hematodermic neoplasm' (blastic NK-cell lymphoma) originates from a population of CD56+ precursor cells related to plasmacytoid monocytes. Am J Surg Pathol 2002;26(7):852–62.

7. Chaperot L, Bendriss N, Manches O, et al. Identification of a leukemic counterpart of the plasmacytoid dendritic cells. Blood 2001;97(10):3210–7.

8. Chaperot L, Perrot I, Jacob MC, et al. Leukemic plasmacytoid dendritic cells share phenotypic and functional features with their normal counterparts. Eur J Immunol 2004;34(2):418–26.

9. Jegalian AG, Facchetti F, Jaffe ES. Plasmacytoid dendritic cells: physiologic roles and pathologic states. Adv Anat Pathol 2009;16(6):392–404.

10. Petrella T, Facchetti F. Tumoral aspects of plasmacytoid dendritic cells: what do we know in 2009? Autoimmunity 2010;43(3):210–4.

11. Reichard KK, Burks EJ, Foucar MK, et al. CD4(+) CD56(+) lineage-negative malignancies are rare tumors of plasmacytoid dendritic cells. Am J Surg Pathol 2005;29(10):1274–83.

12. Dalle S, Beylot-Barry M, Bagot M, et al. Blastic plasmacytoid dendritic cell neoplasm: is transplantation the treatment of choice? Br J Dermatol 2010; 162(1):74–9.

13. Dietrich S, Andrulis M, Hegenbart U, et al. Blastic plasmacytoid dendritic cell neoplasia (BPDC) in elderly patients: results of a treatment algorithm employing allogeneic stem cell transplantation with moderately reduced conditioning intensity. Biol Blood Marrow Transplant 2011;17(8):1250–4.

14. Male HJ, Davis MB, McGuirk JP, et al. Blastic plasmacytoid dendritic cell neoplasm should be treated with acute leukemia type induction chemotherapy and allogeneic stem cell transplantation in first remission. Int J Hematol 2010;92(2):398–400.

15. Roos-Weil D, Dietrich S, Boumendil A, et al. Stem cell transplantation can provide durable disease control in blastic plasmacytoid dendritic cell neoplasm: a retrospective study from the European Group for Blood and Marrow Transplantation. Blood 2013;121(3):440–6.

16. Unteregger M, Valentin A, Zinke-Cerwenka W, et al. Unrelated SCT induces long-term remission in patients with blastic plasmacytoid dendritic cell neoplasm. Bone Marrow Transplant 2013;48(6): 799–802.

17. Jegalian AG, Buxbaum NP, Facchetti F, et al. Blastic plasmacytoid dendritic cell neoplasm in children: diagnostic features and clinical implications. Haematologica 2010;95(11):1873–9.

18. Cota C, Vale E, Viana I, et al. Cutaneous manifestations of blastic plasmacytoid dendritic cell neoplasm-morphologic and phenotypic variability in a series of 33 patients. Am J Surg Pathol 2010; 34(1):75–87.

19. Julia F, Petrella T, Beylot-Barry M, et al. Blastic plasmacytoid dentritic cell neoplasm: clinical features in 90 patients. Br J Dermatol 2013;169(3):579–86.

20. Pileri A, Delfino C, Grandi V, et al. Blastic plasmacytoid dendritic cell neoplasm (BPDCN): the cutaneous sanctuary. G Ital Dermatol Venereol 2012; 147(6):603–8.

21. Hwang K, Park CJ, Jang S, et al. Immunohistochemical analysis of CD123, CD56 and CD4 for the diagnosis of minimal bone marrow involvement by blastic plasmacytoid dendritic cell neoplasm. Histopathology 2013;62(5):764–70.

22. Garnache-Ottou F, Feuillard J, Ferrand C, et al. Extended diagnostic criteria for plasmacytoid dendritic cell leukaemia. Br J Haematol 2009;145(5): 624–36.

23. Herling M, Teitell MA, Shen RR, et al. TCL1 expression in plasmacytoid dendritic cells (DC2s) and the related CD4+ CD56+ blastic tumors of skin. Blood 2003;101(12):5007–9.

24. Jaye DL, Geigerman CM, Herling M, et al. Expression of the plasmacytoid dendritic cell marker BDCA-2 supports a spectrum of maturation among CD4+ CD56+ hematodermic neoplasms. Mod Pathol 2006;19(12):1555–62.

25. Marafioti T, Paterson JC, Ballabio E, et al. Novel markers of normal and neoplastic human plasmacytoid dendritic cells. Blood 2008;111(7):3778–92.

26. Petrella T, Meijer CJ, Dalac S, et al. TCL1 and CLA expression in agranular CD4/CD56 hematodermic neoplasms (blastic NK-cell lymphomas) and leukemia cutis. Am J Clin Pathol 2004;122(2):307–13.

27. Pilichowska ME, Fleming MD, Pinkus JL, et al. CD4+/CD56+ hematodermic neoplasm ("blastic

natural killer cell lymphoma"): neoplastic cells express the immature dendritic cell marker BDCA-2 and produce interferon. Am J Clin Pathol 2007; 128(3):445–53.

28. Facchetti F, Pileri SA, Agostinelli C, et al. Cytoplasmic nucleophosmin is not detected in blastic plasmacytoid dendritic cell neoplasm. Haematologica 2009;94(2):285–8.

29. Angelot-Delettre F, Biichle S, Ferrand C, et al. Intracytoplasmic detection of TCL1–but not ILT7–by flow cytometry is useful for blastic plasmacytoid dendritic cell leukemia diagnosis. Cytometry A 2012; 81(8):718–24.

30. Defays A, David A, de Gassart A, et al. BAD-LAMP is a novel biomarker of nonactivated human plasmacytoid dendritic cells. Blood 2011;118(3):609–17.

31. Dzionek A, Fuchs A, Schmidt P, et al. BDCA-2, BDCA-3, and BDCA-4: three markers for distinct subsets of dendritic cells in human peripheral blood. J Immunol 2000;165(11):6037–46.

32. Montes-Moreno S, Ramos-Medina R, Martínez-López A, et al. SPIB, a novel immunohistochemical marker for human blastic plasmacytoid dendritic cell neoplasms: characterization of its expression in major hematolymphoid neoplasms. Blood 2013; 121(4):643–7.

33. Rizvi H, Paterson JC, Tedoldi S, et al. Expression of the CD2AP adaptor molecule in normal, reactive and neoplastic human tissue. Pathologica 2012; 104(2):56–64.

34. Garnache-Ottou F, Chaperot L, Biichle S, et al. Expression of the myeloid-associated marker CD33 is not an exclusive factor for leukemic plasmacytoid dendritic cells. Blood 2005;105(3): 1256–64.

35. Reichard KK. Blastic plasmacytoid dendritic cell neoplasm. In: F MK, editor. Diagnostic pathology; blood and bone marrow. 1st edition. Manitobe (Canada): Amirsys Publishing; 2012;9:208–13.

36. Reineks EZ, Osei ES, Rosenberg A, et al. CD22 expression on blastic plasmacytoid dendritic cell neoplasms and reactivity of anti-CD22 antibodies to peripheral blood dendritic cells. Cytometry B Clin Cytom 2009;76(4):237–48.

37. Dijkman R, van Doorn R, Szuhai K, et al. Gene-expression profiling and array-based CGH classify CD4+CD56+ hematodermic neoplasm and cutaneous myelomonocytic leukemia as distinct disease entities. Blood 2007;109(4):1720–7.

38. Leroux D, Mugneret F, Callanan M, et al. CD4(+), CD56(+) DC2 acute leukemia is characterized by recurrent clonal chromosomal changes affecting 6 major targets: a study of 21 cases by the Groupe Francais de Cytogenetique Hematologique. Blood 2002;99(11):4154–9.

39. Lucioni M, Novara F, Fiandrino G, et al. Twenty-one cases of blastic plasmacytoid dendritic cell neoplasm: focus on biallelic locus 9p21.3 deletion. Blood 2011;118(17):4591–4.

40. Oiso N, Tatsumi Y, Arao T, et al. Loss of genomic DNA copy numbers in the p18, p16, p27 and RB loci in blastic plasmacytoid dendritic cell neoplasm. Eur J Dermatol 2012;22(3):393–4.

41. Wiesner T, Obenauf AC, Cota C, et al. Alterations of the cell-cycle inhibitors p27(KIP1) and p16(INK4a) are frequent in blastic plasmacytoid dendritic cell neoplasms. J Invest Dermatol 2010;130(4):1152–7.

42. Jardin F, Ruminy P, Parmentier F, et al. TET2 and TP53 mutations are frequently observed in blastic plasmacytoid dendritic cell neoplasm. Br J Haematol 2011;153(3):413–6.

43. Fiandrino G, Arra M, Riboni R, et al. Absence of MYD88 L265P mutation in blastic plasmacytoid dendritic cell neoplasm. Br J Dermatol 2013; 168(4):883–4.

44. Treon SP, Xu L, Yang G, et al. MYD88 L265P somatic mutation in Waldenstrom's macroglobulinemia. N Engl J Med 2012;367(9):826–33.

45. Bénet C, Gomez A, Aguilar C, et al. Histologic and immunohistologic characterization of skin localization of myeloid disorders: a study of 173 cases. Am J Clin Pathol 2011;135(2):278–90.

46. Cronin DM, George TI, Reichard KK, et al. Immunophenotypic analysis of myeloperoxidase-negative leukemia cutis and blastic plasmacytoid dendritic cell neoplasm. Am J Clin Pathol 2012;137(3):367–76.

47. Klco JM, Welch JS, Nguyen TT, et al. State of the art in myeloid sarcoma. Int J Lab Hematol 2011;33(6): 555–65.

48. Muñoz L, Nomdedéu JF, López O, et al. Interleukin-3 receptor alpha chain (CD123) is widely expressed in hematologic malignancies. Haematologica 2001;86(12):1261–9.

49. Rollins-Raval M, Pillai R, Warita K, et al. CD123 immunohistochemical expression in acute myeloid leukemia is associated with underlying FLT3-ITD and NPM1 mutations. Appl Immunohistochem Mol Morphol 2013;21(3):212–7.

50. Chen YC, Chou JM, Ketterling RP, et al. Histologic and immunohistochemical study of bone marrow monocytic nodules in 21 cases with myelodysplasia. Am J Clin Pathol 2003;120(6):874–81.

51. Dargent JL, Delannoy A, Pieron P, et al. Cutaneous accumulation of plasmacytoid dendritic cells associated with acute myeloid leukemia: a rare condition distinct from blastic plasmacytoid dendritic cell neoplasm. J Cutan Pathol 2011;38(11):893–8.

52. Rollins-Raval MA, Marafioti T, Swerdlow SH, et al. The number and growth pattern of plasmacytoid dendritic cells vary in different types of reactive lymph nodes: an immunohistochemical study. Hum Pathol 2013;44(6):1003–10.

53. Vermi W, Facchetti F, Rosati S, et al. Nodal and extranodal tumor-forming accumulation of plasmacytoid

monocytes/interferon-producing cells associated with myeloid disorders. Am J Surg Pathol 2004; 28(5):585–95.

54. Vitte F, Fabiani B, Bénet C, et al. Specific skin lesions in chronic myelomonocytic leukemia: a spectrum of myelomonocytic and dendritic cell proliferations: a study of 42 cases. Am J Surg Pathol 2012;36(9):1302–16.

55. An HJ, Yoon DH, Kim S, et al. Blastic plasmacytoid dendritic cell neoplasm: a single-center experience. Ann Hematol 2013;92(3):351–6.

56. Pagano L, Valentini CG, Facchetti F. Reply to "A combination treatment approach and cord blood stem cell transplant for blastic plasmacytoid dendritic cell neoplasm" and to "A low-grade B-cell lymphoma with prolymphocytic/paraimmunoblastic proliferation and IRF4 rearrangement" dendritic cell leukemia. Haematologica 2013;98(3):e37.

57. Pagano L, Valentini CG, Pulsoni A, et al. Blastic plasmacytoid dendritic cell neoplasm with leukemic presentation: an Italian multicenter study. Haematologica 2013;98(2):239–46.

58. Rauh MJ, Rahman F, Good D, et al. Blastic plasmacytoid dendritic cell neoplasm with leukemic presentation, lacking cutaneous involvement: Case series and literature review. Leuk Res 2012;36(1):81–6.

59. Kharfan-Dabaja MA, Lazarus HM, Nishihori T, et al. Diagnostic and therapeutic advances in blastic plasmacytoid dendritic cell neoplasm: a focus on hematopoietic cell transplantation. Biol Blood Marrow Transplant 2013;19(7):1006–12.

60. Reimer P, Rüdiger T, Kraemer D, et al. What is CD4+CD56+ malignancy and how should it be treated? Bone Marrow Transplant 2003;32(7): 637–46.

61. Reichard KK. Blastic plasmacytoid dendritic cell neoplasms in bone marrow. In: RK, Foucar MK, Czuchlewski D, editors. Bone marrow pathology, vol. 1, 3rd edition. Chicago: ASCP Press; 2010. p. 433–8.

The Differential Diagnosis of Eosinophilia in Neoplastic Hematopathology

Ryan C. Johnson, MD[a],*, Tracy I. George, MD[b]

KEYWORDS

- Eosinophilia • *PDGFRA* • *PDGFRB* • *FGFR1* • Systemic mastocytosis • *KIT*
- Chronic eosinophilic leukemia • Hypereosinophilic syndrome • Myeloproliferative neoplasms

KEY POINTS

- Secondary causes of eosinophilia are far more common than primary (clonal) causes of eosinophilia.
- Patients with an elevated absolute eosinophil count, either sustained and/or with end-organ damage, should be evaluated for primary (clonal) causes of eosinophilia after exclusion of secondary causes.
- Evaluation for primary (clonal) causes of eosinophilia starts with peripheral blood analysis for *PDGFRA* mutation by FISH or PCR, bone marrow aspirate and biopsy, and cytogenetic karyotyping performed on the bone marrow specimen, with additional ancillary tests as indicated after morphologic review.
- Mast cell proliferations may be seen in myeloid and lymphoid neoplasms associated with *PDGFRA*, *PDGFRB*, and *FGFR1*; WHO criteria must be applied when diagnosing systemic mastocytosis.

ABSTRACT

Eosinophilia in the peripheral blood is classified as primary (clonal) hematologic neoplasms or secondary (nonclonal) disorders, associated with hematologic or nonhematologic disorders. This review focuses on the categories of hematolymphoid neoplasms recognized by the 2008 World Health Organization *Classification of Tumours and Haematopoietic and Lymphoid Tissues* that are characteristically associated with eosinophilia. We provide a systematic approach to the diagnosis of these neoplastic proliferations via morphologic, immunophenotypic, and molecular-based methodologies, and provide the clinical settings in which these hematolymphoid neoplasms occur. We discuss recommendations that eosinophilia working groups have published addressing some of the limitations of the current classification scheme.

OVERVIEW

Eosinophils are produced in the bone marrow, derived initially from a granulocyte-macrophage progenitor differentiating to a lineage restricted granulocyte progenitor, to a common basophil-eosinophil progenitor, and finally to the terminally differentiated eosinophil.[1,2] Eosinophils represent 1% to 5% of peripheral blood leukocytes in healthy adults, and the normal range of eosinophils for an adult is 0.30 to 0.50 $\times$ 10^9/L.[2] Eosinophilic differentiation occurs as a response to specific cytokines and growth factors, namely interleukin (IL)-3, IL-5, and GM-CSF.[3,4] Of these,

Disclosures: None (R.C. Johnson); Consultant, Novartis (T.I. George).
[a] Department of Pathology, Stanford University School of Medicine, 300 Pasteur Drive, L235 MC 5324, Stanford, CA 94305, USA; [b] Department of Pathology, University of New Mexico School of Medicine, 1 University of New Mexico, MSC08 4640, Albuquerque, NM 87131-0001, USA
* Corresponding author.
E-mail address: ryancj@stanford.edu

Surgical Pathology 6 (2013) 767–794
http://dx.doi.org/10.1016/j.path.2013.08.008
1875-9181/13/$ – see front matter © 2013 Elsevier Inc. All rights reserved.

IL-5 is thought to be the most specific for eosinophil recruitment and originates via the TH2 arm of cell-mediated immunity.[2] Helminthic infections remain the most common cause of eosinophilia in nonindustrialized nations,[2] and atopy is the most common cause of eosinophilia in industrialized nations.[5] A workup for secondary causes should include a detailed travel history, family or personal history of asthma or atopy, directed laboratory studies including stool ova and parasites, and serologic or urine antigen studies for specific parasitic diseases (eg, *Schistosoma* urine antigen, *Strongyloides* serum antibodies), and other serologic tests as needed (**Box 1**, **Fig. 1**).[6] Imaging studies may also be necessary.

Less commonly, an underlying hematopoietic or nonhematopoietic neoplasm may be responsible for the peripheral eosinophilia. Among hematolymphoid neoplasms, eosinophilia may or may not be part of the neoplastic clone. A short list of examples in which eosinophilia is nonclonal includes Hodgkin lymphoma, mature T-cell lymphomas, including angioimmunoblastic T-cell lymphoma, and acute lymphoblastic leukemia (ALL) with t(5;14)(q31;q32) (**Box 2**, **Fig. 2**). In the cases of B-ALL with t(5;14)(q31;q32), this translocation leads to constitutive overproduction of IL-3.[7] In Hodgkin lymphoma[8] or various mature T-cell lymphomas,[9] IL-5 or, less commonly, GM-CSF overproduction is responsible for the peripheral eosinophilia.

A subset of hematologic neoplasms with associated eosinophilia has their origins in molecular mutational abnormalities and the eosinophilic clone is the same as the underlying neoplastic clone (see **Box 2**). As these causes of eosinophilia are relatively rare, screening for the mutational abnormality should be performed after exclusion of reactive causes, when clinical suspicion is high, or the degree of eosinophilic-related pathology is substantial. In myeloid and lymphoid neoplasms with *PDGFRA* or *PDGFRB* rearrangements, their exquisite sensitivity to imatinib allows for reasonable consideration to perform cytogenetic testing via fluorescence in situ hybridization (FISH) on the peripheral blood.[10] If testing thus far has been negative, further investigation requires morphologic and cytogenetic analysis of the bone marrow aspirate and biopsy.[6,11] Assessment for dysplasia, increased absolute counts in other lineages, and presence of circulating lymphoblasts or myeloblasts should be recorded. It is important to note that dysplasia in the eosinophil lineage is not a proxy for clonality, as abnormal morphology may be seen in reactive and clonal eosinophilia and normal morphology may be seen in neoplastic conditions. Targeted flow

> **Box 1**
> **Secondary nonhematolymphoid causes of eosinophilia**
>
> Helminthic infections (eg, *Strongyloides*, *Toxocara*, filariasis)
>
> Fungal and protozoal infections
>
> Allergic disease, including atopy and drug hypersensitivity
>
> Drugs (eg, GM-CSF, IL-2, penicillin, cephalosporin, NSAIDS, beta blockers)
>
> DRESS syndrome (rash, fever, eosinophilia, lymphocytosis, lymphadenopathy)
>
> Skin disease (eg, bullous pemphigoid, eczema)
>
> Gastrointestinal disease, including allergic gastroenteritis
>
> Asthma (both allergic and nonallergic)
>
> Collagen vascular disease (eg, Churg-Strauss syndrome, granulomatosis with polyangiitis, systemic lupus erythematosus)
>
> Rheumatic diseases (eg, rheumatoid arthritis, systemic sclerosis, Sjögren syndrome)
>
> Other autoimmune/immunologic disorders (eg, polyarteritis nodosa, sarcoidosis, Kimura disease)
>
> Eosinophilia-myalgia syndrome
>
> Immunodeficiency (eg, HIV infection,[a] Omenn syndrome, Hyperimmunoglobulin E syndrome)
>
> Carcinomas (eg, non–small cell lung carcinoma, squamous carcinoma, gastric and large bowel adenocarcinoma)
>
> Metabolic diseases, including adrenal insufficiency
>
> [a] HIV infection does not cause eosinophilia per se, but associated infections may lead to an eosinophilia. *Abbreviation:* NSAIDS, nonsteroidal anti-inflammatory drugs.

cytometric and/or immunohistochemical analysis may also be performed to evaluate for increased numbers of myeloblasts or lymphoblasts, assess for a neoplastic T-cell or B-cell population, or evaluate for the presence of mast cell infiltrates.

Cytogenetic analysis of the bone marrow is a critical component of this evaluation, as specific cytogenetic abnormalities, that is, t(8;21)(q22;q22), t(5;14)(q31;q32), inv(16)(p13.1q22), t(16;16)(p13.1;q22), and t(9;22)(q34;q11.2), may be evidence for a World Health Organization (WHO) cytogenetically defined abnormality, such as acute myeloid leukemia (AML), ALL, or chronic

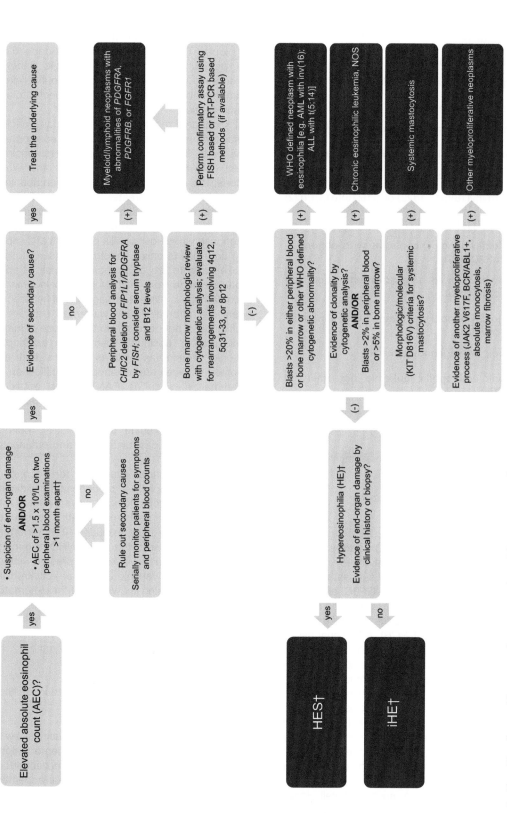

Fig. 1. Algorithm for working up patients presenting with eosinophilia. † The 2008 WHO requires a 6-month sustained eosinophil count for the diagnosis of hypereosinophilic syndrome. (+), present; (−), absent. (*Adapted from* Gotlib J. World Health Organization-defined eosinophilic disorders: 2012 update on diagnosis, risk stratification, and management. Am J Hematol 2012;87;907; with permission.)

Box 2
Primary (clonal) hematolymphoid causes of eosinophilia

Hodgkin lymphoma

Angioimmunoblastic T-cell lymphoma

Sezary syndrome

Lymphocyte variant hypereosinophilia[a]

B-lymphoblastic leukemia with t(5;14)(q31;q32)

Acute myeloid leukemia

   With inv(16)(p13.1q22) or t(16;16)(p13.1;q22)

   With t(8;21)(q22;q22)

Myeloid/lymphoid neoplasms with abnormalities of *PDGFRA*

Myeloid/lymphoid neoplasms with abnormalities of *PDGFRB*

Myeloid/lymphoid neoplasms with abnormalities of *FGFR1*

Chronic myelogenous leukemia

Chronic eosinophilic leukemia, not otherwise specified

Systemic mastocytosis

Hypereosinophilic syndrome

Myeloproliferative neoplasms or myelodysplastic syndromes

   [a] Presence of aberrant T-cell clone.

---

myelogenous leukemia (CML). Cytogenetic analysis may also reveal translocations involving chromosomes 4, 5, or 8, and may suggest neoplasms associated with *PDGFRA*, *PDGFRB*, and *FGFR1*, which should be followed up with confirmatory testing via FISH or reverse transcriptase polymerase chain reaction (RT-PCR). Mutational assessment for *KIT* D816V, *JAK2* V617F, or *BCR-ABL1* may also be necessary given the specific findings noted on morphologic and immunophenotypic review of the bone marrow, and may suggest a diagnosis of systemic mastocytosis (SM) or a myeloproliferative neoplasm (MPN). Cytogenetic analysis may also be important for establishing a diagnosis of chronic eosinophilic leukemia (CEL), if criteria for other WHO diagnostic entities are not met.

Other ancillary testing, such as T-cell clonality studies, serum tryptase, serum B12, and serum IL-5, may also be useful. Lymphadenopathy may

be evaluated with immunohistochemistry and T-cell or B-cell clonality studies in cases in which lymph nodes are prominent and readily accessible for biopsy. These ancillary studies will depend on the particular clinical and pathologic findings noted and, although not part of the routine algorithm, may be useful for specific suspected diagnostic entities.

If secondary reactive causes and malignancies associated with a clonal or nonclonal eosinophilia have been excluded, a diagnosis of hypereosinophilia (HE) may be entertained. Per the WHO criteria, this requires the presence of an absolute eosinophil count of greater than 1.5×10^9/L for longer than 6 months, although eosinophil working groups have recently proposed that HE may be diagnosed when eosinophilia is present at 2 separate time points only 1 month apart (see **Fig. 1**). These patients are at an increased risk of end-organ damage from infiltration of eosinophils; if such damage is evident, a diagnosis of hypereosinophilic syndrome (HES) is warranted. Damage is multifactorial but occurs from the release of major basic protein, eosinophil peroxidase, eosinophil cationic protein, as well as proteins that are involved in T-cell and eosinophil amplification of inflammation, such as RANTES and eotaxin.[2] Eosinophilic-related damage has been reported to occur in essentially every organ system in the human body, including cardiovascular, pulmonary, neurologic, gastrointestinal, and cutaneous systems.[12]

Although the initial evaluation for secondary causes of eosinophilia is predominantly clinically driven, the hematopathologist plays a central role once secondary nonhematopoietic causes of eosinophilia have been excluded. It is important to note that in some cases, these WHO diagnostic entities mentioned previously may present without eosinophilia or a variable degree of eosinophilia. Thus, a solid working knowledge of these hematolymphoid conditions, along with a high index of suspicion, is essential for the hematopathologist.

MYELOID AND LYMPHOID NEOPLASMS ASSOCIATED WITH *PDGFRA* REARRANGEMENTS

CLINICAL FEATURES

Myeloid and lymphoid neoplasms associated with platelet-derived growth factor receptor alpha (*PDGFRA*) rearrangements are a collection of MPNs that all share the same rearrangement involving the gene *PDGFRA* on chromosome locus 4q12. The most common presentation of these rearrangements is as a CEL-like presentation. Some

Fig. 2. B-lymphoblastic leukemia with t(5;14)(q31;q32) and eosinophilia. The peripheral blood of a 3-year-old boy showed a white blood cell (WBC) count of greater than 100×10^9/L. (*A*) Peripheral blood examination reveals that most leukocytes are eosinophils, with occasional lymphoblasts. Eosinophils are morphologically abnormal, including nuclear hyperlobation and ring nuclei (Wright Giemsa, ×60). (*B*) The bone marrow aspirate revealed an increase in mature eosinophils, eosinophilic myelocytes, and greater than 20% blasts. Blasts showed a B-lymphoblast phenotype, and cytogenetic analysis revealed the presence of a t(5;14)(q31;q32). The eosinophilia is nonclonal and secondary to overproduction of IL-3 (Wright Giemsa, ×60).

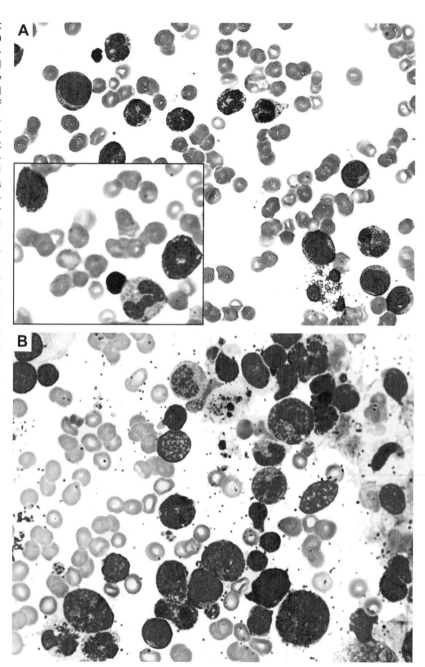

patients, however, may present with AML and/or T-lymphoblastic lymphoma (LBL). This disease is rare, and most patients are male (M:F ratio; 17:1).[13] The etiology of the specific rearrangement is uncertain in these cases, although in some patients a history of cytotoxic chemotherapy was noted.[14–16]

Patients with this entity typically present with constitutional symptoms, including fatigue, myalgias, weight loss, and low-grade fevers. Splenomegaly is present in most patients, with hepatomegaly present in a smaller subset. Symptomatology may be end-organ specific and may include skin, cardiac, neurologic, pulmonary, and gastrointestinal manifestations.[12,13,17,18]

Laboratory parameters that may be elevated at presentation include a mildly elevated serum tryptase (>12 ng/mL); this is generally not as high as in patients with systemic mastocytosis.[19] Serum B12 levels may also be elevated and thought to be related to increased serum B12 binding protein production, a nonspecific finding in MPNs. A recent study of cases with HE revealed that serum B12 levels of 2000 pg/mL were associated only with patients having the *PDGFRA* rearrangement.[20] The combination of splenomegaly, elevated serum B12, and elevated serum tryptase levels in a patient with moderate eosinophilia may serve as highly suspicious evidence for the *PDGFRA* rearrangement when molecular testing is not available.[6,19,20] Confirmatory testing should be sent to reference laboratories in these cases.

Key Features
OF MYELOPROLIFERATIVE NEOPLASMS WITH EOSINOPHILIA (PDGFRA, PDGFRB, FGFR1-ASSOCIATED NEOPLASMS)

1. Blood and marrow eosinophilia

2. Hypercellular bone marrow

3. Fibrotic bone marrow

4. Can see involvement of other myeloid lineages

MICROSCOPIC FEATURES

The peripheral blood will show a CEL-like picture with an overwhelming predominance of mature eosinophils (**Fig. 3**). Eosinophilic myelocytes and promyelocytes may also be increased. Eosinophils may show abnormal morphology, including abnormal granulation or tinctorial quality, and nuclear hyposegmentation or hypersegmentation; eosinophils can also show normal morphology.[13,18,21] Abnormalities in other cell counts may include neutrophilia, neutropenia, anemia, and thrombocytopenia. Basophils and monocytes, however, are generally not increased.[22] Depending on the degree of progression, blasts may be increased in the bone marrow and/or peripheral blood. Blasts may be myeloblasts, T-lymphoblasts, B-lymphoblasts (rarely), or a combination of each; flow cytometry of the blood or bone marrow would show the expected immunophenotype for each population.

The bone marrow will be hypercellular and dominated by mature eosinophils and eosinophilic precursors (see **Fig. 3**). Maturation and localization of eosinophilic precursors is generally maintained, and blasts in such cases are not increased. An increase in blasts indicates a progression of disease toward leukemia. An absolute increase in neutrophils and mast cells may also be present. The mast cell aggregates in cases of *PDGFRA* rearrangements do not show the degree of tight cluster formation as is typical of SM.[6,19,23] These mast cells may show abnormal morphology. Fibrosis may or may not be present.

ANCILLARY STUDIES

It is typically unnecessary to perform immunohistochemistry to highlight eosinophils. If performed, immunohistochemistry will show major basic protein deposition in bone marrow or other tissues involved by eosinophilia.[24] Increased mast cells, both singly and in loose aggregates, are best highlighted by CD117 or tryptase immunohistochemistry. These mast cells may also express CD25, but unlike SM there is no evidence of a *KIT* mutation. Fibrosis will be evident on reticulin and trichrome stains.

The unifying molecular abnormality in this neoplasm is the presence of the *FIP1L1-PDGFRA* rearrangement. Because both of these genes lie on the same gene locus of chromosome 4q12, this gene deletion is cryptic and will not be detected on routine karyotype analysis. Thus, this genetic abnormality is detected either by FISH or by PCR (**Fig. 4**).

Other variant translocations involving the *PDGFRA* gene have been reported but are much less common and include ins(9;4)(q33q12q25) *CDK5RAP2-PDGFRA*, t(2;4)(p24;q12) *STRN-PDGFRA*, t(4;12) *ETV6-PDGFRA*, and t(4;1) (q12;q11) *KIF5B-PDGFRA*. These patients presented with CEL and all were responsive to imatinib.[25–28] There have also been several case reports of a t(4;22)(q12;q11) resulting in a *BCR-PDGFRA* fusion product. Interestingly, these patients have presented with significant leukocytosis resembling CML with eosinophilia either in the peripheral blood or bone marrow. These patients also showed progression to an "accelerated phase" or "blast phase," with AML, T-LBL, or B-LBL.[16,29–31]

DIFFERENTIAL DIAGNOSIS

As most cases of myeloid neoplasms with *PDGFRA* mutations present as a CEL-like proliferation, the differential diagnosis includes myeloid neoplasms associated with *PDGFRB* or *FGFR1* rearrangements, CML with prominent eosinophilia, and CEL not otherwise specified (NOS).

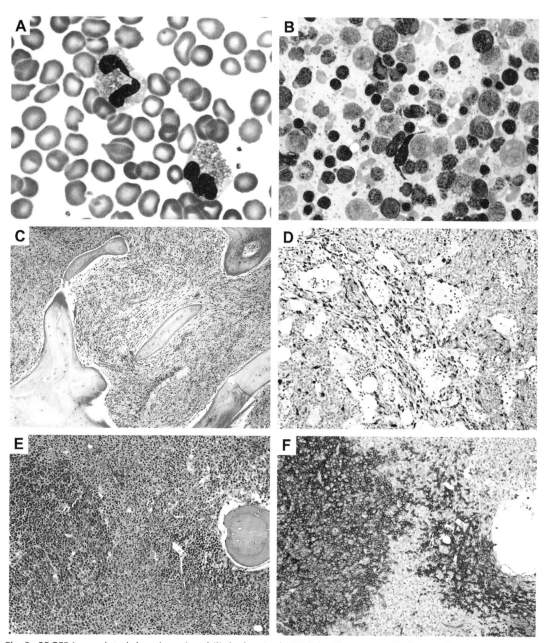

Fig. 3. PDGFRA-associated chronic eosinophilic leukemia. (*A*; Wright Giemsa, ×100) The peripheral blood showed a leukoerythroblastic smear with an eosinophil count of 2.7 × 10⁹/L, and a neutropenia. Other parameters included WBC count: 7.6 × 10⁹/L; hemoglobin (Hgb) 13.3 g/dL, platelets 128 × 10⁹/L. (*B*; Wright Giemsa, ×60) The bone marrow aspirate review revealed an increase in mature eosinophils as well as mast cells, more than 25% of which showed spindle-shaped morphology. Blasts were fewer than 5% of nucleated cells. (*C*; H&E, ×20) Areas of the bone marrow trephine on low-power magnification show a hypercellular marrow with areas of fibrosis and an infiltrative process. (*D*; Tryptase, ×20) Tryptase immunohistochemistry reveals loose clustering and an interstitial increase in mast cells, which aberrantly express CD25 (not shown). (*E*; H&E, ×20) This case also showed an unusual feature of large clusters of proerythroblasts, supported by immunohistochemistry for glycophorin (*F*; Glycophorin, ×20).

PDGFRA-related neoplasms enter the differential diagnosis when cases presenting like CML with eosinophilia are negative for the *BCR-ABL1* translocation or show a translocation involving chromosome 4. FISH or molecular studies for the *PDGFRA* rearrangement will be positive in these cases. Karyotype analysis would demonstrate chromosomal rearrangements involving

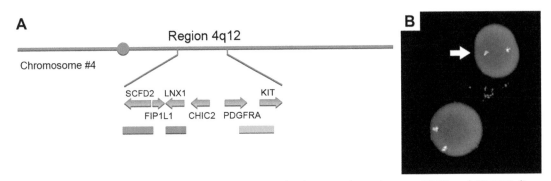

Fig. 4. Diagram of *FIP1L1-PDGFRA* fusion gene. (*A*) Two closely approximated genes, *FIP1L1* and *PDGFRA*, lie on the same chromosome locus 4q12 and are separated by several genes, including the *CHIC2* gene. *FIP1L1-PDGFRA* gene rearrangements cannot be detected by routine cytogenetic karyotype analysis; either FISH analysis to examine for loss of the intervening gene segments or RT-PCR to examine for *PDGFRA* fusion transcripts must be used to detect this abnormality. *CHIC2* gene loss serves as a surrogate marker for the *FIP1L1-PDGFRA* gene rearrangement. (*B*) An example of a *PDGFRA* gene rearrangement (same patient as shown in **Fig. 3**) is indicated here by the loss of the orange probe (specific for *LNX1*, which lies adjacent to *CHIC2*) with apposition of probes for the *PDGFRA* gene (*aqua*) and *SCFD2* gene (*green*), which flank the *FIP1L1* gene (*arrow*). (*Courtesy of* Stanford University Cytogenetics Laboratory, Stanford, CA.)

chromosomes 8 or 5, respectively, for *FGFR1* and *PDGFRB* rearrangements. Cases of CEL NOS may show clonal cytogenetic rearrangements, but would be negative for FISH-based or RT-PCR–based assays for the *PDGFRA* rearrangement. Thus, confirmatory testing following an aberrant karyotype is recommended for definitive assessment.

Finally, SM can be associated with either a reactive or clonal eosinophilia in the bone marrow and/or peripheral blood. Most SM cases are positive for the D816V mutation in exon 17 of the *KIT* proto-oncogene. It is postulated that the presence of the D816V *KIT* mutation is mutually exclusive from rearrangements involving *PDGFRA*.[32] Other characteristics, such as a markedly elevated serum B12 level, mildly elevated serum tryptase level, or loose clustering of mast cells on bone marrow core biopsy, are suggestive of *PDGFRA* rearrangements as opposed to SM (**Table 1**), but

Table 1
Laboratory and clinical differences noted between myeloid neoplasms associated with *PDGFRA* rearrangements and systemic mastocytosis

	Myeloid/Lymphoid Neoplasms With *PDGFRA* Abnormalities	Systemic Mastocytosis
Gender distribution	M ≫ F	M ≈ F
BM mast cell aggregates	Loose clusters/interstitial	Dense aggregates
AEC/tryptase ratio	>100	<100
Treatment	Imatinib-sensitive	Imatinib-resistant; 2nd generation TKIs; cladribine
Symptom profile	Cardiac/pulmonary	GI/UP/vascular
Vitamin B12 level	Elevated	Normal
Tryptase level	+	++/+++
Genetic mutation	*PDGFRA*	D816V *KIT*

Abbreviations: +, mildly elevated; ++, moderately elevated; +++, markedly elevated; AEC, absolute eosinophil count; BM, bone marrow; F, female; GI, gastrointestinal; M, male; TKI, tyrosine kinase inhibitor; UP, urticaria pigmentosa.

Adapted from Maric I, Robyn J, Metcalfe DD, et al. KIT D816V-associated systemic mastocytosis with eosinophilia and FIP1L1/PDGFRA-associated chronic eosinophilic leukemia are distinct entities. J Allergy Clin Immunol 2007:120;685; with permission.

molecular and cytogenetic studies must be performed for confirmation.

PROGNOSIS

Before the discovery of the *FIP1L1-PDGFRA* rearrangement, trials of imatinib therapy were conducted in patients with elevated eosinophil counts and myeloproliferative features, with many of these patients showing a complete hematologic response.[29,33,34] The rearrangement was discovered subsequently, and cultured cells containing the fused gene protein product were also shown to be sensitive to imatinib in vitro.[18,35] Imatinib monotherapy of 100 to 400 mg per day is currently recommended for patients with *FIP1L1-PDGFRA* rearrangements to attain a complete hematologic and molecular response.[6] Patients with increased numbers of blasts in the peripheral blood or bone marrow must be watched more closely with serial peripheral blood differential counts to examine for impending transformation.

Resistance to imatinib and second-generation tyrosine kinase inhibitors (TKIs) nilotinib and sorafenib, has been reported. Although rare, the most frequent mutation reported in patients treated with imatinib is T674I, resulting from a point mutation in the ATP-binding pocket of the *PDGFRA* portion of the fusion gene.[18,36] This mutation is homologous to the T315I mutations that develop in the *ABL* gene in imatinib-resistant CML.[37] The T674I mutation is also thought to confer some resistance to second-generation TKIs, although case reports of treatment success and in vitro activity to second-generation TKIs have been reported in patients bearing this mutation.[36,38,39]

Although the overall prognosis associated with *PDGFRA* rearranged neoplasms is improved in the era of TKI therapy, those patients who present or develop signs and symptoms of eosinophilic cardiomyopathy have a much more guarded prognosis.[21,23] Such patients who present acutely or have significant end-organ damage may also be placed on corticosteroid therapy to reduce the degree of inflammation in the end organ involved. Patients may also present with or progress to leukemia or lymphoblastic lymphoma. It is unknown whether additional mutational abnormalities are required for this progression, or the time course from onset of the transformation. However, treatment outcome data for this rare neoplasm shows that, independent of presentation as CEL, leukemia, or LBL, patients may achieve complete molecular remission with imatinib monotherapy or combination chemotherapy including imatinib.[29,31,33,34]

MYELOID AND LYMPHOID NEOPLASMS ASSOCIATED WITH *PDGFRB* REARRANGEMENTS

CLINICAL FEATURES

This neoplasm was first reported by Keene and colleagues[40] in 1987 and described 2 cases with peripheral blood findings of CEL and a concurrent t(5;12)(q33.1;p13). Several other studies followed showing the identical cytogenetic abnormality in patients whose morphologic presentations range from chronic myelomonocytic leukemia (CMML) with eosinophilia to myelodysplastic syndrome (MDS)-like features with increased marrow fibrosis, to rare presentations of de novo AML.[41–45]

The age of presentation is variable with a recent review showing an average age of presentation in the fifth decade with a range from 6 to 72 years.[45,46] Most patients who carry the t(5;12)(q33.1;p13) are male (M:F ratio, 2:1).[45] The presentation is similarly variable. Patients may be completely asymptomatic at diagnosis, presenting only with an elevated leukocyte count. Generalized systemic symptoms include night sweats, low-grade fever, weight loss, and fatigue. Most patients present with or develop splenomegaly; hepatomegaly has been reported in a smaller subset.[45] Gastrointestinal manifestations may also occur and are similar to those seen in other hypereosinophilic conditions and include diarrhea; skin findings may include generalized erythema and or erythematous plaques that can progress to marked surface ulceration.[46] Cardiac manifestations have also been reported and may be severe with subsequent valvular abnormalities and ventricular failure.[40]

MICROSCOPIC FEATURES

Most patients will show a leukocytosis at diagnosis; a concurrent anemia and thrombocytopenia may also be present. The appearance of the peripheral blood is that of an MPN or mixed MDS/MPN syndrome (**Fig. 5**). Most patients will show eosinophilia; a recent review showed a range of eosinophil counts from 3% to 94%.[45] However, eosinophilia is not always present. An accompanying neutrophilia and/or monocytosis may also be seen. Basophilia has also been reported.[28] Thus, depending on the relative peripheral blood counts, peripheral blood findings resemble CMML with eosinophilia, atypical CML with eosinophilia, CEL, or juvenile myelomonocytic leukemia (JMML), depending on the age of presentation.[47] Rarely, patients may present with or develop AML.[45,48]

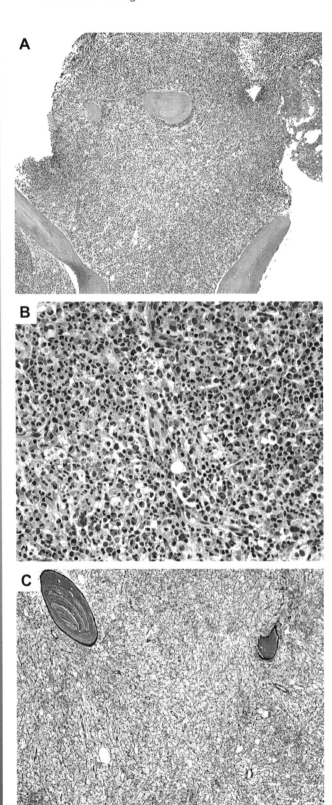

Fig. 5. Myeloid neoplasms with *PDGFRB* re-arrangement. A 72-year-old man presented with chronic anemia with a rising WBC count while on hydroxyurea. Laboratory values included WBC 15.1 × 10⁹/L; Hgb 10.0 g/dL; 77% neutrophils (absolute neutrophil count [ANC] = 12.1 × 10⁹/L), 7% eosinophils (AEC = 1.1 × 10⁹/L), 3% monocytes. (*A*) The bone marrow biopsy is hypercellular and shows increased fibrosis (H&E, ×10). (*B*) Higher-power examination of the marrow shows increased myeloid precursors and a marked increase in eosinophils. Blasts comprised 0.5% of events on flow cytometry (H&E, ×20). (*C*) A reticulin stain demonstrated extensive intersections of reticulin fibrosis. *JAK2* V617F testing was negative. Cytogenetic analysis revealed a t(5;12) translocation, and confirmatory FISH testing was positive for a *PGDFRB* rearrangement. This patient was placed on imatinib 200 mg daily and demonstrated a complete hematologic and cytogenetic response (Reticulin, ×20).

Bone marrow findings show a hypercellular marrow comprised predominantly of mature eosinophils, neutrophils, and/or monocytes. In cases that present as CEL, eosinophils in various stages of maturation may be evident.[40] Rarely, mast cells may be increased and can show atypical morphology; these cases may show a concomitantly elevated serum tryptase level.[28] Bone marrow fibrosis has been reported[28,48] and may resemble primary myelofibrosis.

ANCILLARY STUDIES

The t(5;12)(q33.1;p13) is the most common abnormality seen in these neoplasms. This usually results in the translocation of the platelet-derived growth factor receptor beta (PDGFRB) gene on chromosome 5q33 to the ETV6 gene located on chromosome 12p13. More than 20 variant translocations have been described thus far incorporating a variety of chromosomes (Table 2).[47,49] All cases reported to date have shown readily apparent abnormalities detectable in standard cytogenetic karyotype analysis (ie, unlike most PDGFRA rearrangements, PDGFRB rearrangements are not cryptic). However, FISH break-apart probes for the PDGFRB gene and RT-PCR methods for detection of the ETV6-PDGFRB fusion gene are available.[50] In addition, not all cases of t(5;12)(q33.1;p13) with an associated MPN or AML will possess the PDGFRB gene fusion and thus will not be responsive to imatinib therapy,[45] highlighting the importance of FISH or RT-PCR studies for confirmation.[13,27,45] If such testing is not available, trial therapy with imatinib may be indicated.

DIFFERENTIAL DIAGNOSIS

In most cases, based on the presence of an absolute increase in eosinophils, neutrophils, and/or monocytes in the peripheral blood and similar evidence of an MPN in the bone marrow, a diagnosis of CMML or atypical CML may be entertained.

Table 2
PDGFRB-associated fusion genes and corresponding morphology

Fusion Gene	Translocation	Diagnosis at Presentation
ETV6–PDGFRB[a]	t(5;12)(q33.1;p13)[a]	CMML with eosinophilia or CEL
WDR48–PDGFRB	t(1;3;5)(p36;p21.33;q33.1)	CEL
CAPRIN1–PDGFRB	der(1)t(1;5)(p34;q33.1), der(5) t(1;5)(p34;q15), der(11) ins(11;5)(p13;q15q33.1)	CEL
TPM3–PDGFRB	t(1;5)(q21.2;q33.1)	CEL
PDE4DIP–PDGFRB	t(1;5)(q21.1;q33.1)	MDS/MPN with eosinophilia
PRKG2–PDGFRB	t(4;5;5)(q13.1-q21.1;q31;q33.1)	Chronic basophilic leukemia
GOLGA4–PDGFRB	t(3;5)(p22–21.3;q33.1)	aCML with eosinophilia, MPN with eosinophilia
CEP85L–PDGFRB	t(5;6)(q33.1;q22.31)	MPN with eosinophilia
HIP1–PDGFRB	t(5;7)(q33.1;q11.23)	CMML with eosinophilia
KANK1–PDGFRB	t(5;9)(q33.1;p24.3)	Essential thrombocythemia
CCDC6–PDGFRB	t(5;10)(q33.1;q21.2)	aCML with eosinophilia, MPN with eosinophilia
GIT2–PDGFRB	t(5;12)(q33.1;q24.1)	CEL
NIN–PDGFRB	t(5;14)(q33.1;q21-q22)	aCML with eosinophilia
CCDC88C–PDGFRB	t(5;14)(q33.1;q32.12)	CMML with eosinophilia
TP53BP1–PDGFRB	t(5;15)(q33.1;q15-q21)	aCML with eosinophilia
NDE1–PDGFRB	t(5;16)(q33.1;p13.11)	CMML
RABEP1–PDGFRB	t(5;17)(q33.1;p13.2)	CMML
SPECC1–PDGFRB	t(5;17)(q33.1;p11.2)	JMML

Please see Bain and colleagues (2007)[47] and Savage and colleagues (2013)[102] for additional references.

Abbreviations: aCML, atypical chronic myeloid leukemia; CEL, chronic eosinophilic leukemia; CMML, chronic myelomonocytic leukemia; JMML, juvenile myelomonocytic leukemia; MDS, myelodysplastic syndrome; MPN, myeloproliferative neoplasm.

[a] Most common genetic abnormality within this group of neoplasms.
Modified from Refs.[13,47,102]

JMML may enter the differential diagnosis in pediatric patients. In the case of atypical CML, consideration for other diagnoses may be made once PCR analysis for the *BCR-ABL1* gene transcript is negative. It is important to be aware of the association of translocations involving chromosome 5q, especially in cases in which eosinophilia is prominent, to ensure that such cases have subsequent FISH or PCR testing for the gene fusion product involving *PDGFRB*.

In cases with a CEL-like proliferation with or without end-organ damage, CEL NOS, HES, and myeloid neoplasms with *PDGFRA* rearrangements become higher in the differential diagnosis. Cases showing *PDGFRA* gene rearrangements may be detected either by FISH analysis of the peripheral blood to examine for the loss of the *CHIC2* gene on chromosome 4q12 or via RT-PCR for the rearranged *PDGFRA* gene transcript. Cases with *FGFR1* rearrangements may less commonly present as CEL, but these cases are identified on karyotype analysis showing a translocation involving chromosome locus 8p12. In addition, progression to, or the concomitant presence of AML or T-LBL is more often reported in cases of *PDGFRA* and *FGFR1* rearrangements, as compared with *PDGFRB* rearrangements.

Immunohistochemistry for tryptase may be necessary in cases with associated fibrosis to evaluate for atypical mast cell populations (coexpression of CD25 and/or CD2 may be seen). Thus, the differential diagnosis could include SM.[51] Cases of SM would be positive for D816V *KIT*; it appears that cases with concomitant *PDGFRB* rearrangements and *KIT* mutations are mutually exclusive, although such a study has not been conducted to date. Cases without a mast cell proliferation may resemble primary myelofibrosis.

PROGNOSIS

The *PDGFRB* fusion gene results in constitutive tyrosine kinase therapy, which renders this neoplasm particularly sensitive to imatinib. Thus, the drug regimen is similar to patients with the *FIP1L1-PDGFRA* rearrangement and consists of imatinib, from 100 to 400 mg daily, although some sources advocate dosing at the higher end of this range.[6,49] These patients will usually experience complete morphologic and molecular remissions. Responses to imatinib have been reported in the variant translocations other than the classic t(5;12)(q33.1;p13).[47] Remissions may be monitored with karyotypic analysis, FISH, or RT-PCR.[50] Maintenance therapy usually consists of a similar or lower dose of imatinib therapy.

As this neoplasm is rare, determining the true survival rate is challenging. However, patients who are diagnosed at an early time course in disease are less likely to have end-organ manifestations of disease (eg, eosinophil-related cardiomyopathy) and show an improved prognosis. In patients in whom more severe manifestations of disease have already occurred, adjunct therapy with corticosteroids may be used.

MYELOID AND LYMPHOID NEOPLASMS WITH *FGFR1* ABNORMALITIES

CLINICAL FEATURES

Myeloid and lymphoid neoplasms with fibroblast growth factor receptor 1 (*FGFR1*) abnormalities are known by several names, including 8p11 myeloproliferative syndrome/8p11 stem cell syndrome (although the gene is now known to be mapped to 8p12), and stem cell leukemia/lymphoma syndrome. The first description of the entity was made in 1977 when Manthorpe and colleagues[52] described a case of a 41-year-old man with persistent blood eosinophilia and a concomitant T-cell lymphoma; the term 8p11 myeloproliferative syndrome (abbreviated here as 8p12 MPS) was coined by a review of 13 cases by Macdonald and colleagues.[53] As the clinical presentation shows overlap with MPNs with abnormalities of *PDGFRA* and *PDGFRB*, these were placed within the same category within the 2008 WHO classification. It is important to remember, however, that eosinophilia does not present in all cases, and neoplasms with *FGFR1* rearrangements are not sensitive to imatinib therapy.

The 8p12 MPS is a rare hematolymphoid neoplasm that occurs in a variety of ages, with reports ranging from 3 to 84 years of age with a median age of onset in the fifth decade of life.[53,54] The presentation is heterogeneous, including AML, T-ALL or B-ALL, or as an MPN. The 8p12 MPS presents with only a slight male predominance.[54] Although a subset of patients are asymptomatic at presentation, those that are symptomatic present with fatigue, weight loss, night sweats, or fever.[47] Asymptomatic patients are usually detected by abnormalities of a complete blood count. Approximately 90% of all patients have blood or bone marrow eosinophilia at presentation, with monocytosis and thrombocytopenia occurring in approximately three-fourths and one-half of patients, respectively.[53,54]

The presentation of neoplasms with *FGFR1* abnormalities seems to be dependent on the fusion partner that is associated with the 8p12 translocation. Cases showing the most common translocation t(8;13)(p12;q11-12) typically present with concurrent lymphadenopathy due to T-LBL; cases with t(8;9)(p12;q33.2) may present with tonsillar enlargement and a monocytosis[55]; cases with t(6;8)(q27;p12) may present with eosinophilia and polycythemia[56]; whereas cases with t(8;22)(p12;q11) may show basophilia.[57]

MICROSCOPIC FEATURES AND ANCILLARY STUDIES

Given the heterogeneous presentation at diagnosis, peripheral blood, bone marrow, and lymph node biopsies will show a varied appearance. Most cases will show a concomitant eosinophilia in the bone marrow and/or peripheral blood and is part of the neoplastic clone (Fig. 6). When lymphoblastic lymphoma is present (Fig. 7), these cases will show a hypercellular marrow with either myeloproliferative features or acute leukemia. Nearly all cases reported appear to represent de novo disease with no associated therapy-related etiology or underlying MDS; one case was stated to have arisen from an underlying MDS 5 years prior.[58]

To date, 13 distinct translocations and 1 insertion have been reported, all of which involve the FGFR1 gene on chromosome 8 (Table 3). The t(8;13)(p12;q11-12) ZMYM2(ZNF198)-FGFR1 is the most commonly reported translocation seen in cases of 8p12 MPS, and occurs in approximately one-half of all cases of 8p12 MPS.[54] This subset of patients may present with lymphadenopathy involved by T-LBL or less frequently B-LBL. Lymph node biopsy will demonstrate complete effacement of the lymph node with capsular involvement, cells with immature features, with interspersed eosinophils in most cases, and a prominent high endothelial vessel network. Bone marrow may show concurrent involvement. These patients may also present with an MPN characterized by circulating left shifted granulocytes and an absolute eosinophilia. The myeloproliferative component eventually advances to AML or a mixed phenotype acute leukemia. The t(8;13)(p12;q11-12) or variant translocation involving chromosome 8p12 will be identified by routine karyotype analysis.

Basophilia and concurrent eosinophilia in 8p12 MPS is often reported with the t(8;22)(p12;q11) BCR-FGFR1 translocation, which may also show concurrent LBL in the bone marrow or lymph nodes. Most of these cases reported present as MPNs with a subset evolving to AML.[57,59,60] Cases may also present as mixed phenotype acute

Table 3
FGFR1-associated fusion genes and corresponding morphology

Fusion Gene	Translocation	Diagnosis at Presentation
ZMYM2–FGFR1[a]	t(8;13)(p12;q11-q12)[a]	Variable, including CEL, AML, T-LBL, B-ALL
CNTRL–FGFR1	t(8;9)(p12;q33.2)	Variable, including aCML, MPN with tonsillar T-LBL, AML
FGFR1OP–FGFR1	t(6;8)(q27;p12)	Variable, including PV, aCML, AML, B-ALL
BCR–FGFR1	t(8;22)(p12;q11)	aCML
TRIM24–FGFR1	t(7;8)(q32-q34;p12)	AML
MYO18A–FGFR1	t(8;17)(p12;q11.2)	MDS/MPN with eosinophilia and basophilia
ERVK3-1–FGFR1	t(8;19)(p12;q13.43)	AML secondary to MDS/MPN
FGFR1OP2–FGFR1	ins(12;8)(p12.1;p12)	T-LBL with eosinophilia
LRRFIP1–FGFR1	t(2;8)(q37.3;p12)	MDS
CPSF6–FGFR1	t(8;12)(p12;q15)/dic(8;12)(p12;p11)	MDS/MPN with eosinophilia
NUP98–FGFR1	t(8;11)(p12;p15)	AML
TPR–FGFR1	t(1;8)(q25;p12)	aCML
CUX1–FGFR1	t(7;8)(q22.1;p12)	T-ALL

Please see Bain and colleagues (2007)[47] and Savage and colleagues (2013)[102] for additional references.
Abbreviations: aCML, atypical chronic myeloid leukemia; AML, acute myeloid leukemia; B-ALL, B-acute lymphoblastic leukemia; CEL, chronic eosinophilic leukemia; MDS, myelodysplastic syndrome; MPN, myeloproliferative neoplasm; PV, polycythemia vera; T-ALL, T-acute lymphoblastic leukemia; T-LBL, T-lymphoblastic lymphoma.
[a] Most common genetic abnormality within this group of neoplasms.
Data from Refs.[13,47,102]

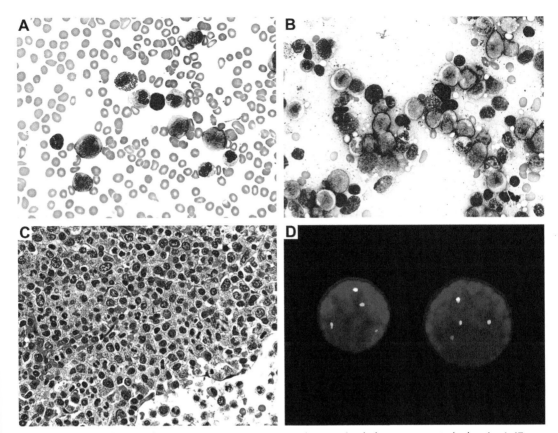

Fig. 6. Myeloid neoplasm with *FGFR1* rearrangement presenting as mixed phenotype acute leukemia. A 47-year-old man presented with neck swelling, massive lymphadenopathy, low-grade fevers, WBC count of 132×10^9/L, Hgb 11.1 g/dL; platelets 117×10^9/L; 36% neutrophils (ANC = 59.6×10^9/L), 8% metamyelocytes, 4% monocytes (absolute monocyte count [AMC] = 5.3×10^9/L), and 42% blasts. (*A*) The peripheral blood reveals increased numbers of blasts with an absolute neutrophilia and monocytosis (Wright Giemsa, ×60). (*B*) The bone marrow aspirate revealed a similar increase in blasts with increased numbers of neutrophils, eosinophils, and mast cells. Flow cytometry of the bone marrow core biopsy revealed a T/B/myeloid mixed phenotype acute leukemia (Wright Giemsa, ×60). (*C*) The bone marrow core biopsy was expectedly hypercellular with sheets of blasts and mature neutrophils and eosinophils (H&E, ×40). (*D*) Karyotype revealed a t(8;22) translocation, with other minor cytogenetic abnormalities, and subsequent FISH testing using a break-apart probe for *FGFR1* revealed one split red-and-green signal consistent with a rearrangement involving *FGFR1*. The patient has since received multiagent chemotherapy in preparation for bone marrow transplantation.

leukemia (see **Fig. 6**). Routine karyotype analysis will reveal the t(8;22)(p12;q11). The t(6;8)(q27;p12) in 8p12 MPS results in the fusion of genes *FGFR1OP1* and *FGFR1* that leads to dimerization of and the constitutive activation of the tyrosine kinase product.[61] Several cases have been reported thus far in the literature, a subset of which have presented or subsequently developed polycythemia.[56,62] These patients all eventually developed AML, ALL, or myeloid sarcoma.

DIFFERENTIAL DIAGNOSIS

Given the markedly varied presentation at diagnosis, the differential diagnosis is broad. It is important to have a high index of suspicion when eosinophilia is present with lymphadenopathy or if LBL presents concomitantly with leukemia.

Although a correct diagnosis of T-ALL/LBL or B-ALL/LBL may be made in a patient with lymphadenopathy, the presence of a prominent eosinophilic infiltrate or a concomitant myeloid hyperplasia in a peripheral blood or bone marrow trephine study should raise consideration of a diagnosis of 8p12 MPS. Karyotypic analysis will reveal a variant 8p12 translocation. Other neoplastic conditions that may show diffuse lymph node involvement and eosinophilia include angioimmunoblastic T-cell lymphoma (AITL) and peripheral T-cell lymphoma, not otherwise specified (PTCL). The morphology in these cases tends to appear more mature than in T-LBL, and these mature T-cell lymphomas lack TdT by immunohistochemistry. However, TdT is not positive in all cases of T-LBL and other markers of immaturity, such as CD1a, CD99, and CD34, may also need to be performed.[63]

The chronic phase of 8p12 MPS shows a significant amount of morphologic overlap with MPNs or MDS/MPNs. Cases of t(8;9)(p12;q33.2) may originally be diagnosed as polycythemia vera, even when the JAK2 V617F mutation is not detected. Similarly, the presence of significant monocytosis, especially those cases in the chronic phase demonstrating the t(8;9)(p12;q33.2), may show similarities to CMML. Thus, conventional cytogenetic analysis, FISH studies, and other molecular genetic studies are all important in narrowing the differential diagnosis to 8p12 MPS.

The acute phase of 8p12 MPS may present as AML, T-ALL, a mixed phenotype acute leukemia, or rarely B-ALL. Even when in the acute phase, increased numbers of maturing granulocytes, eosinophils, or basophils may be present in the peripheral blood and thus the case may be mistaken for blast phase of CML. Correlation with other findings, such as lymphadenopathy and cytogenetic studies, will serve the pathologist well in making a diagnosis of 8p12 MPS. As these cases may look similar to those in the myeloproliferative umbrella category to which PDGFRA and PDGFRB belong, molecular testing for PDGFRA and PDGFRB rearrangements may also be necessary to exclude these imatinib-sensitive neoplasms.

PROGNOSIS

The prognosis of 8p12 MPS is poor. Regardless of the translocation and fusion gene formed, all cases encode for an aberrant tyrosine kinase. However, unlike the cases of myeloid and lymphoid neoplasms with PDGFRA and PDGFRB rearrangements, 8p12 MPS is not responsive to imatinib. A recent case review showed that approximately two-thirds of patients present with AML/myeloid sarcoma, one-fifth with LBL, and one-tenth with a MPN.[54] Directed therapies have been attempted based on presentation with limited success. Stem cell transplantation has shown a relative success in management of this disorder, with extension of the median survival to approximately 24 months as compared with 12 months. Furthermore, transplantation should be considered even at the MPN stage of diagnosis, although the mean time to transformation is approximately 4 months (range 0–24).[54] Interferon-α and midostaurin have been used in a small

subset of patients and reported to show reduction in leukocytosis, and lymphadenopathy, although in these cases the patients were treated in the chronic phase and subsequently went on to receive bone marrow transplantation.[64,65] Recently, agents that had been originally intended for the native and mutated BCR-ABL1 tyrosine kinase fusion proteins (eg, ponatinib) have been shown to prolong survival in murine models with FGFR1 rearrangements.[66] It is to be determined whether these agents will show similar efficacy in humans.

CEL NOS

CLINICAL FEATURES

CEL NOS is characterized by a clonal proliferation of eosinophils with evidence of an underlying MPN that is related to the eosinophilic clone. CEL NOS is a diagnosis of exclusion, requiring the absence of other mutations or rearrangements that may be associated with eosinophilia, including BCR-ABL1 and rearrangements of PDGFRA, PDGFRB, and FGFR1; however, evidence of clonality should be established in these cases. If clonality cannot be established, a defined increase in either peripheral and/or bone marrow blasts should be present, but fewer than 20% in either site. The peripheral eosinophil count is greater than 1.5×10^9/L.[67] Due to the change in the 2008 WHO classification now distinguishing CEL NOS, HES, and eosinophilia associated with rearrangements of PDGFRA, determination of the true incidence of CEL NOS is challenging. However, it is thought that CEL NOS is an exceptionally rare entity with a greater incidence in males.[6,67]

Patients eventually diagnosed with CEL NOS may be identified asymptomatically after workup for peripheral eosinophilia. Those who are symptomatic at diagnosis will show manifestations of end-organ–related symptomatology, including fever, fatigue, night sweats, dyspnea, pruritus, weakness or other musculoskeletal complaints, or gastrointestinal symptoms, including diarrhea. End-organ involvement may resemble that of HES and neoplasms with PDGFRA rearrangements and similarly thought to be due to the release of contents within eosinophilic granules in the cardiac, pulmonary, gastrointestinal, and central and peripheral nervous systems.

MICROSCOPIC FEATURES

The sine qua non feature of this neoplasm is eosinophilia, which is usually represented by predominantly mature eosinophils, with fewer numbers of

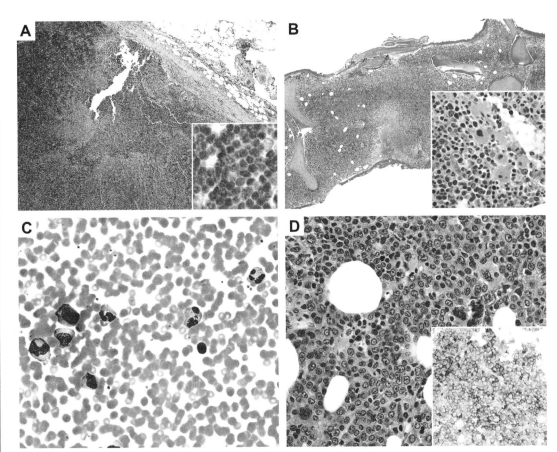

Fig. 7. Myeloid neoplasms with *FGFR1* rearrangements presenting as T-lymphoblastic lymphoma (originally described by Savage and colleagues[103]). A 46-year-old man presented with cervical and abdominal lymphadenopathy. (*A*) A biopsy of an inguinal lymph node revealed an effaced lymph node replaced by lymphoblasts. Eosinophils were also interspersed throughout the lymph node. Immunohistochemistry revealed the infiltrate was positive for TdT (*A*; H&E, ×10, *inset*; Tdt, ×40); flow cytometry studies performed on the lymph node were consistent with T-lymphoblastic lymphoma. (*B*; H&E, ×10) Concurrent bone marrow was hypercellular with myeloproliferative features including clusters of atypical megakaryocytes (*inset*; H&E, ×20). (*C*) Concurrent peripheral blood showed an elevated WBC count of 33.2 × 10^9 and a peripheral eosinophilia (8% eosinophils, AEC = 2.73 × 10^9); occasional circulating blasts were also noted (Wright Giemsa, ×60). (*D*) Following a preparatory regimen for allogeneic bone marrow transplantation, the patient developed pancytopenia. The bone marrow biopsy revealed sheets of proerythroblasts (acute erythroid leukemia), which was confirmed by immunohistochemistry for glycophorin B (*D*; H&E, ×40, *inset*; Glycophorin, ×20).

left-shifted eosinophilic precursors (**Fig. 8**). Eosinophils may show normal morphology or may show hypogranulation, hypolobation or hyperlobation, ring eosinophils, or cytoplasmic vacuolization.[68–71] Abnormal morphology, however, should not be regarded as a proxy for clonality, as reactive eosinophilias may show similar findings and normal morphology may be seen in neoplastic eosinophils.[72–74] Eosinophilia predominates but may be associated with absolute increases in other cells, including neutrophils and monocytes. A subtle or appreciable increase in blasts may also be seen, but should not exceed 20% in either the peripheral blood or bone marrow.

In the bone marrow, a similar increase in eosinophils and eosinophilic precursors is appreciated. Because of this increase, the marrow is generally hypercellular. Other findings include the presence of increased blasts, abnormal localization of immature precursors, as well as dysplasia in multiple lineages, including eosinophils. An increase in blasts is defined as greater than 2% blasts in the peripheral blood and/or greater than 5% blasts in the bone marrow. The increase in eosinophils may also lead to marrow fibrosis that may be appreciable at diagnosis.[69] Other accompanying findings may include the presence of Charcot-Leyden crystals, as well as fibrosis.[3,68,75] Biopsy

Fig. 8. CEL NOS. (*A*) A peripheral blood smear of a 60-year-old woman with eosinophilia includes a leukocytosis consisting predominantly of mature eosinophils. Eosinophils show hypogranular, vacuolated, and hyperlobated forms (Wright Giemsa, ×100). (*B*) The bone marrow aspirate showed predominantly mature eosinophils; examination of the other lineages showed moderate megaloblastoid changes in the erythroid lineage and hypolobated neutrophils (Wright Giemsa, ×100). (*C*) The bone marrow findings were reflective of the bone marrow aspirate with a predominance of mature eosinophils (H&E, ×40).

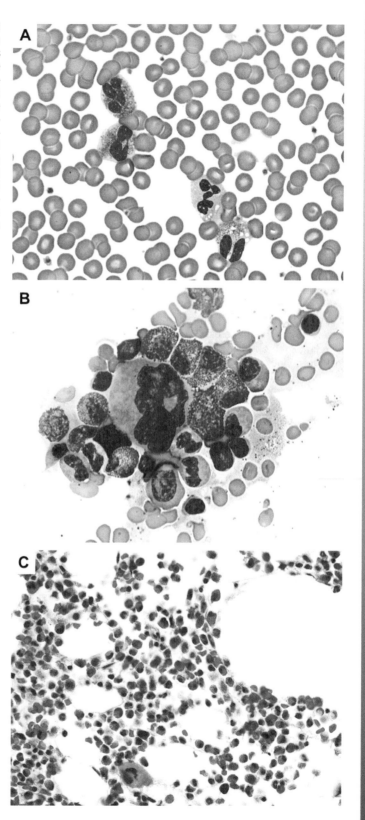

of tissues with end-organ involvement may reveal significant eosinophil infiltration.

ANCILLARY STUDIES

Detection of increased blasts in blood or marrow in CEL NOS may be established by morphology or immunophenotypic studies. If no increase in blasts is noted, demonstration of eosinophil clonality must be made to distinguish this entity from idiopathic hypereosinophilia (iHE) and HES.[67] Isolation of eosinophils by cell culture or cell-sorting techniques with subsequent molecular analysis[76,77] or FISH[78] have been performed. Clonality can be established in female patients with molecular analysis of X chromosome genes such as *PGK*, *HUMARA*, or *G6PD*.[76,79] Some groups advocate that isolation of and detection of a clonal cytogenetic abnormality in the eosinophil population is unnecessary for the diagnosis of CEL NOS, as these techniques are often cumbersome and mainly of historical interest. Isochromosome 17q or gain of chromosome 8 have been reported most frequently in the literature.[73,79]

DIFFERENTIAL DIAGNOSIS

After reactive causes for eosinophilia have been excluded, the differential diagnosis for CEL NOS is broad and reflective of other clonal hematopoietic neoplasms that may also demonstrate eosinophilia. Other myeloid neoplasms that may show a mild or marked increased in blasts and show accompanying eosinophilia include AML with t(8;21)(q22;q22) and AML with inv(16)(p13.1q22)/(16;16)(p13.1;q22).[5,80] AML with inv(16)(p13.1q22) may show similar morphologic overlap that may include nuclear hypolobation and abnormal granulation. In addition, cases of AML with inv(16)(p13.1q22) are defined by the translocation and thus may have fewer than 20% blasts in the peripheral blood and bone marrow[80] and lead to initial diagnostic difficulty.

Other MPNs may similarly be accompanied by eosinophilia, including CML and CMML. Myeloid and lymphoid neoplasms associated with *PDGFRA* rearrangements present similarly with peripheral eosinophilia and symptoms related to end-organ damage. Although routine karyotypic studies may appear normal, assessment for the cryptic del(4q) either by molecular or FISH techniques will be positive in myeloid neoplasms with *PDGFRA* rearrangements. Neoplasms associated with *PDGFRB* rearrangements show features similar to CMML with a concomitant absolute eosinophilia in the peripheral blood along with a hypercellular marrow with increased mature eosinophils. These cases may also be accompanied by a mast cell infiltrate. Cytogenetic studies in these cases would show a translocation involving chromosome 5q31~33, the locus of *PDGFRB*. Finally, although patients with *FGFR1* rearrangements may show a predominance of eosinophils in the blood and bone marrow, most of these patients will also show or eventually develop AML, T-LBL, or B-LBL as well as the presence of a rearrangement involving chromosome locus 8p12, the site of the *FGFR1* gene. This underscores the importance and necessity of molecular and cytogenetic analysis in distinguishing CEL NOS from myeloid and lymphoid neoplasms with abnormalities of *PDGFRA*, *PDGRFB*, and *FGFR1*.

PROGNOSIS

The prognosis of CEL NOS is variable. Previous studies examining the prognosis of eosinophilic disease were likely not homogeneous and included patients with HES, neoplasms associated with *PDGFRA* rearrangements, and CEL NOS.[6,18] Thus, although these studies had noted a 5-year survival rate of approximately 80%,[68,70,75] this heterogeneity limits determination of the true prognosis of CEL NOS. However, in general, those patients with more severe end-organ damage, including those with cardiac damage, are thought to carry a worse prognosis.

HES

CLINICAL FEATURES

The term hypereosinophilic syndrome (HES) was originally used by Hardy and Anderson in 1968 to refer to patients with hypereosinophilia causing significant pulmonary and cardiovascular end-organ damage not the result of parasitic or allergic disease.[81,82] Chusid and colleagues[68] performed a large review of cases from the literature, as well as from their own set of 14 patients. Most patients in their review were middle-aged men who presented with end-organ damage, eosinophilia, and a short time-course to death. Criteria that were proposed and subsequently adopted for HES included a persistent eosinophilia greater than 1.5×10^9/L for longer than 6 months, a lack of evidence of known secondary causes of eosinophilia, and signs and symptoms of organ involvement.[67,82,83] In the current WHO classification, the criteria also include exclusion of a primary hematolymphoid neoplastic cause of eosinophilia and a lack of evidence of eosinophil clonality.[67,84]

Individuals may present with evidence of end-organ involvement and biopsy may reveal increased eosinophils in tissues markedly beyond that expected for location. Some working groups also regard these patients as having a diagnosis of HE when the peripheral blood or bone marrow does not reveal an elevated eosinophil count. These working groups have further subdivided cases with a letter subscript to specify the underlying cause of eosinophilia when known (f = familial, n = neoplastic, r = reactive) or unknown (us = undetermined significance).[24,85] Other proposed refinements to the diagnosis include duration of eosinophilia of greater than 1.5×10^9/L for only 1 month instead of 6.[6,85]

In the review by Chusid and colleagues,[68] the male-to-female ratio was 9:1. These patients had generally presented in their fourth or fifth decade of life with end-organ damage, with the age of onset ranging from 5 to 80 years of age.[68,81] Recent studies have reported a male-to-female ratio of 11:8 when exclusion of eosinophilia associated with *FIP1L1-PDGFRA* rearrangement is made,[20] and may more closely approximate the incidence of iHE and HES.

The organ systems most commonly affected in HES include cardiovascular, cutaneous, and nervous systems.[83,84,86] Patients may present with nonspecific systemic symptoms, including fatigue, weight loss, fever, and shortness of breath.[75] Signs and symptoms that may point to more specific end-organ involvement may also be evident on history and physical examination. Mucocutaneous findings include pruritus, cutaneous rash, diaphoresis, angioedema, erythema, and eczema.[24,75,83] Early cardiac manifestations may include shortness of breath, chest pain, or cough, with eventual progression to congestive heart failure, including orthopnea and peripheral edema.[70,84] Peripheral and central nervous system complications include altered behavior and cognition, ataxia, sensory polyneuropathy, and mononeuritis multiplex, as well as manifestations related to emboli of cardiac origin.[83,86] Gastrointestinal, hepatobiliary, renal, and pulmonary involvement occurs, but is less common.

MICROSCOPIC FEATURES

Cardiac manifestations are the most well characterized and thus prototypical demonstration of pathogenesis in patients with HES (**Fig. 9**). Cardiac pathogenesis progresses in 3 phases, with an early necrotic phase, followed by a thrombotic stage involving thrombus formation along the damaged endocardium, and finally by a fibrotic phase that may take years to develop.[20,75,83] The necrosis seen is due to tissue infiltration of eosinophils, with subsequent degranulation and granule deposition. This necrosis eventually leads to damage of the endocardial lining, predisposing patients to develop endocardial thrombus formation that may lead to splinter hemorrhages or symptoms related to cerebral or peripheral vascular embolic events. Eventually the endocardial surface and myocardium become replaced with collagen fibrosis, leading to diastolic heart failure.[20,47] Pulmonary involvement presents as a

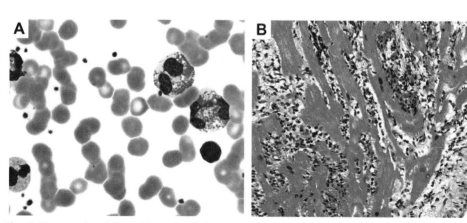

Fig. 9. Hypereosinophilia with eosinophilic myocarditis. A 45-year-old woman presented with a diffuse rash, altered mental status changes, blurred vision, and myocardial infarction. Laboratory values included WBC count 23.8×10^9/L, Hgb 9.8, platelet count 500×10^9/L, ANC: 17.5×10^9/L, AEC 1.98×10^9/L. (*A*) The peripheral blood smear showed eosinophils with normal morphology (Wright Giemsa, ×100). (*B*) A cardiac biopsy shows a dense infiltrate of eosinophils with interstitial edema and extensive myocyte damage. *PDGFRA, BCR-ABL1, JAK2*, and T-cell clonality studies were negative. The patient was placed on high-dose corticosteroid therapy and showed improvement in mental status, cardiac function, and normalization of eosinophil counts while on steroid therapy (H&E, ×20). ([*B*] *Courtesy of* Gerald Berry, MD, Department of Pathology, Stanford University School of Medicine.)

nonspecific interstitial and alveolar space infiltration of eosinophils that may be associated with other inflammatory cells, including lymphocytes and plasma cells, as well as a fibrinous exudate. Eosinophils may or may not be degranulated, and Charcot-Leyden crystals could be in severe cases.[87,88] Similar findings may be seen in other organ systems. If eosinophils are not evident in tissues due to degranulation, immunohistochemistry for major basic protein or other eosinophil granular proteins may be performed.[17,24]

Bone marrow involvement in cases of HES is characterized by a variably cellular, but often hypercellular, marrow predominated by mature eosinophils with occasional eosinophil myelocytes and metamyelocytes. Blasts are expected to be fewer than 5% of cells on a manual differential count. Mature eosinophils are generally normal in morphology, although some may show degranulation. Increases in other myeloid lineages are not expected. Peripheral blood shows an absolute eosinophilia with predominantly mature forms; blasts are expected to be fewer than 2% of cells on a manual differential count. The absolute eosinophil count must be sustained higher than 1.5×10^9/L for the diagnosis of HE.

ANCILLARY STUDIES

By definition, patients with HES will have a normal karyotype and no evidence of rearrangements in PDGFRA, PDGFRB, FGFR1, or mutations in KIT, JAK2, or BCR-ABL1. Cytogenetic and molecular testing must be performed for this diagnosis to be made.

DIFFERENTIAL DIAGNOSIS

At initial diagnosis, symptomatic patients with an elevated eosinophil count should have a series of diagnostic tests before the early initiation of therapy when possible (see Fig. 1). The minimum evaluation for presumed HES includes a complete blood count with manual differential and morphologic review and a complete metabolic panel with focus on liver enzymes, cardiac enzymes, or renal function tests to determine if serum marker evidence of liver cardiac, or kidney end-organ damage is present. A serum B12 level and serum tryptase should be performed; if levels are elevated, this may be suggestive of an MPN, especially myeloid neoplasms with rearrangements involving the PDGFRA gene or SM, respectively.[23,49,89] Serum antineutrophil cytoplasmic antibodies, antinuclear antibodies, rheumatoid factor, or other antibody levels should also be performed if the differential diagnosis includes collagen vascular disease or other autoimmune conditions. Stool ova and parasite testing and serology testing may also be indicated if the clinical and travel history are suggestive of an infectious agent. Imaging studies, such as chest and abdomen computed tomography or echocardiography, may be required depending on the presenting symptoms.

Hematopoietic neoplasms should be ruled out once secondary causes have been excluded. These additional tests should be attempted before initiation of therapy that usually comprises intravenous corticosteroids.[6] T-cell and B-cell receptor gene rearrangement studies, as well as flow cytometry, may be performed on the peripheral blood to evaluate the T-lymphocyte or B-lymphocyte compartments. Approximately 10% to 14% of cases with findings suggestive of HES are more appropriately categorized as myeloid or lymphoid neoplasms with rearrangements of PDGFRA when such testing is performed.[17,18,20,89] BCR-ABL1 testing on peripheral blood may reveal rare cases of chronic-phase CML with prominent eosinophilia.[24,90] Finally JAK2 V617F mutation testing may be performed if an absolute thrombocytosis is present.

A bone marrow biopsy and aspirate with cytogenetic karyotyping should be performed before therapy initiation. AML with inv(16)(p13.1q22)/t(16;16)(p13.1;q22) may also present with few myeloblasts and a marrow eosinophil predominance (so called oligoblastic AML). Eosinophils in AML with inv(16)(p13.1q22) often are dysplastic appearing with abnormal basophilic granules; blasts present may show monocytic differentiation. B-ALL with t(5;14)(q31;q32) characteristically shows peripheral and bone marrow eosinophilia (see Fig. 2). Karyotype analysis may also reveal chromosomal rearrangements involving either the PDGFRB gene at chromosome locus 5p33.1 or the FGFR1 gene at locus 8p12. In addition, rearrangements of PDGFRA may not show the cryptic deletion but may show an overt karyotypic abnormality involving locus 4q12.

PROGNOSIS

The overall prognosis of HES is variable. Few studies have been conducted on HES since the distinction with other neoplasms associated with HE had been made in the 2008 WHO classification. Before these changes, one of the first large studies of hypereosinophilic patients in 1975 comprising 14 patients showed a 3-year survival rate of approximately 10%[68] with a subsequent review of 40 patients conducted 14 years later revealing a 5-year survival rate of 80%.[91] Early therapy generally consisted of corticosteroids with the addition of cytotoxic agents, such as hydroxyurea, busulfan, or 6-mercaptopurine if recalcitrant to steroid therapy.[82] The reasons for the improved outcome rates are unknown but may include earlier detection and definitive therapy. However, many studies conducted were retrospective reviews that may have included patients with more severe disease manifestations. A recent international review by Ogbogu and colleagues[20] of 188 patients revealed a higher frequency of cutaneous, gastrointestinal, and pulmonary involvement with fewer numbers of patients with cardiac and neurologic manifestations of disease. Although only 4 deaths were noted in this retrospective study, which spanned 6 years, 11% of patients had *PDGFRA* rearrangements and 17% of patients tested showed a clonal T-cell population, not further specified. Prospective studies of patients who meet the current criteria for HES are needed to obtain a more homogeneous population of patients and establish appropriate outcome data.

The most recent study of patients with HES assessed 23 patients and reviewed 21 patients from the literature who died from HES; the most common cause of death was due to cardiac dysfunction, including myocarditis, cardiomyopathy, and conduction abnormalities, but other causes included thromboembolic disease, cerebral hemorrhage, and sepsis related to high-dose immunosuppressive therapy. Corticosteroids, interferon alpha, and hydroxyurea were the most common agents used, with occasional patients on cytotoxic therapy, such as vincristine and cladribine.[92] Another study of HES performed in 2006 showed that most patients managed with prednisone showed a 55% morphologic response rate after 1 month. A smaller set of patients were treated with antibodies to IL-5 (mepolizumab) with an 80% complete drug response rate after 1 month of therapy.[20]

SM

CLINICAL FEATURES

SM is the result of a clonal proliferation of mast cells present in one or multiple extracutaneous organ systems with or without skin involvement. The 2008 WHO *Classification of Tumours of Haematopoietic and Lymphoid Tissues* requires either 1 major and 1 minor criterion, or 3 minor criteria for the diagnosis of SM. The major criterion is the presence of multiple dense aggregates of mast cells composed of at least 15 mast cells per aggregate. The 4 minor criteria include (1) abnormal mast cell morphology, (2) D816V *KIT* mutation,

(3) expression of CD25 and/or CD2 on mast cells, and (4) an elevated serum tryptase level[93]; the last criterion cannot be used if an associated hematologic non–mast cell disorder (AHD) is present. Cases of SM are further delineated based on the presence of laboratory and clinical findings (eg, indolent, aggressive).[93,94] In a subset of cases, SM is associated with eosinophilia (SM-eo). This eosinophilia may be reactive, associated with the neoplastic mast cell clone, or reflect a separate neoplastic process associated with an AHD.

Depending on the site of involvement and burden of disease, patient presentation may be heterogeneous, including generalized systemic symptoms and/or localized symptoms.[95] Systemic manifestations may include low-grade fever, fatigue, and weight loss. Bone marrow involvement may lead to cytopenias. Cutaneous manifestations include multiple maculopapular cutaneous lesions, diffuse erythema with skin thickening and edema, as well as pruritus. Musculoskeletal signs and symptoms may include generalized muscle or bone pain, osteoporosis with pathologic facture, and joint pain. Nonspecific symptoms, such as abdominal pain, may indicate hepatic and/or splenic involvement by SM or extramedullary hematopoiesis.

The exact frequency of SM-eo within the larger category of SM is not completely known. A study by Pardanani and colleagues[23] reviewed 123 patients with "SM with an associated myeloid non mast cell neoplasm" and reported that eosinophilia was present in 34% of patients. This study is now known to include both patients with SM and those with myeloid neoplasms with *PDGFRA*; the latter category can also include mast cell proliferations but should not be regarded as SM.

MICROSCOPIC FEATURES

Peripheral blood findings for SM-eo include a peripheral eosinophilia that may be either mild or marked (**Figs. 10** and **11**). In most cases, the eosinophils show normal nuclear morphology and appropriate granulation. Other indices, such as an absolute monocytosis and absolute neutrophilia, may be present and resemble an MPN. In some cases, eosinophils may be the only index that is elevated, leading to a differential diagnosis that includes CEL. If the burden in the bone marrow is significant, circulating mast cells in the peripheral blood may also be identified on thorough morphologic review. Dysplasia in the neutrophil lineage, such as hypogranular neutrophils or neutrophils with Pelgeroid nuclei, may also be seen. An associated anemia and thrombocytopenia are invariably present. A subset of patients

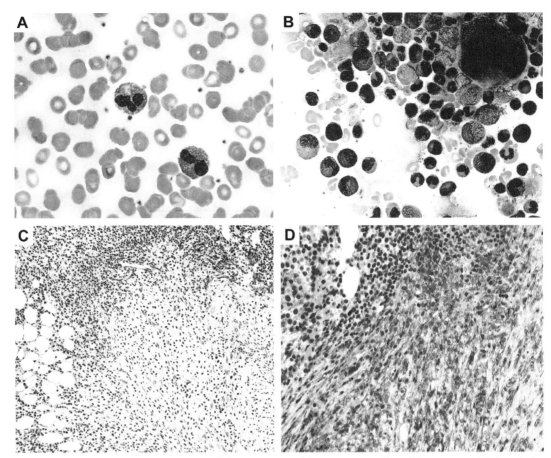

Fig. 10. Systemic mastocytosis with eosinophilia. A 68-year-old woman was referred from an outside hospital to evaluate for systemic mastocytosis. Her laboratory parameters included WBC count 13.4×10^9/L, Hgb 10 g/dL, AEC 7.8×10^9/L, absolute monocytes 1.04×10^9/L; serum tryptase 274 ng/mL. (*A*) A peripheral blood smear revealed normal eosinophil morphology (Wright Giemsa, ×100). (*B*) A bone marrow aspirate revealed predominantly eosinophilic myelocytes and mature eosinophils (31%) with mast cells accounting for 2% of nucleated cells (Wright Giemsa, ×60). (*C*) The bone marrow core biopsy demonstrated a hypercellular marrow with aggregates of mast cells present in large dense clusters; eosinophils are seen at the periphery (H&E, ×40). (*D*) A tryptase stain confirmed the major criterion for SM; the bone marrow was positive for the D816V *KIT* mutation. D816V was negative in the peripheral blood and serum IL-5 levels were elevated (70 pg/mL). The elevated IL-5 level and lack of D816V *KIT* mutation in the peripheral blood support a nonclonal reactive eosinophilia (Tryptase, ×40).

may also have concurrent systemic findings that may warrant a diagnosis of aggressive systemic mastocytosis (ASM).

In the current WHO classification, 1 major criterion and 1 minor criterion or 3 minor criteria must be met for the diagnosis of SM. The major criterion is the presence of multiple dense aggregates of mast cells composed of at least 15 cells per aggregate.[93] These aggregates may be paratrabecular, perivascular, or perisinusoidal in location. Associated fibrosis is typically present and may be the first clue to the presence of mast cell involvement.

Mast cell morphology is most appropriately assessed in the bone marrow aspirate slides, where spindle-shaped forms (atypical type 1 mast cells) may even be seen in clusters within aspirate spicules. Promastocyte forms (atypical type 2 mast cells) contain bilobed or indented nuclei and hypogranular cytoplasm that does not obscure the nucleus as compared with appropriately granulated, round normal mast cells.[96]

Other findings in the bone marrow include an eosinophilia, which may be the predominant component in the trephine biopsy. Eosinophils tend to be predominantly mature, but a range in maturation may be identified. Clustering of eosinophils may be seen, but cases usually show an interstitial population of eosinophils even within

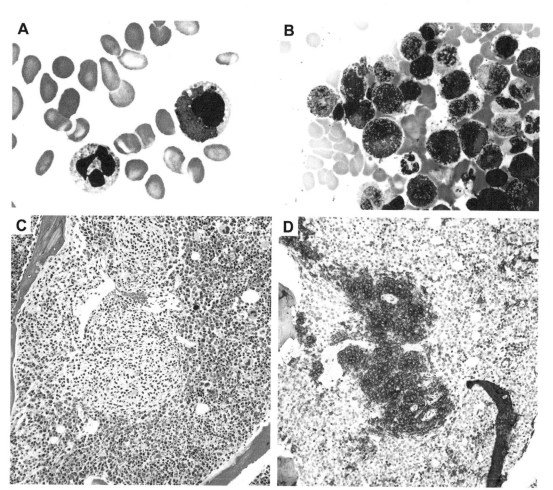

Fig. 11. Aggressive systemic mastocytosis associated with chronic eosinophilic leukemia. A 74-year-old man presented with splenomegaly and weight loss. Laboratory parameters included WBC count 8.1×10^9/L, Hgb 10 g/dL, platelet count 56×10^9/L, AEC: 3.9×10^9/L; serum tryptase 338 ng/mL. (*A*) Peripheral blood examination revealed a leukoerythroblastic smear with a subset of hypogranular neutrophils and hypolobated eosinophils (Wright Giemsa, ×100). (*B*) The bone marrow aspirate showed predominantly mature eosinophils (20%); mast cells were not increased (1%), but were hypogranular and spindle shaped (Wright Giemsa, ×100). (*C*) The bone marrow biopsy revealed a hypercellular marrow with dense mast cell aggregates. Additionally, dysplastic megakaryocytes were identified in the background (H&E, ×40). (*D*) A tryptase stain confirmed the major criterion for SM; this case was also positive for the D816V *KIT* mutation (Tryptase, ×40).

areas of clustered mast cells. These eosinophils may be reactive or part of the neoplastic clone. Due to the proliferation of eosinophils, mast cells, and other cell types, the bone marrow biopsy is predictably hypercellular. Although elevated serum IL-5 levels may suggest immune dysregulation leading to a reactive eosinophilic population, cytogenetic and/or mutational analysis is most appropriate for making the distinction between a clonal or reactive eosinophil population.

ANCILLARY STUDIES

CD117 and tryptase immunohistochemistry will serve to demonstrate mast cell aggregates on bone marrow trephine biopsy or in extramedullary locations. Immunophenotyping either by flow cytometry or immunohistochemistry can demonstrate aberrant expression of CD25[97]; CD2 coexpression is best seen by flow cytometry. Expression of CD25 may also be seen on eosinophils in some cases.

KIT mutations are usually performed on bone marrow aspirate material, but can also be performed on formalin-fixed, EDTA decalcified bone marrow biopsy material. Some institutions perform flow cytometry sorting of mast cells or microdissection of mast cells from biopsy material to determine the *KIT* mutation status of the mast cells in contrast to an AHD, if present. If mast cells are not circulating and an AHD is present, *KIT* mutation testing can be performed on peripheral blood to determine if the AHD carries the *KIT* mutation.[98] Although the D816V *KIT* mutation is most common in SM, other *KIT* mutations have been reported.[98,99]

DIFFERENTIAL DIAGNOSIS

Primary considerations in the differential diagnosis of SM-eo include cases in which mastocytosis and an associated eosinophilia are evident. These include myeloid neoplasms with rearrangements involving the *PDGFRA*, *PDGFRB*, and *FGFR1*. These cases usually present with peripheral and bone marrow eosinophilia, and an underlying neoplastic mast cell population may be evident on review of the bone marrow aspirate and/or biopsy. Of these 3 categories, neoplasms associated with *PDGFRA* rearrangements most closely resemble SM-eo. However, several criteria, including the density of mast cell infiltration, relative elevation of serum B12, and tryptase measurements, may help in favoring one of these diagnoses (see **Table 1**. As mentioned previously, karyotypic analysis of the bone marrow and FISH/PCR for *PDGFRA* detection is necessary to exclude myeloid neoplasms with rearrangements involving *PDGFRA*, *PDGFRB*, and *FGFR1*.

Perhaps the most challenging issue seen with SM-eo cases is determining if the eosinophilic component of the disorder is reactive, neoplastic, and associated with the SM component of the disease, or a separate neoplastic process (an AHD may or may not carry the *KIT* mutation). In the authors' experience, rare SM-eo cases are reactive to elevated IL-5 levels. The AHD most commonly seen with eosinophilia in these patients with SM is a CMML with eosinophilia; most SM-CMML cases carry the D816V *KIT* mutation in both the SM and CMML compartments.[97] SM-CEL is not infrequently found; the CEL may or may not carry the D816V *KIT* mutation.

PROGNOSIS

Few studies have established the prognosis of SM-eo. In a study by Böhm and colleagues,[51] the presence of eosinophilia was associated with decreased overall survival and event-free survival as compared with patients with SM without eosinophilia. Patients with SM-eo were more likely to also have hepatomegaly and splenomegaly, and lack cutaneous lesions at or subsequent to diagnosis. However, 2 of the patients in their study with "SM with associated CEL" had deletions of the *CHIC2* gene and would be more appropriately diagnosed with *PDGFRA* rearrangement-associated myeloid neoplasms. No cardiomyopathy was found in patients with SM-eo and the *KIT* D816V mutation even when a diagnosis of aggressive SM was most appropriate.[51] In a subsequent study by Pardanani and colleagues,[23] the presence of eosinophilia did not significantly alter the prognosis of patients with SM, but this study also included patients with *PDGFRA*-associated neoplasms. Further studies using a well-defined cohort of patients are needed to establish the true prognosis of patients with SM-eo.

Regarding therapeutic choices for managing SM-eo, patients generally start on glucocorticoid and or interferon-alpha therapy. Cladribine can also be considered. Recalcitrant patients may be placed on trials including midostaurin[100] or second-generation tyrosine kinase inhibitors, such as dasatinib. Cytoreductive therapy, such as hydroxyurea or cytarabine, may be used in patients with an associated MPN or disease that does not respond to one of the previously mentioned agents.[101]

> **Pitfalls**
> OF MYELOPROLIFERATIVE NEOPLASMS
> WITH EOSINOPHILIA
>
> ! Abnormal eosinophil morphology is *not* a surrogate for clonality, and may be seen in reactive eosinophilia.
>
> ! Loose collections of CD25+ aberrant mast cells may be seen in myeloid neoplasms associated with *PDGFRA*, *PDGFRB*, and *FGFR1*, and thus do not always indicate systemic mastocytosis.
>
> ! *PDGFRA* mutations are cryptic and *not* detected by standard cytogenetic karyotype; FISH or PCR testing must be performed.

REFERENCES

1. Seita J, Weissman IL. Hematopoietic stem cell: self-renewal versus differentiation. Wiley Interdiscip Rev Syst Biol Med 2010;2:640–53.
2. Rothenberg ME. Eosinophilia. N Engl J Med 1998; 338:1592–600.
3. Sanderson CJ. Interleukin-5, eosinophils, and disease. Blood 1992;79:3101–9.
4. Horie S, Okubo Y, Hossain M, et al. Interleukin-13 but not interleukin-4 prolongs eosinophil survival and induces eosinophil chemotaxis. Intern Med 1997;36:179–85.

5. Brito-Babapulle F. The eosinophilias, including the idiopathic hypereosinophilic syndrome. Br J Haematol 2003;121:203–23.

6. Gotlib J. World Health Organization-defined eosinophilic disorders: 2012 update on diagnosis, risk stratification, and management. Am J Hematol 2012;87:903–14.

7. Catovsky D, Bernasconi C, Verdonck PJ, et al. The association of eosinophilia with lymphoblastic leukaemia or lymphoma: a study of seven patients. Br J Haematol 1980;45:523–34.

8. Endo M, Usuki K, Kitazume K, et al. Hypereosinophilic syndrome in Hodgkin's disease with increased granulocyte-macrophage colony-stimulating factor. Ann Hematol 1995;71:313–4.

9. Murata K, Yamada Y, Kamihira S, et al. Frequency of eosinophilia in adult T-cell leukemia/lymphoma. Cancer 1992;69:966–71.

10. Greipp PT, Dewald GW, Tefferi A. Prevalence, breakpoint distribution, and clinical correlates of t(5;12). Cancer Genet Cytogenet 2004;153:170–2.

11. Klion AD. How I treat hypereosinophilic syndromes. Blood 2009;114:3736–41.

12. Gotlib J, Cools J, Malone JM, et al. The FIP1L1-PDGFRalpha fusion tyrosine kinase in hypereosinophilic syndrome and chronic eosinophilic leukemia: implications for diagnosis, classification, and management. Blood 2004;103:2879–91.

13. Bain BJ, Gilliland DG, Horny HP, et al. Myeloid and lymphoid neoplasms with eosinophilia and abnormalities of PDGFRA, PDGFRB, or FGFR1. In: Swerdlow SH, Campo E, Harris NL, et al, editors. WHO classification of tumours of haematopoietic and lymphoid tissues. Lyon (France): IARC; 2008. p. 68–73.

14. Ohnishi H, Kandabashi K, Maeda Y, et al. Chronic eosinophilic leukaemia with FIP1L1-PDGFRA fusion and T6741 mutation that evolved from Langerhans cell histiocytosis with eosinophilia after chemotherapy. Br J Haematol 2006;134:547–9.

15. Tanaka Y, Kurata M, Togami K, et al. Chronic eosinophilic leukemia with the FIP1L1-PDGFRalpha fusion gene in a patient with a history of combination chemotherapy. Int J Hematol 2006;83:152–5.

16. Safley AM, Sebastian S, Collins TS, et al. Molecular and cytogenetic characterization of a novel translocation t(4;22) involving the breakpoint cluster region and platelet-derived growth factor receptor-alpha genes in a patient with atypical chronic myeloid leukemia. Genes Chromosomes Cancer 2004;40:44–50.

17. Pardanani A, Brockman SR, Paternoster SF, et al. FIP1L1-PDGFRA fusion: prevalence and clinicopathologic correlates in 89 consecutive patients with moderate to severe eosinophilia. Blood 2004;104:3038–45.

18. Cools J, DeAngelo DJ, Gotlib J, et al. A tyrosine kinase created by fusion of the PDGFRA and FIP1L1 genes as a therapeutic target of imatinib in idiopathic hypereosinophilic syndrome. N Engl J Med 2003;348:1201–14.

19. Klion AD, Robyn J, Akin C, et al. Molecular remission and reversal of myelofibrosis in response to imatinib mesylate treatment in patients with the myeloproliferative variant of hypereosinophilic syndrome. Blood 2004;103:473–8.

20. Ogbogu PU, Bochner BS, Butterfield JH, et al. Hypereosinophilic syndrome: a multicenter, retrospective analysis of clinical characteristics and response to therapy. J Allergy Clin Immunol 2009;124:1319–25.

21. Vandenberghe P, Wlodarska I, Michaux L, et al. Clinical and molecular features of FIP1L1-PDGFRA (+) chronic eosinophilic leukemias. Leukemia 2004;18:734–42.

22. Robyn J, Lemery S, McCoy JP, et al. Multilineage involvement of the fusion gene in patients with FIP1L1/PDGFRA-positive hypereosinophilic syndrome. Br J Haematol 2006;132:286–92.

23. Pardanani A, Lim KH, Lasho TL, et al. Prognostically relevant breakdown of 123 patients with systemic mastocytosis associated with other myeloid malignancies. Blood 2009;114:3769–72.

24. Valent P, Klion AD, Horny HP, et al. Contemporary consensus proposal on criteria and classification of eosinophilic disorders and related syndromes. J Allergy Clin Immunol 2012;130:607–12.

25. Score J, Curtis C, Waghorn K, et al. Identification of a novel imatinib responsive KIF5B-PDGFRA fusion gene following screening for PDGFRA overexpression in patients with hypereosinophilia. Leukemia 2006;20:827–32.

26. Tashiro H, Shirasaki R, Noguchi M, et al. Molecular analysis of chronic eosinophilic leukemia with t(4;10) showing good response to imatinib mesylate. Int J Hematol 2006;83:433–8.

27. Curtis CE, Grand FH, Waghorn K, et al. A novel ETV6-PDGFRB fusion transcript missed by standard screening in a patient with an imatinib responsive chronic myeloproliferative disease. Leukemia 2007;21:1839–41.

28. Walz C, Metzgeroth G, Haferlach C, et al. Characterization of three new imatinib-responsive fusion genes in chronic myeloproliferative disorders generated by disruption of the platelet-derived growth factor receptor beta gene. Haematologica 2007;92:163–9.

29. Trempat P, Villalva C, Laurent G, et al. Chronic myeloproliferative disorders with rearrangement of the platelet-derived growth factor alpha receptor: a new clinical target for STI571/Glivec. Oncogene 2003;22:5702–6.

30. Baxter EJ, Hochhaus A, Bolufer P, et al. The t(4;22)(q12;q11) in atypical chronic myeloid

leukaemia fuses BCR to PDGFRA. Hum Mol Genet 2002;11:1391–7.

31. Metzgeroth G, Walz C, Score J, et al. Recurrent finding of the FIP1L1-PDGFRA fusion gene in eosinophilia-associated acute myeloid leukemia and lymphoblastic T-cell lymphoma. Leukemia 2007;21:1183–8.

32. Maric I, Robyn J, Metcalfe DD, et al. KIT D816V-associated systemic mastocytosis with eosinophilia and FIP1L1/PDGFRA-associated chronic eosinophilic leukemia are distinct entities. J Allergy Clin Immunol 2007;120:680–7.

33. Ault P, Cortes J, Koller C, et al. Response of idiopathic hypereosinophilic syndrome to treatment with imatinib mesylate. Leuk Res 2002;26:881–4.

34. Gleich GJ, Leiferman KM, Pardanani A, et al. Treatment of hypereosinophilic syndrome with imatinib mesilate. Lancet 2002;359:1577–8.

35. Griffin JH, Leung J, Bruner RJ, et al. Discovery of a fusion kinase in EOL-1 cells and idiopathic hypereosinophilic syndrome. Proc Natl Acad Sci U S A 2003;100:7830–5.

36. Von Bubnoff N, Gorantla SP, Engh RA, et al. The low frequency of clinical resistance to PDGFR inhibitors in myeloid neoplasms with abnormalities of PDGFRA might be related to the limited repertoire of possible PDGFRA kinase domain mutations in vitro. Oncogene 2011;30:933–43.

37. Jabbour E, Kantarjian H, Jones D, et al. Characteristics and outcomes of patients with chronic myeloid leukemia and T315I mutation following failure of imatinib mesylate therapy. Blood 2008;112:53–5.

38. Von Bubnoff N, Gorantla SP, Thöne S, et al. The FIP1L1-PDGFRA T674I mutation can be inhibited by the tyrosine kinase inhibitor AMN107 (nilotinib). Blood 2006;107:4970–2.

39. Lierman E, Folens C, Stover EH, et al. Sorafenib is a potent inhibitor of FIP1L1-PDGFRalpha and the imatinib-resistant FIP1L1-PDGFRalpha T674I mutant. Blood 2006;108:1374–6.

40. Keene P, Mendelow B, Pinto MR, et al. Abnormalities of chromosome 12p13 and malignant proliferation of eosinophils: a nonrandom association. Br J Haematol 1987;67:25–31.

41. Srivastava A, Boswell HS, Heerema NA, et al. KRAS2 oncogene overexpression in myelodysplastic syndrome with translocation 5;12. Cancer Genet Cytogenet 1988;35:61–71.

42. Berkowicz M, Rosner E, Rechavi G, et al. Atypical chronic myelomonocytic leukemia with eosinophilia and translocation (5;12). A new association. Cancer Genet Cytogenet 1991;51:277–8.

43. Lerza R, Castello G, Sessarego M, et al. Myelodysplastic syndrome associated with increased bone marrow fibrosis and translocation (5;12)(q33;p12.3). Br J Haematol 1992;82:476–7.

44. Wessels JW, Fibbe WE, Van der Keur D, et al. t(5;12)(q31;p12): a clinical entity with features of both myeloid leukemia and chronic myelomonocytic leukemia. Cancer Genet Cytogenet 1993;65:7–11.

45. Steer EJ, Cross NC. Myeloproliferative disorders with translocations of chromosome 5q31-35: role of the platelet-derived growth factor receptor Beta. Acta Haematol 2002;107:113–22.

46. Apperley JF, Gardembas M, Melo JV, et al. Response to imatinib mesylate in patients with chronic myeloproliferative diseases with rearrangements of the platelet-derived growth factor receptor beta. N Engl J Med 2002;347:481–7.

47. Bain BJ, Fletcher SH. Chronic eosinophilic leukemias and the myeloproliferative variant of the hypereosinophilic syndrome. Immunol Allergy Clin North Am 2007;27:377–88.

48. Tokita K, Maki K, Tadokoro J, et al. Chronic idiopathic myelofibrosis expressing a novel type of TEL-PDGFRB chimaera responded to imatinib mesylate therapy. Leukemia 2007;21:190–2.

49. Noel P. Eosinophilic myeloid disorders. Semin Hematol 2012;49:120–7.

50. David M, Cross NC, Burgstaller S, et al. Durable responses to imatinib in patients with PDGFRB fusion gene-positive and BCR-ABL-negative chronic myeloproliferative disorders. Blood 2007;109:61–4.

51. Böhm A, Födinger M, Wimazal F, et al. Eosinophilia in systemic mastocytosis: clinical and molecular correlates and prognostic significance. J Allergy Clin Immunol 2007;120:192–9.

52. Manthorpe R, Egeberg J, Hesselvik M, et al. Unique eosinophil granules in a case of T-cell lymphoma. Scand J Haematol 1977;19:129–44.

53. Macdonald D, Aguiar RC, Mason PJ, et al. A new myeloproliferative disorder associated with chromosomal translocations involving 8p11: a review. Leukemia 1995;9:1628–30.

54. Jackson CC, Medeiros LJ, Miranda RN. 8p11 myeloproliferative syndrome: a review. Hum Pathol 2010;41:461–76.

55. Mozziconacci MJ, Carbuccia N, Prebet T, et al. Common features of myeloproliferative disorders with t(8;9)(p12;q33) and CEP110-FGFR1 fusion: report of a new case and review of the literature. Leuk Res 2008;32:1304–8.

56. Vizmanos JL, Hernández R, Vidal MJ, et al. Clinical variability of patients with the t(6;8)(q27;p12) and FGFR1OP-FGFR1 fusion: two further cases. Hematol J 2004;5:534–7.

57. Demiroglu A, Steer EJ, Heath C, et al. The t(8;22) in chronic myeloid leukemia fuses BCR to FGFR1: ransforming activity and specific inhibition of FGFR1 fusion proteins. Blood 2001;98:3778–83.

58. Soler G, Nusbaum S, Varet B, et al. LRRFIP1, a new FGFR1 partner gene associated with 8p11 myeloproliferative syndrome. Leukemia 2009;23: 1359–61.

59. Fioretos T, Panagopoulos I, Lassen C, et al. Fusion of the BCR and the fibroblast growth factor receptor-1 (FGFR1) genes as a result of t(8;22)(p11;q11) in a myeloproliferative disorder: the first fusion gene involving BCR but not ABL. Genes Chromosomes Cancer 2001;32:302–10.

60. Kim SY, Oh B, She CJ, et al. 8p11 myeloproliferative syndrome with BCR-FGFR1 rearrangement presenting with T-lymphoblastic lymphoma and bone marrow stromal cell proliferation: a case report and review of the literature. Leuk Res 2011; 35:30–4.

61. Guasch G, Ollendorff V, Borg JP, et al. 8p12 stem cell myeloproliferative disorder: the FOP-fibroblast growth factor receptor 1 fusion protein of the t(6;8) translocation induces cell survival mediated by mitogen-activated protein kinase and phosphatidylinositol 3-kinase/Akt/mTOR pathways. Mol Cell Biol 2001;21:8129–42.

62. Popovici C, Zhang B, Grégoire MJ, et al. The t(6;8)(q27;p11) translocation in a stem cell myeloproliferative disorder fuses a novel gene, FOP, to fibroblast growth factor receptor 1. Blood 1999; 93:1381–9.

63. Borowitz MJ, Chan JK. T lymphoblastic leukemia/lymphoma. In: Swerdlow SH, Campo E, Harris NL, et al, editors. WHO classification of tumours of haematopoietic and lymphoid tissues. Lyon (France): IARC; 2008. p. 176–8.

64. Chen J, Deangelo DJ, Kutok JL, et al. PKC412 inhibits the zinc finger 198-fibroblast growth factor receptor 1 fusion tyrosine kinase and is active in treatment of stem cell myeloproliferative disorder. Proc Natl Acad Sci U S A 2004;101: 14479–84.

65. Martinez-Climent JA, Vizcarra E, Benet I, et al. Cytogenetic response induced by interferon alpha in the myeloproliferative disorder with eosinophilia, T cell lymphoma and the chromosomal translocation t(8;13)(p11;q12). Leukemia 1998;12: 999–1000.

66. Ren M, Qin H, Ren R, et al. Ponatinib suppresses the development of myeloid and lymphoid malignancies associated with FGFR1 abnormalities. Leukemia 2013;27:32–40.

67. Bain BJ, Gilliland DG, Vardiman JW, et al. Chronic eosinophilic leukemia, not otherwise specified. In: Swerdlow SH, Campo E, Harris NL, et al, editors. WHO classification of tumours of haematopoietic and lymphoid tissues. Lyon (France): IARC; 2008. p. 51–3.

68. Chusid MJ, Dale DC, West BC, et al. The hypereosinophilic syndrome: analysis of fourteen cases with review of the literature. Medicine (Baltimore) 1975;54:1–27.

69. Flaum MA, Schooley RT, Fauci AS, et al. A clinicopathologic correlation of the idiopathic hypereosinophilic syndrome: I: hematologic manifestations. Blood 1981;58:1012–20.

70. Schooley RT, Flaum MA, Gralnick HR, et al. A clinicopathologic correlation of the idiopathic hypereosinophilic syndrome: II: clinical manifestations. Blood 1981;58:1021–6.

71. Hernández P, Cabrera H, Espinosa E, et al. Ring eosinophils in human haematological malignancies. Br J Haematol 1989;72:597.

72. Bain BJ. The significance of ring eosinophils in humans. Br J Haematol 1989;73:579–81.

73. Bain BJ. Eosinophilic leukaemias and the idiopathic hypereosinophilic syndrome. Br J Haematol 1996;95:2–9.

74. Caulfield JP, Hein A, Rothenberg ME, et al. A morphometric study of normodense and hypodense human eosinophils that are derived in vivo and in vitro. Am J Pathol 1980;137:27–41.

75. Weller PF, Bubley GJ. The idiopathic hypereosinophilic syndrome. Blood 1994;83:2759–79.

76. Chang HW, Leong KH, Koh DR, et al. Clonality of isolated eosinophils in the hypereosinophilic syndrome. Blood 1999;93:1651–7.

77. Goldman JM, Najfeld V, Th'ng KH. Agar culture and chromosome analysis of eosinophilic leukaemia. J Clin Pathol 1975;28:956–61.

78. Forrest DL, Horsman DE, Jensen CL, et al. Myelodysplastic syndrome with hypereosinophilia and a nonrandom chromosomal abnormality dic(1;7): confirmation of eosinophil clonal involvement by fluorescence in situ hybridization. Cancer Genet Cytogenet 1998;107:65–8.

79. Parreira L, Tavares de Castro J, Hibbin JA, et al. Chromosome and cell culture studies in eosinophilic leukaemia. Br J Haematol 1986;62: 659–69.

80. Arber DA, Brunning RD, Le Beau MM, et al. Acute myeloid leukemia with recurrent cytogenetic abnormalities. In: Swerdlow SH, Campo E, Harris NL, et al, editors. WHO classification of tumours of haematopoietic and lymphoid tissues. Lyon (France): IARC; 2008. p. 110–23.

81. Hardy WR, Anderson RE. The hypereosinophilic syndromes. Ann Intern Med 1968;68:1220–9.

82. Gleich GJ, Leiferman KM. The hypereosinophilic syndromes: still more heterogeneity. Curr Opin Immunol 2005;17:679–84.

83. Fauci AS, Harley JB, Roberts WC, et al. NIH conference. The idiopathic hypereosinophilic syndrome. Clinical, pathophysiologic, and therapeutic considerations. Ann Intern Med 1982;97:78–92.

84. Roufosse F, Cogan E, Goldman M. Recent advances in pathogenesis and management of

hypereosinophilic syndromes. Allergy 2004;59: 673–89.

85. Valent P, Gleich GJ, Reiter A, et al. Pathogenesis and classification of eosinophil disorders: a review of recent developments in the field. Expert Rev Hematol 2012;5:157.

86. Moore PM, Harley JB, Fauci AS. Neurologic dysfunction in the idiopathic hypereosinophilic syndrome. Ann Intern Med 1985;102:109–14.

87. Wechsler ME. Pulmonary eosinophilic syndromes. Immunol Allergy Clin North Am 2007;27:477–92.

88. Cottin V, Cordier JF. Eosinophilic pneumonias. Allergy 2005;60:841–7.

89. Simon HU, Klion A. Therapeutic approaches to patients with hypereosinophilic syndromes. Semin Hematol 2012;49:160–70.

90. Vardiman JW, Melo JV, Baccarani M, et al. Chronic myelogenous leukemia, BCR-ABL1 positive. In: Swerdlow SH, Campo E, Harris NL, et al, editors. WHO classification of tumours of haematopoietic and lymphoid tissues. Lyon (France): IARC; 2008. p. 32–7.

91. Lefebvre C, Bletry O, Degoulet P, et al. Prognostic factors of hypereosinophilic syndrome: study of 40 cases. Ann Med Interne (Paris) 1989;140: 253–7.

92. Podjasek JC, Butterfield JH. Mortality in hypereosinophilic syndrome: 19 years of experience at Mayo Clinic with a review of the literature. Leuk Res 2013; 37:392–5.

93. Horny HP, Metcalfe DD, Bennett JM, et al. Mastocytosis. In: Swerdlow SH, Campo E, Harris NL, et al, editors. WHO classification of tumours of haematopoietic and lymphoid tissues. Lyon (France): IARC; 2008. p. 54–63.

94. Valent P, Sperr WR, Schwartz LB, et al. Diagnosis and classification of mast cell proliferative disorders: delineation from immunologic diseases and non-mast cell hematopoietic neoplasms. J Allergy Clin Immunol 2004;114:3–12.

95. George TI. Mastocytosis. Curr Cancer Ther Rev 2012;8(1):35–43.

96. George TI, Horny HP. Systemic mastocytosis. Surg Path Clinics 2010;3(4):1185–202.

97. Sotlar K, Horny HP, Simonitsch I, et al. CD25 indicates the neoplastic phenotype of mast cells: a novel immunohistochemical marker for the diagnosis of systemic mastocytosis in routinely processed bone marrow biopsy specimens. Am J Surg Pathol 2004;28(10):1319–25.

98. Sotlar K, Colak S, Bache A, et al. Variable presence of KITD816V in clonal haematological non-mast cell lineage diseases associated with systemic mastocytosis (SM-AHNMD). J Pathol 2010;220(5):586–95.

99. Feger F, Ribadeau DA, Lerich L, et al. Kit and c-kit mutations in mastocytosis: a short overview with special reference to novel molecular and diagnostic concepts. Int Arch Allergy Immunol 2002; 127(2):110–4.

100. Gotlib J, Berube C, Growney JD, et al. Activity of the tyrosine kinase inhibitor PKC412 in a patient with mast cell leukemia with the D816V KIT mutation. Blood 2005;106(8):1865–2870.

101. Valent P, Sperr WR, Akin C. How I treat patients with advanced systemic mastocytosis. Blood 2010;116: 5812–7.

102. Savage N, George TI, Gotlib J. Myeloid neoplasms associated with eosinophilia and rearrangement of PDGFRA, PDGFRB, and FGFR1: a review. Int J Lab Hematol 2013;35(5):491–500.

103. Savage NM, Johnson RC, Gotlib J, et al. Myeloid and lymphoid neoplasms with FGFR1 abnormalities: diagnostic and therapeutic challenges. Am J Hematol 2013;88:427–30.

Challenges in Consolidated Reporting of Hematopoietic Neoplasms

Robert S. Ohgami, MD, PhD*, Daniel A. Arber, MD

KEYWORDS

- Comprehensive pathology reports • Consolidated pathology reports • Integrated pathology reports
- Synthesized reports • Molecular pathology • Bone marrow • Hematopathology

KEY POINTS

- Comprehensive hematopathology reports require careful incorporation of multiple studies and findings, often over an extended period of time.
- Pathologists need to be up to date with current diagnostic classifications in hematopathology, which depend heavily on genetic and molecular findings.
- Future pathologic diagnoses will depend even more heavily on integration of advanced technologic findings, which require an efficient data infrastructure.

ABSTRACT

This article focuses on the challenges of generating comprehensive diagnostic reports in hematopathology. In particular, two main challenges that diagnosticians face are (1) interpreting and understanding the rapid advances in molecular and genetic pathology, which have gained increasing importance in classifications of hematopoietic neoplasms, and (2) managing the logistics of reporting ancillary studies and incorporating them effectively into a final synthesized report. This article summarizes many important genetic findings in hematopoietic neoplasms, which are required for accurate diagnoses, and discusses practical issues to generating accurate and complete hematopathology reports.

OVERVIEW

Hematopathologic neoplastic diagnoses are multifaceted, requiring integration of diverse sources of data (clinical, morphologic, immunophenotypic, molecular, and genetic). Multiple guidelines for a comprehensive report with regards to bone marrow and lymph node specimens, in hematopathology, have been published over the years from a variety of organizations,[1,2] including the College of American Pathologists.[3–5]

A complete hematopathology neoplasm report should include

- Specimen and site
- Procedure (eg, biopsy, aspirate, excision, resection)
- Histologic type (based on 2008 World Health Organization [WHO] criteria) and extent of tumor
- Immunophenotyping and additional pathologic findings
- Clinical prognostic factors and indices
- Cytogenetic and molecular findings
- Other ancillary tests

Although the majority of pathology reports are issued in a few days from the time a specimen is collected, complexity often arises from the

Disclosure Statement: The authors have no conflicts of interest to disclose.
Department of Pathology, Stanford University Medical Center, 300 Pasteur Drive, Room L235, Stanford, CA 94305, USA
* Corresponding author.
E-mail address: rohgami@stanford.edu

Surgical Pathology 6 (2013) 795–806
http://dx.doi.org/10.1016/j.path.2013.08.001
1875-9181/13/$ – see front matter © 2013 Elsevier Inc. All rights reserved.

Acronyms and Abbreviations for Hematopoietic Neoplasms Reporting	
ALCL	Anaplastic large cell lymphoma
ALK	Anaplastic lymphoma kinase
AML	Acute myeloid leukemia
AML-MRC	Acute myeloid leukemia with myelodysplasia-related changes
AML-RGA	Acute myeloid leukemia with recurrent genetic abnormalities
B-ALL	B-lymphoblastic leukemia/ lymphoma
B-ALL RGA	B-lymphoblastic leukemia/ lymphoma with recurrent genetic abnormalities
BL	Burkitt lymphoma
CLL/SLL	Chronic lymphocytic leukemia/ small lymphocytic lymphoma
CML	Chronic myelogenous leukemia
DLBCL	Diffuse large B-cell lymphoma
FL	Follicular lymphoma
IPSS-R	Revised International Prognostic Scoring System
LCH	Langerhans cell histiocytosis
MCL	Mantle cell lymphoma
MDS	Myelodysplastic syndrome
MM	Plasma cell myeloma
MLNE	Myeloid and lymphoid neoplasms with eosinophilia
NOS	Not otherwise specified
PCN	Plasma cell neoplasm
T-ALL	T-lymphoblastic leukemia
WHO	World Health Organization

integration of advanced genetic and molecular data, which may not be available until long after the initial morphologic and immunophenotypic analyses are complete; however, such data are often essential to a correct and final diagnosis.

Additionally, cases of bone marrow studies offer a unique challenge because they typically do, and should, include evaluation of peripheral blood as well as bone marrow aspirate and bone marrow core biopsy specimens. Occasionally, immunophenotypic, cytogenetic, and molecular studies are performed on both peripheral blood and bone marrow specimens. As such, without a specialized pathologist reviewing all the testing performed, individual pieces of data and reports may lead to incorrect diagnoses or multiple vague ones, when instead collective summation of all facets of information would have yielded a clear answer.

Given the increasingly paramount importance of genetics in the diagnosis of hematolymphoid neoplasms,[6] some of the key genetic features of hematolymphoid neoplasms are first reviewed, with areas of complexity discussed briefly. The final section addresses some of the data consolidation issues with regards to incorporating findings into a comprehensive report.

GENETIC FEATURES OF MYELOID NEOPLASMS AND ACUTE LEUKEMIAS

In 2008, the updated classification of the WHO on hematolymphoid neoplasms included several myeloid neoplasms and acute leukemias for which the diagnosis specifically is defined by cytogenetic data.[6] These groups and subtypes include acute myeloid leukemia with recurrent genetic abnormalities (AML-RGA); acute myeloid leukemia with myelodysplasia-related changes (AML-MRC); myelodysplastic syndrome (MDS) with isolated 5q deletion; myeloid and lymphoid neoplasms with eosinophilia (MLNE) and PDGFRA, PDGFRB, or FGFR1 abnormalities; chronic myelogenous leukemia (CML); and B-lymphoblastic leukemia/lymphoma with recurrent genetic abnormalities (B-ALL RGA) (Table 1). As a result of the critical nature of cytogenetic data, all other categories of myeloid neoplasms and acute leukemias, by default, require cytogenetic information. For instance, the diagnosis of acute myeloid leukemia (AML) not otherwise specified (NOS) can only be definitively made after ruling out the subgroups of AML-RGA and AML-MRC; the latter 2 can be or are defined by cytogenetic abnormalities.[6,7] Similarly, in B-lymphoblastic leukemia/lymphoma (B-ALL), cytogenetics plays a key role in not only identifying patients with RGA but also subtyping them within this group.

The importance of such cytogenetic analysis is in conferring prognostic and therapeutic significance in most myeloid neoplasms and acute leukemias, even if not forming a formal diagnostic group in the 2008 WHO classification. For instance, AMLs are stratified by cytogenetic risk status into favorable risk, intermediate risk, and unfavorable risk categories (Table 2), and these categories play important roles in treatment decisions according to the National Comprehensive Cancer Network guidelines.[8,9] In MDS, the only subtype that is defined by cytogenetics is MDS with isolated 5q deletion; however, other chromosomal abnormalities are nonetheless important and have been incorporated into prognostic scoring systems, such as the Revised International Prognostic Scoring System (IPSS-R)[10]

Table 1
Select cytogenetic and molecular findings in myeloid neoplasms and acute leukemias

Neoplasm	WHO Subgroup	WHO Subtype	Key Cytogenetic/Molecular Findings	Cytogenetic/Molecular Notes
AML	AML-RGA	AML with t(8;21)(q22;q22); *RUNX1-RUNXT1*	t(8;21)(q22;q22); RUNX1-RUNXT1	Required for diagnosis, good prognosis
		AML with inv(16)(p13.1q22) or t(16;16)(p13.1;q22); *CBFBMYH11*	inv(16)(p13.1q22) or t(16;16)(p13.1.q22); CBFB-MYH11	Required for diagnosis, good prognosis
		AML with t(15;17)(q22;q12); *PML-RARA*	t(15;17)(q22;q12); PML-RARA	Required for diagnosis, good prognosis
		AML with t(9;11)(p22;q23); *MLLT3-MLL*	t(9;11)(p22;q23); MLLT3-MLL	Required for diagnosis, intermediate prognosis
		AML with t(6;9)(p23;q24); *DEK-NUP214*	t(6;9)(p23;q24); DEK-NUP214	Required for diagnosis, poor prognosis
		AML with inv(3)(q21q26.2) or t(3;3)(q21;q26.2); *RPN1-EVI1*	inv(3)(q21q26.2) or t(3;3)(q21;q26.2); RPN1-EVI1	Required for diagnosis, poor prognosis
		AML with t(1;22)(p13;q13); *RBM15-MKL1*	t(1;22)(p13;q13); RBM15-MKL1	Required for diagnosis, poor to intermediate prognosis
		*AML with mutated NPM1	NPM1 mutations	Required for diagnosis
		*AML with mutated CEPBA	CEBPA mutations	*Provisional entities
	AML, NOS	AML with minimal differentiation	Many gene mutations, including FLT3 (see Fig. 1)	—
		AML without maturation		
		AML with maturation		
		Acute myelomonocytic leukemia		
		Acute monoblastic/monocytic leukemia		
		Acute erythroid leukemia		
		Acute megakaryoblastic leukemia		
		Acute basophilic leukemia		
		Acute panmyelosis with myelofibrosis		

(continued on next page)

Table 1
(Continued)

Neoplasm	WHO Subgroup	WHO Subtype	Key Cytogenetic/Molecular Findings	Cytogenetic/Molecular Notes
		AML-MRC	Balanced t(11;16)(q23;p13.3), t(3;21)(q26.2;q22.1), t(1;3)(p36.3;q21.1), t(2;11)(p21;q23), t(5;12)(q33;p12), t(5;7)(q33;q11.2), t(5;17)(q33;p13), t(5;10)(q33;q21), t(3;5)(q25;q34) Unbalanced −7/del(7q), −5/del(5q), i(17q)/t(17p), −13/del(13q), del(11q), del(12p)/t(12p), del(9q), idic(X)(q13) Complex cytogenetics ≥3 unrelated abnormalities	One balanced, or one unbalanced cytogenetic change, or a complex cytogenetic change can define this subgroup of AML
		MS	del(7), 8+, t(v;11q23) MLL rearranged, inv(16), 4+, del(16), 16q−, 5q−, 20q−, 11+	—
MN-T		AML-T	Often abnormalities of 11q23 and del(5q)/−5, del(7q)/−7	Not required for diagnosis; this entire group is poor prognosis
		MDS-T		
MP-DS		TAM	Constitutional trisomy 21, GATA1 mutations	Constitutional trisomy 21 required for diagnosis
		ML-DS	Constitutional trisomy 21, GATA1 mutations	Constitutional trisomy 21 required for diagnosis
BPDCN		BPDCN	9p21.3 (CDKN2A/CDKN2B), 13q13.1-q14.3 (RB1), 12p13.2-p13.1 (CDKN1B), 13q11-q12 (LATS2), and 7p12.2 (IKZF1)[39]	Not required for diagnosis
MDS		RCUD	Group 1: normal, −Y, del(5q), del(20q)	Group 1: good prognosis
		RARS	Group 2: complex (≥3 abnormalities) or chromosome 7 abnormalities	Group 2: poor prognosis
		MDS with isolated del(5q)	Group 3: other abnormalities	Group 3: intermediate prognosis
		RCMD		
		RAEB		
		MDS, U		
		C-MDS	Monosomy 7	
MPN		CML	t(9;22)(q34;q11.2); BCR-ABL1	100% of cases with t(9;22)
		MCD	KIT mutations	>95% of cases with mutations
		PV	JAK2 mutations	>95% of cases with mutations
		ET	JAK2 or MPL mutations	60%–70% of cases with mutations
		PMF	JAK2 or MPL mutations	60%–70% of cases with mutations
		CNL	SETBP1 and CSF3R mutations[40,41]	—
		CEL, NOS	—	—
		MPN, U	—	—

MLNE	MLNE PDGFRA	Cryptic deletion at 4q12, FIP1L1-PDGFRA	These cytogenetic abnormalities alone define these neoplasms
	MLNE PDGFRB	Abnormalities of PDGFRB on 5q33	
	MLNE FGFR1	Abnormalities of FGFR1 on 8p11	
MDS/MPN	CMML	−7, ASXL1, SRSF2, CBL, IDH2[42]	These cytogenetic and mutational findings are often seen in these myeloid neoplasms
	JMML	−7	
	aCML	SETBP1 and CSF3R mutations[40,41]	
	MDS/MPN U	JAK2, MPL	
ALAL	AUL	—	—
	MPAL with t(9;22)(q34;q11.2); *BCR-ABL1*	t(9;22)(q34;q11.2); BCR-ABL1	Required for diagnosis
	MPAL with t(v;11q23)/*MLL* rearrangement	Various translocations with MLL on 11q23	Required for diagnosis
	MPAL, B-myeloid, NOS	—	—
	MPAL, T-myeloid, NOS	—	—
	*NKL	—	*Provisional entity
B-ALL	B-ALL with hyperdiploidy	Hyperdiploidy >50 chromosomes	Required for diagnosis, good prognosis
RGA	B-ALL with t(12;21)(p12;q23); *ETV6-RUNX1*	t(12;21)(p12;q23); ETV6-RUNX1	Required for diagnosis, good prognosis
	B-ALL with t(9;22)(q34;q11.2); *BCR-ABL1*	t(9;22)(q34;q11.2); BCR-ABL1	Required for diagnosis, poor prognosis
	B-ALL with t(1;19)(q23;p13.3); *TCF3-PBX1*	t(1;19)(q23;p13.3); TCF3-PBX1	Required for diagnosis, limited prognostic impact with current therapy
	B-ALL with t(v;11q23); *MLL* rearranged	t(v;11q23); MLL rearranged	Required for diagnosis, poor prognosis
	B-ALL with hypodiploidy	Hypodiploidy <46 chromosomes	Required for diagnosis, poor prognosis
	B-ALL with t(5;14)(q31;q32); *IL3-IGH@*	t(5;14)(q31;q32); IL3-IGH@	Required for diagnosis, poor prognosis
	B-ALL, NOS	Various mutations in genes, such as IKZF1, and other abnormalities, such as iAMP(21)	—
T-ALL	T-ALL	Abnormalities of 14q11.2, 7q35, 7p14-15, 10q24, 5q35	

Abbreviations: aCML, atypical CML; ALAL, acute leukemia of ambiguous lineage; AML-T, therapy-related AML; AUL, acute undifferentiated leukemia; BPDCN, blastic plasmacytoid dendritic cell neoplasm; C-MDS, childhood MDS; CEL, chronic eosinophilic leukemia; CNL, chronic myelomonocytic leukemia; NOS; CMML, chronic neutrophilic leukemia; ET, essential thrombocythemia; JMML, juvenile myelomonocytic leukemia; MCD, mastocytosis; MDS, U, MDS, unclassifiable; MDS-T, therapy-related MDS; ML-DS, myeloid leukemia associated with Down syndrome; MN-T, therapy-related myeloid neoplasm; MPN, U, myeloproliferative neoplasm, unclassifiable; MS, myeloid sarcoma; NKL, NK lymphoblastic leukemia/lymphoma; PMF, primary myelofibrosis; PV, polycythemia vera; RAEB, refractory anemia with excess blasts; RARS, refractory anemia with ring sideroblasts; RCMD, refractory cytopenia with multilineage dysplasia; RCUD, refractory cytopenia with unilineage dysplasia; TAM, transient abnormal myelopoiesis.

Table 2
Criteria for cytogenetic risk classification in acute myeloid leukemia

AML Cytogenetic Prognostic Subgroup	Cytogenetic Abnormality
Favorable	t(15;17) + any other abnormality inv(16)/t(16;16)/del(16q) + any other abnormality t(8;21) without del(9q) or complex karyotype
Intermediate	+8, −Y, +6, del(12p) Normal karyotype
Unfavorable	−5/del(5q), −7/del(7q) t(8;21) with del(9q) inv(3q), abnormal 11q23, 20q 21q, del(9q), t(6;9) t(9;22), abnormal 17p Complex karyotypes (≥3 abnormalities)

Based on the Southwest Oncology Group karyotype stratification.
Data from Slovak ML, Kopecky KJ, Cassileth PA, et al. Karyotypic analysis predicts outcome of preremission and postremission therapy in adult acute myeloid leukemia: a southwest oncology group/eastern cooperative oncology group study. Blood 2000;96(13):4075–83.

Table 3
IPSS-R cytogenetic risk stratification

MDS Cytogenetic Prognostic Subgroup	Cytogenetic Abnormality
Very good	del(11q), −Y
Good	Normal, del(20q), isolated del(5q), del(12p), double including del(5q)
Intermediate	+8, del(7q), i(17q), +19, any other single/double clones
Poor	inv(3)/t(3q)/del(3q), −7, double including −7/del(7q), complex: 3 abnormalities
Very poor	Complex: >3 abnormalities

From Greenberg PL, Tuechler H, Schanz J, et al. Revised international prognostic scoring system for myelodysplastic syndromes. Blood 2012;120(12):2457; with permission.

or the WHO Prognostic Scoring System (see **Table 1**; **Table 3**).[6] These numeric systems are used to estimate survival as well as to assist in determining which chemotherapies patients receive.

Although the increased incorporation of cytogenetic data into diagnoses has allowed patients to enter clinical trials and led to newer and more efficient therapies and more tailored follow-up, the complexity of understanding and incorporating these findings into classification schemes has offered new challenges for pathologists.

In addition, single-gene and panel-based gene mutational analyses have also become important in both diagnosis and prognosis of patients. Two provisional entities in AML rely on the identification of gene mutations (*NPM1* and *CEBPA*) for subclassification and have become increasingly validated as useful for determining which chemotherapy regimens patients should receive.[11–14] Although not included as diagnostic categories or provisional entities, testing for *FLT3*, especially in normal karyotype AML, and for *KIT* in core binding factor AML (AML with t[8;21][q22;q22]; *RUNX1-RUNXT1* and AML with inv[16][p13.1q22]

or t[16;16][p13.1;q22]; *CBFB-MYH11*) are also important in providing prognostic information and in some instances are used to select therapies, such as when FLT3 inhibitors are used.[15] Beyond these genetic mutations recognized by the 2008 WHO, other mutations, for instance in *DNMT3A* and *IDH1/2*,[16,17] are increasingly recognized as important in myeloid neoplasms (**Fig. 1**). Specific gene mutations are also critical in B-ALL, such as *IKZF1* deletions, seen in 15% of B-ALLs, which are associated with poorer prognosis, and mutations in *JAK1/2* (25% of B-ALLs), *PAX5* (30% of B-ALLs), and *TP53* (12% of B-ALLs).[18,19]

Finally, epigenetic changes, such as aberrant DNA methylation and altered micro-RNA expression patterns, are additionally being recognized in disease. Although not yet included in diagnostic classifications or in most therapeutic trials or formal stratification schemas, alterations in genome-wide methylation[20] as well as in individual genes, such as *GSTM1* and *ALOX12*, have been reported in AML[21] and offer prognostic and diagnostic utility in some instances. Micro-RNAs have been reported as altered in AML as well as in other leukemias, such as T-lymphoblastic leukemia (T-ALL) (*miR-19b, miR-20a, miR-26a, miR-92,* and *miR-223*).[22]

With such rapid advances in the genetic and epigenetic landscape of myeloid neoplasms and acute leukemias, understanding, diagnosing, and incorporating these findings into these entities

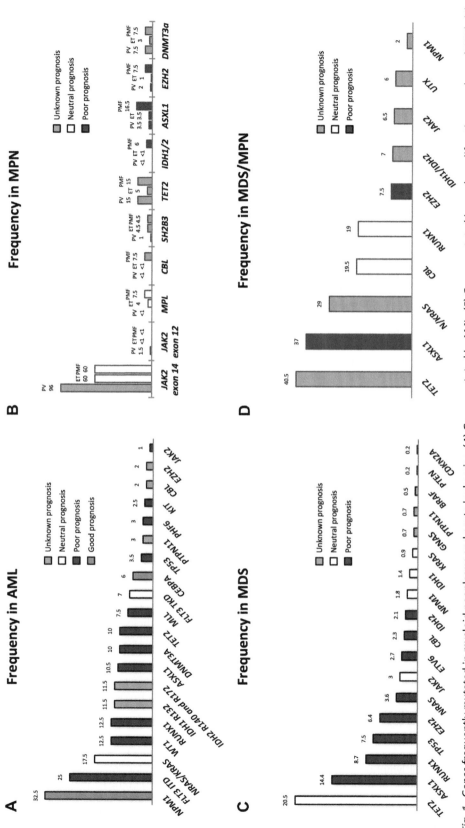

Fig. 1. Genes frequently mutated in myeloid neoplasms and acute leukemias. (*A*) Genes mutated in AML. (*B*) Genes mutated in myeloproliferative neoplasms (MPN). (*C*) Genes mutated in MDS. (*D*) Genes mutated in MDS/MPN. (*Adapted from* Refs.[45–47]; with permission.)

will only become more difficult without appropriate preparedness.

GENETIC FEATURES OF MATURE LYMPHOID AND OTHER HEMATOPOIETIC NEOPLASMS

The genetic and molecular landscape of mature lymphoid neoplasms is no less complex. In the 2008 WHO classification of hematolymphoid neoplasms,[6] cytogenetic data play an important role in the diagnosis of many mature lymphomas including: follicular lymphoma (FL), mantle cell lymphoma (MCL), Burkitt lymphoma (BL), and ALK+ anaplastic large cell lymphoma (ALCL). Unlike myeloid neoplasms and acute leukemias, however, a single cytogenetic abnormality is neither required nor specific for a given diagnosis (Table 4). For instance, although most MCLs show a t(11;14)(q13;32), CCND1-IGH@, a small subset do not and instead have translocations of CCND2 or CCND3 or, in some rare cases, none of these genetic abnormalities.[23] In addition, many abnormalities are not specific to one subtype of neoplasm but instead seen commonly in others. Again, with reference to t(11;14)(q13;32), this abnormality is seen not only in MCL but also in plasma cell neoplasm (PCNs).[24]

Without appropriate understanding of these genetic findings and complete and correct information, erroneous conclusions can be drawn from singular pieces of data. For instance, lack of awareness of t(11;14) in PCNs might lead to assuming that a positive result on its own, without other data, indicates a diagnosis of MCL. This potential for misinterpretation demonstrates the necessity of a knowledgeable pathologist to review and consolidate findings into a full report with bone marrow or lymph node specimen studies in order to convey a correct comprehensive diagnosis.

In addition, in some instances, cytogenetic findings change their prognostic significance depending on which neoplasm they are seen in. For instance, del(13q14) is seen in both chronic lymphocytic leukemia/small lymphocytic lymphoma (CLL/SLL)[25] and plasma cell myelomas (MMs)[26]; however, in CLL/SLL, this genetic abnormality is associated with good prognosis whereas in MM it is an unfavorable prognostic marker. Other abnormalities preserve their prognostic implications across different diseases. For instance, deletions of 17p13 (TP53) can be seen in CLL/SLL, FL, and diffuse large B-cell lymphoma (DLBCL) and are known to be a marker of poor prognosis in all 3 lymphoma subtypes.[27-29] Although these cytogenetic findings do not change the bottom-line diagnosis in cases, they can affect the therapy a clinician ultimately administers and, thus, incorporation of this information into reports becomes of paramount importance.

Complicating current diagnoses are emerging genetic mutational data from next-generation sequencing studies, which have identified some gene mutations as closely linked to known diagnostic entities; for instance, MYD88 L265P mutations in more than 90% of lymphoplasmacytic lymphomas,[30-32] BRAF V600E mutations in virtually all cases of hairy cell leukemia,[33] and STAT3 mutations in T-cell large granular lymphocytic leukemia.[34,35] Even though these mutational changes are not formally recognized by the 2008 WHO as diagnostic criteria in these diseases, pathologists must be aware of their utility as well as caveats: 4% of CLL/SLL cases have MYD88 mutations, BRAF V600E mutations are seen in 60% of Langerhans cell histiocytosis (LCH),[36] and STAT3 mutations are also seen in subsets of cases of ALK− ALCLs and other CD30+ peripheral T-cell lymphomas.[34]

Lymphoid neoplasms have an additional level of complexity, the ability to determine clonality by B-cell or T-cell receptor rearrangement studies. Although not required for any diagnosis, these tests are frequently ordered and, without careful correlation with clinical, laboratory, immunophenotypic, and other molecular findings, can lead to an incorrect diagnosis. For instance, errors can occur when positive T-cell receptor gene rearrangement studies are incorrectly interpreted, on their own, as diagnostic of a T-cell lymphoma when it is well known that T-cell clones are not infrequent in reactive tissues and are even seen in precursor B-cell neoplasms.

These complex diagnoses coupled with a rapidly evolving genetic landscape of hematolymphoid neoplasms make both understanding and incorporation of these findings into reports a potential diagnostic nightmare; however, this complexity affords a unique and challenging opportunity for pathologists to be able to insert themselves more centrally into the care of patients.

UNIQUE CHALLENGES TO COMPREHENSIVE REPORTING IN PATHOLOGY

Before asking how pathologists incorporate all data comprehensively into a single report, the question must first be asked, should pathologists be responsible for integrating and interpreting such diverse and complex information?

Some investigators argue that it is not necessarily the responsibility of pathologists to consolidate information for others and that treating

Table 4

Cytogenetic and mutational findings seen in select mature lymphoid and histiocytic and dendritic cell neoplasms[a]

Neoplasm	WHO Subtype	Key Cytogenetic/Molecular Findings	Cytogenetic/Molecular Notes
Mature B-cell neoplasms	CLL/SLL	del(17p) (*TP53*), del(11q) (*ATM*), del(13q) (miR-15a and miR-16-1), trisomy 12, somatic hypermutation *IGHV@*	These abnormalities are not disease defining but offer prognostic information
	HCL	*BRAF* V600E[33]	100% of cases
	LPL	*MYD88* L265P[30–32,43]	>90% of cases
	PCN	−13/del(13q), t(4;14)(p16;q32), t(11;14)(q13;32)	These abnormalities are not disease defining but offer prognostic information
	ENMZL	t(11;18)(q21;21) (*BIRC3-MALT1*), t(14;18)(q32;21) (*IGH@MALT1*), t(1;14)(p22;q32) (*IGH@-FOXP1*), t(11;18)(q21;q21), trisomy 3, trisomy 18, *TNFAIP3*	Disease defining in correct context
	FL	t(14;18)(q32;q21) (*IGH@-BCL2*), t(2;18)(p12;q21), t(18;22)(q21;q11), 3q27 (*BCL-6*), del(17p), chromosome 1, 6, 10 and others	BCL2 and BCL6 abnormalities can be disease defining in the correct context
	MCL	t(11;14)(q13;q32) (*CCND1-IGH@*), t(2;12)(p12;p13) (*CCND2-IGK@*), t(6;14)(p21;q32)(*CCND3-IGH@*)	Disease defining in correct context
	DLBCL	t(14;18)(q32;q21) (*IGH@-BCL2*), t(8;14)(q24.1;q32) (*MYC-IGH@*), der(1q21), del(6q), del(17p), +7	These abnormalities are not disease defining but offer prognostic information
	BL	t(8;14)(q24.1;q32) (*MYC-IGH@*), t(2;8)(p12;q24.1) (*IGK@-MYC*), t(8;22)(q24.1;q11) (*MYC-IGL@*)	100% of cases
	BCLU-DLBCL vs BL	t(8;14)(q24.1;q32) (*MYC-IGH@*), t(14;18)(q32;q21) (*IGH@-BCL2*), t(v;3)(q27) (*BCL6* translocated)	These abnormalities are not disease defining but offer prognostic information
Mature T-cell neoplasms	T-PLL	Chromosome abnormalities of Xq28 (*MTCP1*) or 14q32.1 (*TCL1* and *TCL1b*)	90% of cases
	T-LGL	*STAT3* activating mutations[34,35]	Variable frequency, 20%–90%
	CLNK	*STAT3* activating mutations[44]	60%
	HSTL	Isochromosome 7q	50%–100%
	EATL	+9q31.3 or −16q12.1	>80% of cases
	ALCL, ALK+	t(2;5)(p23;q35), *ALK-NPM*, other 2p23 abnormalities/translocations	Disease defining
	ALCL, ALK−	Complex cytogenetic abnormalities in most cases, *STAT3* SH2 domain mutations[34]	Significance of *STAT3* mutations unknown
	PTCL, NOS	Complex cytogenetic abnormalities in most cases, *STAT3* SH2 domain mutations[34]	*STAT3* mutations seen in a subset of CD30+ cases
Histiocytic and dendritic cell neoplasms	LCH	*BRAF* V600E[36]	60% of cases

Abbreviations: BCLU-DLBCL vs BL, B-cell lymphoma, unclassifiable, with features intermediate between DLBCL and BL; CLNK, chronic lymphoproliferative disorder of natural killer cells; EATL, enteropathy-associated T-cell lymphoma; ENMZL, extranodal marginal zone lymphoma; HCL, hairy cell leukemia; HSTL, hepatosplenic γδ T-cell lymphoma; LPL, lymphoplasmacytic lymphoma; PTCL, peripheral T-cell lymphoma; T-LGL, T-cell large granular lymphocytic leukemia; T-PLL, T-cell prolymphocytic leukemia.
[a] This table is not a comprehensive review of all subtypes of lymphoid neoplasms or histiocytic and dendritic cell neoplasms but rather selected groups.

clinicians can, and do, review individual diagnostic reports and molecular/genetic and laboratory findings on their own. As such, it could be said that consolidation and collation of data by pathologists are repetitive. Given the importance of a complete picture and integration of clinical, laboratory, morphologic, immunophenotypic, genetic, and molecular data for any definitive hematopathologic diagnosis, however, it does seem that it is by necessity and self-interest the responsibility of the diagnosing pathologist to accurately interpret and integrate all these aspects of data into a comprehensive report.

HOW CAN PATHOLOGISTS INCORPORATE RELEVANT DATA INTO A COMPLETE SYNTHESIZED REPORT?

At most pathology centers, multiple initial, amended, or addended reports are issued over a length of time, slowly incorporating additional molecular and cytogenetic data as they become available (**Fig. 2**). Most centers rely heavily on an ordering pathologist to act as a hub and integrator of information, collecting necessary pieces of data from different and independent information systems. Generally, these information systems are not designed to interface effectively together and this manual work can be time consuming and frustrating. On occasion, a pathologist is unaware of

additional testing that has been ordered by a treating physician and duplicate tests may be inadvertently performed, or, worse, a pathologist is unaware of the results when they are, in fact, relevant to a patient's diagnosis. This excessive testing not only generates unnecessary costs but also creates the possibility of introducing confusing and potentially conflicting diagnoses.

At some centers,[37] however, pathologists have taken the lead to ensure that the proper tests are performed and reported in a comprehensive way, collaborating with the treating service to implement standard algorithms of tests to be ordered for frequently diagnosed diseases. Additionally, the primary pathologist involved in the diagnosis orders ancillary testing as a case evolves, minimizing confusion. This approach can result in more efficient, comprehensive reports as well as cost savings for the involved institution. At other centers, computer programs have been designed to interface with the laboratory information system to pull data from multiple sources into larger worksheets[38] or even assemble the data into released pathology reports. Many of these computer programs, however, are generally "home-grown" and not immediately expandable to different information systems. Nonetheless, the theme and message that such integrated information systems are and will be critical to pathologists are clear.

Finally, a future complication arises with the already imminent inclusion of next-generation

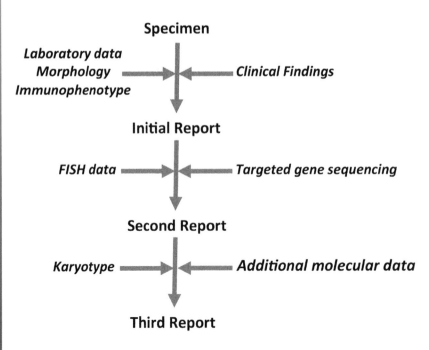

Fig. 2. Standard scheme for integrating ancillary data into hematopathology reports. FISH, fluorescence in situ hybridization.

sequencing data and the explosion of studies demonstrating significance of individual genes or combinations of gene mutations in many hemato-lymphoid diseases. Genetic findings that were deemed insignificant or unknown mere months ago may suddenly become newly significant in a patient's diagnosis and therapy. This raises an even more convoluted problem for pathologists; that is, will pathologists need to go back to very recent reports and incorporate this newly significant information?

In many regards, the central role of pathologists in efficiently communicating diagnoses by generating comprehensive elegant reports is a role we have performed in the past. Pathologists typically have been advocates and the impetus behind both developing and practically implementing advanced technologies as well as stewarding their incorporation into medical diagnoses. Such forward thinking is critical to our future and will continue to place pathologists as key players in patient care.

REFERENCES

1. Peterson LC, Agosti SJ, Hoyer JD, et al, Hematology Clinical Microscopy Resource Committee, Members of the Cancer Committee, College of American Pathologists. Protocol for the examination of specimens from patients with hematopoietic neoplasms of the bone marrow: a basis for checklists. Arch Pathol Lab Med 2002;126(9):1050–6.

2. Jaffe ES, Banks PM, Nathwani B, et al. Recommendations for the reporting of lymphoid neoplasms: a report from the association of directors of anatomic and surgical pathology. Mod Pathol 2004;17(1): 131–5.

3. Hussong JW, Arber DA, Bradley KT, et al. Hematopoietic neoplasms involving the bone marrow. CAP Cancer Protocols. 2012.

4. Hussong JW, Arber DA, Bradley KT, et al. Protocol for the examination of specimens from patients with hodgkin lymphoma. CAP Cancer Protocols. 2012.

5. Hussong JW, Arber DA, Bradley KT, et al. Protocol for the examination of specimens from patients with non-hodgkin lymphoma/lymphoid neoplasms. CAP Cancer Protocols. 2012.

6. Swerdlow SH, Campo E, Harris NL, et al. International Agency for Research on Cancer, World Health Organization. WHO classification of tumours of haematopoietic and lymphoid tissues. 4th edition. Lyon (France): International Agency for Research on Cancer; 2008. p. 439.

7. Weinberg OK, Seetharam M, Ren L, et al. Clinical characterization of acute myeloid leukemia with myelodysplasia-related changes as defined by the 2008 WHO classification system. Blood 2009; 113(9):1906–8.

8. Slovak ML, Kopecky KJ, Cassileth PA, et al. Karyotypic analysis predicts outcome of preremission and postremission therapy in adult acute myeloid leukemia: a southwest oncology group/eastern cooperative oncology group study. Blood 2000; 96(13):4075–83.

9. O'Donnell MR, Abboud CN, Altman J, et al. Acute myeloid leukemia. J Natl Compr Canc Netw 2012; 10(8):984–1021.

10. Greenberg PL, Tuechler H, Schanz J, et al. Revised international prognostic scoring system for myelodysplastic syndromes. Blood 2012;120(12): 2454–65.

11. Wouters BJ, Lowenberg B, Erpelinck-Verschueren CA, et al. Double CEBPA mutations, but not single CEBPA mutations, define a subgroup of acute myeloid leukemia with a distinctive gene expression profile that is uniquely associated with a favorable outcome. Blood 2009;113(13):3088–91.

12. Preudhomme C, Sagot C, Boissel N, et al. Favorable prognostic significance of CEBPA mutations in patients with de novo acute myeloid leukemia: a study from the acute leukemia french association (ALFA). Blood 2002;100(8):2717–23.

13. Verhaak RG, Goudswaard CS, van Putten W, et al. Mutations in nucleophosmin (NPM1) in acute myeloid leukemia (AML): association with other gene abnormalities and previously established gene expression signatures and their favorable prognostic significance. Blood 2005;106(12): 3747–54.

14. Thiede C, Koch S, Creutzig E, et al. Prevalence and prognostic impact of NPM1 mutations in 1485 adult patients with acute myeloid leukemia (AML). Blood 2006;107(10):4011–20.

15. Thiede C, Steudel C, Mohr B, et al. Analysis of FLT3-activating mutations in 979 patients with acute myelogenous leukemia: association with FAB subtypes and identification of subgroups with poor prognosis. Blood 2002;99(12):4326–35.

16. Ley TJ, Ding L, Walter MJ, et al. DNMT3A mutations in acute myeloid leukemia. N Engl J Med 2010; 363(25):2424–33.

17. Paschka P, Schlenk RF, Gaidzik VI, et al. IDH1 and IDH2 mutations are frequent genetic alterations in acute myeloid leukemia and confer adverse prognosis in cytogenetically normal acute myeloid leukemia with NPM1 mutation without FLT3 internal tandem duplication. J Clin Oncol 2010;28(22): 3636–43.

18. Mullighan CG. The molecular genetic makeup of acute lymphoblastic leukemia. Hematology Am Soc Hematol Educ Program 2012;2012:389–96.

19. Zhang J, Mullighan CG, Harvey RC, et al. Key pathways are frequently mutated in high-risk childhood

acute lymphoblastic leukemia: a report from the children's oncology group. Blood 2011;118(11): 3080–7.

20. Figueroa ME, Lugthart S, Li Y, et al. DNA methylation signatures identify biologically distinct subtypes in acute myeloid leukemia. Cancer Cell 2010;17(1): 13–27.

21. Ohgami RS, Ma L, Ren L, et al. DNA methylation analysis of ALOX12 and GSTM1 in acute myeloid leukaemia identifies prognostically significant groups. Br J Haematol 2012;159(2):182–90.

22. Mavrakis KJ, Van Der Meulen J, Wolfe AL, et al. A cooperative microRNA-tumor suppressor gene network in acute T-cell lymphoblastic leukemia (T-ALL). Nat Genet 2011;43(7):673–8.

23. Wlodarska I, Dierickx D, Vanhentenrijk V, et al. Translocations targeting CCND2, CCND3, and MYCN do occur in t(11;14)-negative mantle cell lymphomas. Blood 2008;111(12):5683–90.

24. Fonseca R, Blood EA, Oken MM, et al. Myeloma and the t(11;14)(q13;q32); evidence for a biologically defined unique subset of patients. Blood 2002; 99(10):3735–41.

25. Dohner H, Stilgenbauer S, Benner A, et al. Genomic aberrations and survival in chronic lymphocytic leukemia. N Engl J Med 2000;343(26):1910–6.

26. Zojer N, Konigsberg R, Ackermann J, et al. Deletion of 13q14 remains an independent adverse prognostic variable in multiple myeloma despite its frequent detection by interphase fluorescence in situ hybridization. Blood 2000;95(6):1925–30.

27. Stephens DM, Byrd JC. Chronic lymphocytic leukemia with del(17p13.1): a distinct clinical subtype requiring novel treatment approaches. Oncology (Williston Park) 2012;26(11):1044–54.

28. Ott G, Rosenwald A. Molecular pathogenesis of follicular lymphoma. Haematologica 2008;93(12): 1773–6.

29. Stefancikova L, Moulis M, Fabian P, et al. Prognostic impact of p53 aberrations for R-CHOP-treated patients with diffuse large B-cell lymphoma. Int J Oncol 2011;39(6):1413–20.

30. Poulain S, Roumier C, Decambron A, et al. MYD88 L265P mutation in waldenstrom macroglobulinemia. Blood 2013;121(22):4504–11.

31. Treon SP, Xu L, Yang G, et al. MYD88 L265P somatic mutation in waldenstrom's macroglobulinemia. N Engl J Med 2012;367(9):826–33.

32. Xu L, Hunter ZR, Yang G, et al. MYD88 L265P in waldenstrom macroglobulinemia, immunoglobulin M monoclonal gammopathy, and other B-cell lymphoproliferative disorders using conventional and quantitative allele-specific polymerase chain reaction. Blood 2013;121(11):2051–8.

33. Arcaini L, Zibellini S, Boveri E, et al. The BRAF V600E mutation in hairy cell leukemia and other mature B-cell neoplasms. Blood 2012;119(1): 188–91.

34. Ohgami RS, Ma L, Merker JD, et al. STAT3 mutations are frequent in CD30+ T-cell lymphomas and T-cell large granular lymphocytic leukemia. Leukemia 2013. [Epub ahead of print].

35. Koskela HL, Eldfors S, Ellonen P, et al. Somatic STAT3 mutations in large granular lymphocytic leukemia. N Engl J Med 2012;366(20):1905–13.

36. Badalian-Very G, Vergilio JA, Degar BA, et al. Recurrent BRAF mutations in langerhans cell histiocytosis. Blood 2010;116(11):1919–23.

37. Titus K. Lab teams up to curb unnecessary testing. CAP Today 2012;26.

38. Shultz E, Rosenbloom T, Kiepek W, et al. Quill: a novel approach to structured reporting. AMIA Annu Symp Proc 2003;1074.

39. Lucioni M, Novara F, Fiandrino G, et al. Twenty-one cases of blastic plasmacytoid dendritic cell neoplasm: focus on biallelic locus 9p21.3 deletion. Blood 2011;118(17):4591–4.

40. Maxson JE, Gotlib J, Pollyea DA, et al. Oncogenic CSF3R mutations in chronic neutrophilic leukemia and atypical CML. N Engl J Med 2013;368(19): 1781–90.

41. Piazza R, Valletta S, Winkelmann N, et al. Recurrent SETBP1 mutations in atypical chronic myeloid leukemia. Nat Genet 2013;45(1):18–24.

42. Itzykson R, Kosmider O, Renneville A, et al. Prognostic score including gene mutations in chronic myelomonocytic leukemia. J Clin Oncol 2013; 31(19):2428–36.

43. Varettoni M, Arcaini L, Zibellini S, et al. Prevalence and clinical significance of the MYD88 (L265P) somatic mutation in waldenstrom's macroglobulinemia and related lymphoid neoplasms. Blood 2013; 121(13):2522–8.

44. Jerez A, Clemente MJ, Makishima H, et al. STAT3 mutations unify the pathogenesis of chronic lymphoproliferative disorders of NK cells and T-cell large granular lymphocyte leukemia. Blood 2012; 120(15):3048–57.

45. Ofran Y, Rowe JM. Genetic profiling in acute myeloid leukaemia–where are we and what is its role in patient management. Br J Haematol 2013;160(3): 303–20.

46. Cross NC. Genetic and epigenetic complexity in myeloproliferative neoplasms. Hematology Am Soc Hematol Educ Program 2011;2011:208–14.

47. Graubert T, Walter MJ. Genetics of myelodysplastic syndromes: new insights. Hematology Am Soc Hematol Educ Program 2011;2011:543–9.

Index

Note: Page numbers for article titles are in **boldface** type.

A

Acute erythroid leukemia, erythroid/myeloid subtype (acute erythroleukemia). See *Acute erythroleukemia*.
　other types of, autoimmune hemolytic anemia, 655
　　Burkitt lymphoma, 656–657
　　megaloblastic anemia on bone marrow biopsy, 655
Acute erythroleukemia (Erythroleukemia), bone marrow aspirate smear, erythroid elements on, 643, 645
　　pronormoblasts and myeloblasts in, 644–645
　bone marrow biopsy in, hypercelluarity in, 642–643
　　morphologic dysplasia on, 643, 645
　clinical features of, cytopenias, 642
　　evolution from myelodysplastic/myeloproliferative neoplasm, 642
　diagnosis of, bone marrow in, 642–643, 645
　　cytochemistry in, 644–645
　　genetics in, 645–646
　　immunophenotype in, 644–645
　　peripheral blood in, 642
　differential diagnosis of. See also *Myelodysplastic syndrome (MDS), with erythroid predominance*.
　　myelodysplastic syndrome with erythroid predominance, 646–650
　　pure erythroid leukemia, 650–657
　FLT3-ITD mutation in, 646
　GATA1 mutation in, 646
　immunophenotype of, 644–645
　immunostain of, CD34 and CD117, 644–645
　karyotype abnormality in, 645–646
　NPMA mutation in, 646
　prognosis for, 650
　treatment of, 650
　WHO classification of, 641–642
Acute lymphoblastic leukemia/lymphoma, early T-cell precursor. See *Early T-cell precursor acute lymphoblastic leukemia/lymphoma (ETP-ALL)*.
Acute myeloid leukemia with inv(3)/t(3;3) abnormalities, **677–692**
　clinical features of, 679
　diagnosis of, cytogenetic evaluation of bone marrow or peripheral blood, 680–682
　　dyserythropoiesis in, 679, 681
　　dysgranulopoiesis in, 679, 681, 689

　　dysplastic megakaryocytes in, 679–681
　　EVI1 gene rearrangements in, 678–679
　　FISH analysis in, 682–683
　　flow cytometry in, 679–680
　　key pathology features of, 678
　　megakaryocytes in, 679, 683
　　single-nucleotide polymorphism in, 683
　differential diagnosis of, 683–684, 688
　　acute megakaryoblastic leukemia, 486
　　acute panmyelosis with myelofibrosis, 687
　　AML with multilineage dysplasia, 684–686
　　chronic myeloid leukemia, 687–688
　　myeloid dysplasia syndrome with del(5q), 684
　　myeloid proliferations related to Down syndrome, 688
　　myeloproliferative disorder with Down syndrome, 686, 688
　microscopic features of, 679
　prognosis for, molecular studies of, 689–690
　　overall survival, 689

B

Blastic plasmacytoid dendritic cell neoplasm (BPDCN [hematodermic neoplasm]), **743–765**
　clinical features of, skin lesions, 744
　diagnosis of, 752–758
　　CD22 expression in, 752
　　classic immunophenotypic profile for, 752
　　markers for, 752
　　TCL1 in, 752, 755, 757
　differential diagnosis of, 758–761
　　acute myeloid leukemia/monocytic leukemia, 758–759, 761
　　B-cell lymphoblastic leukemia/lymphoma, 759–761
　　lymphoblastic leukemia/lymphoma cutis, 761
　　myelomoid leukemia, 760, 761
　　pDC (plasmacytoid dendritic cell) nodules, 760
　　T-cell lymphoblastic leukemia/lymphoma, 759–761
　　T-cell lymphomas, 760
　distinction from acute myeloid leukemia, 743–744
　genetic alterations in, 758
　immunophenotypic profile of, CD 4, 735, 752, 753
　　CD 56, 753–755
　　CD123, 752, 754–755
　　CD124, 754–755
　microscopic features of, bone marrow involvement, 749

surgpath.theclinics.com

Blastic (*continued*)
cell resemblance to lymphocytes, 752
cell size in, 750–751
cytologic features like immature myeloid cells,
748
in cutaneous involvement, 745–746
in peripheral blood and bone marrow, 745–746
leukemic involvement, 745–746
lymph node involvement, 749–750
lymphoblast-like cytology, 746–747
perivascular and periadnexal pattern, 745–746
resemblance to monocytic cells, 748
splenic red pulp infiltration by, 751
morphology of, cutaneous, 744
interstitial in bone marrow, 744
paracortical expansion in lymph node, 744
prognosis for, in adults, 761–762
in children, 762

C

CEL NOS (chronic eosinophilic leukemia, not
otherwise specified)
clinical features of, 781
differential diagnosis of, acute and chronic
myelogenous leukemia, 784
immunophenotypic studies of, 784
microscopic features of, eosinophilia, 782
in bone marrow aspirate, 782–783
in peripheral blood smear, 783
prognosis for, 5-year survival rate, 784
Classical Hodgkin lymphoma (CHL)
atypical phenotypes in, **729–742**
BCL2, BCL6, 736
CD138, 736
CD15, 730–732, 739, 742
CD20, 733, 736–737, 739–742
CD30, 729–730, 736–742
CD45, 732, 734
CD79a, 733, 735
multiple myeloma oncogene in, 735–736
OCT-2, 734–736, 742
PAX-5, 730, 732–733
Clonal relationships between malignant lymphomas
and histiocytic/dendritic cell tumors, **619–629**
diagnosis of, comparative molecular testing in,
624, 626
comparative PCR molecular testing in, 624,
626
fluorescence in situ hybridization in, 624–627
metachronous presentation in, 623, 625
synchronous presentation in, 620, 624
transdifferentiation in, 621–623
WHO criteria in, 622
differential diagnosis of, 622
lymphoblastic transformation of chronic
myelogenous leukemia, 621

lymphoma and histiocytic/dendritic cell tumors
occuring synchronously, 621
lymphoma with reactive histiocytic/dendritic
cell component, 620–621
summary, 622
examples of, 620
follicular lymphomas, 620, 624
histiocytic sarcoma, 620, 623, 626
Langerhans cell tumors, 620, 625
potential mechanisms for, 620–621
prognosis for, 627

E

Early T-cell precursor acute lymphoblastic leukemia/
lymphoma (ETP-ALL), **661–676**
clinical features of, 663
differential diagnosis of, algorithmic approach to,
667
immunotypic basis of, 666, 668
in blood and bone marrow, 666, 669–671
in extramedullary sites, 667, 669
epidemiology of, 663
flow cytometry in, 663–665
gene expression in, 664
genetic features of, 665
immunophenotype definition of, 663–665
immunophenotypes of, 662
comparison with non-ETP-ALL, for survival and
remission, 663–664
stages of T-cell development and early T-cell
precursor, 662–663
gene expression profiling of, 663
in duodenum, 672, 674
infiltration into bronchial mucosa, 674
lymph node effacement in, 672
micro RNA profiling in, 666
molecular features of, 665–666
prognosis for, 669–675
somatic mutations in, 666
structural genetic rearrangements in, 665–666
T-cell receptor gene rearrangements in, 666
Eosinophilia in neoplastic hematopathology,
algorithm for workup of patients with, 769
causes of eosinophilia, primary hematolymphoid,
768, 770–771
secondary nonhematolymphoid, 768, 770
cytogenetic analysis of bone marrow in, 768, 770
differential diagnosis of, **767–794**
CEL NOS, 781–784
hypereosinophilic syndrome, 784–785
myeloid and lymphoid meoplasms associated
with *PDGFRA* rearrangements, 770–772
myeloid and lymphoid neoplasms associated
with *PDGFRAB rearrangements,* 775–778
myeloid and lymphoid neoplasms with *FGFR1*
abnormalities, 778–781

systemic mastocytosis, 787–790
hematologic neoplasms, molecular mutational
    abnormalities in, 768, 770–771
Erythroleukemia. See *Acute erythroid leukemia
    (Erythroleukemia); Pure erythroid leukemia (PEL).*

H

Hematodermic neoplasm. See *Blastic plasmacytoid
    dendritic cell neoplasm (BPDCN [hematodermic
    neoplasm]).*
Hematopoietic neoplasm reporting, challenges in,
    795–806
    comprehensive, incorporation of relevant data into
        complete synthesized report, 804–805
        unique challenges in, 802, 804
    cytogenetic analysis, importance of, 796
    cytogenetic and molecular findings, in acute
        myeloid leukemia, 799–800
        in myeloid neoplasms, 796–799
    cytogenetic and mutational findings, in mature
        lymphoid neoplasms and histiocytic and
        dendritic cell neoplasms, 802–803
    epigenetic changes and, 800
    gene mutational analyses in, 800
    genetic mutations, in myeloid neoplasms and
        acute leukemias, 801
    hematology neoplasm report, contents of
        complete, 795
    WHO Prognostic Scoring System, 797–800
Hodgkin lymphoma. See *Classical Hodgkin
    lymphoma.*
Hypereosinophilic syndrome (HES), ancillary studies
    in, cytogenetic testing, 786
        molecular testing, 786
    criteria for, 784
    differential diagnosis of, acute myeloid leukemia,
        786
        myeloproliferative neoplasm, 786
    end-organ involvement in, 784–785
    microscopic features of, in bone marrow
        involvement, 786
        in cardiac manifestations, 785
        in pulmonary involvement, 785–786
    organ systems affected in, 785
    prognosis for, death from cardiac dysfunction,
        787
        survival rates, 786
    WHO classification of, 784

M

Myelodysplastic syndromes (MDS), diagnosis of,
    cytogenetic studies in, 719, 721
        diagnostic algorithm for, 719–720
        FISH in, 719
        immunohistochemistry for CD34, 719, 722–723

refractory cytopenia of childhood and CD61
    immunohistochemistry, 719, 723
    WHO 2008 classification in, 719
differential diagnosis of, alcohol as Bm toxin, 708
    autoimmune conditions, 708–709, 712
    congenital causes, 710, 713–716
    Fanconi anemia, 710, 713
    Fanconi anemia dyskeratosis congenita, 710,
        715
    HIV infection-associated, 708, 710
    medication-induced dysplasia, 708, 711
    monocytopenia immunodeficiency, 710, 716
    Pearson sydrome, 710
    systemic lupus erythematosus, 712
    T-cell large granular lymphocyte leukemia/
        hairy cell leukemia, 710, 718
    valproic acid in children, 708, 711
    vitamin B_{12} deficiency, 708
French-American-British classification of, 693
International Prognostic Scoring System-R for, in
    diagnosis, 719–720
    in prognosis, cytogenetic risk groups in, 724
        prognostic risk scores and clinical
            outcomes, 725
        prognostic score values in, 725
microscopic features of, anemia, 694
    blast enumeration, 701, 704–705
    dimorphic red blood cells, 695, 701
    dysgranulopoiesis in peripheral blood, 701
    dysmegakaryopoiesis, 701
    erythroid hyperplasia with megaloblastoid
        maturation, 697, 701
    erythroid maturation abnormalities, 696
    in mimics of MDS, 696
    iron staining for ring sideroblasts, 699, 701
    megakaryocyte abnormalities, 701, 707–708
    megakaryocyte lineage abnormalities, 701,
        707–708
    myeloid lineage in bone marrow aspirate,
        701–702
    neurtrophil abnormalities, 700–701
    nuclear abnormalities, 698, 701
    platelet abnormalities, 701, 706
    poikilocytes in, 694–696
    red blood cell abnormalities in, 684–696
pathophysiology of, 693
update on, **693–728**
with erythroid predominance, acute
    erythroleukemia *vs.,* 646–650
    high-grade myelodysplastic syndromes,
        646–649
    low-grade, refractory cytopenia with
        multilineage dysplasia, 646, 649
    myeloproliferative neoplasms and
        myelodysplastic/myeloproliferative
        neoplasms, 649–650
    reactive conditions in, 646–647, 649

Myelodysplastic (*continued*)
    with refractory anemia with ring sideroblasts,
        646–649
Myeloid and lymphoid neoplasms, *PDGFRA*
    rearrangement-associated, 770–775
        differential diagnosis of, 772–775
            CEL NOS, 772–774
            chronic myeloid leukemia, 773–774
            chronic myeloid leukemia with prominent
                eosinophilia, 772–773
            systemic mastocytosis, 774–775, 778
        immunohistochemistry of, glycophorin, 773
            tryptase, 773
        laboratory parameters of, 771–772
        microscopic features of, in bone marrow, 772
            in peripheral blood, 772
        physical presentation of, 771
        prognosis for, 775
    PDGFRB rearrangement-associated, ancillary
    studies of, 777
        differential diagnosis of, 777–778
        FISH anaylsis of peripheral blood, 778
        fusion genes and corresponding morphology,
            777
        immunohistochemistry for tryptase in, 778
        microscopic features of, 775–777
            hypercellularity on bone marrow biopsy,
                775, 777
            morphologic presentations of, 775
        prognosis for, survival rate, 778
            tyrosine kinase therapy and, 778
    with *FGFR1* abnormalities, 778–781
        8p12 MPS, prognosis for, 781
        8p12 MPS, acute and chronic phases of, 781
        8p12 translocation myeloproliferative
            syndrome, 778–779
        differential diagnosis of, 8p12
            myeloproliferative syndrome, 780
            angioblasticT-cell lymphoma, 780
            T-cell lymphoma, not otherwise specified,
                780–781
        fusion genes and translocations, 779
        microscopic features of, presenting as mixed
            phenotype acute leukemia, 779–780
        presenting as T-lymphoblastic lymphoma, 782
Myeloid neoplasms with inv(3)(q21Q26.2) or
    t(3;3)(q26,2) abnormalities. See under *Acute
    myeloid leukemia.*

P

Pure erythroid leukemia (PEL), clinical features of,
    651

defined, 650–651
diagnosis of, 653
    cytochemistry and immunophenotype in,
        651–654
    genetics in, 654
    peripheral blood and bone marrow
        morphology in, 651–652
differential diagnosis of, Burkitt lymphoma,
    656–657
    myelodysplastic syndromes, 654, 657
    other neoplasms involving bone marrow, 657
    reactive erythroid hyperplasia, 654–657

S

Systemic mastocystitis (SM), clinical presentation of,
    787
differential diagnosis of, 790
genetic studies of, *KIT* mutations, 789–790
immunohistochemistry in, CD117, CD25, and
    tryptase in, 789
microscopic features of, eosinophilia in bone
    marrow biopsy, 788–789
    eosinophilia in peripheral blood, 787–789
    mast cells in bone marrow aspirate, 788
prognosis for, 790
therapeutic choices for, 790
WHO classification and criteria for, 787–788

T

T-cell large granular lymphocytic leukemia (T-LGL),
    differential diagnosis of, flow cytometry in,
    634–636
        hepatosplenic T-cell lymphoma, 633
        malignancies of cytotoxic lymphocytes, 634,
            636
        physiologic cytotoxic T-cell response, 633–634
    distinguishing from reactive conditions, **631–639**
    elements in, 631–632
    gross features of, splenomegaly, 632
    key features of, 633
    microscopic features of, in peripheral smears, 632
        intrasinusoidal infiltrates in bone marrow
            biopsies, 632–633, 638
    on bone marrow biopsy specimen, 632–633, 635,
        637–638
    on peripheral blood smear, 634–635
    prognosis for, 638
    STAT3 gene in, 631, 636
T-cell neoplasms, cytogenetic and mutational
    findings in, 803

United States Postal Service

Statement of Ownership, Management, and Circulation
(All Periodicals Publications Except Requestor Publications)

1. Publication Title	2. Publication Number							3. Filing Date
Surgical Pathology Clinics	0	2	5	-	4	7	8	9/14/13

4. Issue Frequency	5. Number of Issues Published Annually	6. Annual Subscription Price
Mar, Jun, Sep, Dec	4	$191.00

7. Complete Mailing Address of Known Office of Publication (Not printer) (Street, city, county, state, and ZIP+4®)

Elsevier Inc.
360 Park Avenue South
New York, NY 10010-1710

Contact Person
Stephen R. Bushing

Telephone (Include area code)
215-239-3688

8. Complete Mailing Address of Headquarters or General Business Office of Publisher (Not printer)

Elsevier Inc., 360 Park Avenue South, New York, NY 10010-1710

9. Full Names and Complete Mailing Addresses of Publisher, Editor, and Managing Editor (Do not leave blank)

Publisher (Name and complete mailing address)

Linda Belfus, Elsevier, Inc., 1600 John F. Kennedy Blvd. Suite 1800, Philadelphia, PA 19103-2899

Editor (Name and complete mailing address)

Joanne Husovski, Elsevier, Inc., 1600 John F. Kennedy Blvd. Suite 1800, Philadelphia, PA 19103-2899

Managing Editor (Name and complete mailing address)

Barbara Cohen - Kligerman, Elsevier, Inc., 1600 John F. Kennedy Blvd. Suite 1800, Philadelphia, PA 19103-2899

10. Owner (Do not leave blank. If the publication is owned by a corporation, give the name and address of the corporation immediately followed by the names and addresses of all stockholders owning or holding 1 percent or more of the total amount of stock. If not owned by a corporation, give the names and addresses of the individual owners. If owned by a partnership or other unincorporated firm, give its name and address as well as those of each individual owner. If the publication is published by a nonprofit organization, give its name and address.)

Full Name	Complete Mailing Address
Wholly owned subsidiary of	1600 John F. Kennedy Blvd., Ste. 1800
Reed/Elsevier, US holdings	Philadelphia, PA 19103-2899

11. Known Bondholders, Mortgagees, and Other Security Holders Owning or Holding 1 Percent or More of Total Amount of Bonds, Mortgages, or Other Securities. If none, check box. ☐ None

Full Name	Complete Mailing Address
N/A	

12. Tax Status (For completion by nonprofit organizations authorized to mail at nonprofit rates) (Check one)
The purpose, function, and nonprofit status of this organization and the exempt status for federal income tax purposes:
☐ Has Not Changed During Preceding 12 Months
☐ Has Changed During Preceding 12 Months (Publisher must submit explanation of change with this statement)

PS Form 3526, September 2007 (Page 1 of 3 (Instructions Page 3)) PSN 7530-01-000-9931 PRIVACY NOTICE: See our Privacy policy in www.usps.com

13. Publication Title				14. Issue Date for Circulation Data Below
Surgical Pathology Clinics				September 2013

15. Extent and Nature of Circulation			Average No. Copies Each Issue During Preceding 12 Months	No. Copies of Single Issue Published Nearest to Filing Date
a. Total Number of Copies (Net press run)			749	908
b. Paid Circulation (By Mail and Outside the Mail)	(1)	Mailed Outside-County Paid Subscriptions Stated on PS Form 3541. (Include paid distribution above nominal rate, advertiser's proof copies, and exchange copies)	464	522
	(2)	Mailed In-County Paid Subscriptions Stated on PS Form 3541 (Include paid distribution above nominal rate, advertiser's proof copies, and exchange copies)		
	(3)	Paid Distribution Outside the Mails Including Sales Through Dealers and Carriers, Street Vendors, Counter Sales, and Other Paid Distribution Outside USPS®	45	53
	(4)	Paid Distribution by Other Classes Mailed Through the USPS (e.g. First-Class Mail®)		
c. Total Paid Distribution (Sum of 15b (1), (2), (3), and (4))			509	575
d. Free or Nominal Rate Distribution (By Mail and Outside the Mail)	(1)	Free or Nominal Rate Outside-County Copies Included on PS Form 3541	29	3
	(2)	Free or Nominal Rate In-County Copies Included on PS Form 3541		
	(3)	Free or Nominal Rate Copies Mailed at Other Classes Through the USPS (e.g. First-Class Mail)		
	(4)	Free or Nominal Rate Distribution Outside the Mail (Carriers or other means)		
e. Total Free or Nominal Rate Distribution (Sum of 15d (1), (2), (3) and (4))			29	3
f. Total Distribution (Sum of 15c and 15e)			538	578
g. Copies not Distributed (See instructions to publishers #4 (page #3))			211	330
h. Total (Sum of 15f and g)			749	908
i. Percent Paid (15c divided by 15f times 100)			94.61%	99.48%

16. Publication of Statement of Ownership

☐ If the publication is a general publication, publication of this statement is required. Will be printed
in the December 2013 issue of this publication. ☐ Publication not required

17. Signature and Title of Editor, Publisher, Business Manager, or Owner

Stephen R. Bushing

Stephen R. Bushing – Inventory Distribution Coordinator

Date
September 14, 2013

I certify that all information furnished on this form is true and complete. I understand that anyone who furnishes false or misleading information on this form or who omits material or information requested on the form may be subject to criminal sanctions (including fines and imprisonment) and/or civil sanctions (including civil penalties).

PS Form 3526, September 2007 (Page 2 of 3)

Moving?

Make sure your subscription moves with you!

To notify us of your new address, find your **Clinics Account Number** (located on your mailing label above your name), and contact customer service at:

Email: journalscustomerservice-usa@@elsevier.com

800-654-2452 (subscribers in the U.S. & Canada)
314-447-8871 (subscribers outside of the U.S. & Canada)

Fax number: 314-447-8029

Elsevier Health Sciences Division
Subscription Customer Service
3251 Riverport Lane
Maryland Heights, MO 63043

*To ensure uninterrupted delivery of your subscription, please notify us at least 4 weeks in advance of move.

Printed and bound by CPI Group (UK) Ltd, Croydon, CR0 4YY

03/10/2024

01040381-0019